METHODS IN PHARMACOLOGY

Volume 5

Myocardial Biology

General Editor: **Arnold Schwartz**
Baylor College of Medicine, Houston, Texas

Volume 1
Edited by **Arnold Schwartz**

Volume 2: PHYSICAL METHODS
Edited by **Colin F. Chignell**

Volume 3: SMOOTH MUSCLE
Edited by **Edwin E. Daniel** and **David M. Paton**

Volume 4A: RENAL PHARMACOLOGY
Edited by **Manuel Martinez-Maldonado**

Volume 4B: RENAL PHARMACOLOGY
Edited by **Manuel Martinez-Maldonado**

Volume 5: MYOCARDIAL BIOLOGY
Edited by **Arnold Schwartz**

METHODS IN PHARMACOLOGY

Volume 5

Myocardial Biology

Edited by

Arnold Schwartz

University of Cincinnati College of Medicine
Cincinnati, Ohio

SPRINGER SCIENCE+BUSINESS MEDIA, LLC

Library of Congress Catalog Card Number 74-34441
ISBN 978-1-4684-4780-4 ISBN 978-1-4684-4778-1 (eBook)
DOI 10.1007/978-1-4684-4778-1

Originally published by Plenum press, New York in 1984
Softcover reprint of the hardcover 1st edition 1984

Contributors

HENRY R. BESCH, JR.
Krannert Institute of Cardiology
Department of Medicine
and Department of Pharmacology
and Toxicology
Indiana University School of Medicine
Indianapolis, Indiana

ALAN D. CARDIN
Division of Lipoprotein Research
Department of Pharmacology and Cell
Biophysics
University of Cincinnati College of Medicine
Cincinnati, Ohio

DOUGLAS A. FUGMAN
Department of Pharmacology and Cell
Biophysics
University of Cincinnati
College of Medicine
Cincinnati, Ohio
Present Address:
Department of Anatomy and Cell Biology
University of Cincinnati College of Medicine
Cincinnati, Ohio

GUNTER GRUPP
Departments of Pharmacology and Cell
Biophysics, Physiology, and Internal
Medicine (Division of Cardiology)
University of Cincinnati College of Medicine
Cincinnati, Ohio

INGRID L. GRUPP
Departments of Pharmacology and Cell
Biophysics, Physiology, and Internal
Medicine (Division of Cardiology)
University of Cincinnati College of Medicine
Cincinnati, Ohio

GEORGE HOLDSWORTH
Division of Lipoprotein Research
Department of Pharmacology and Cell
Biophysics
University of Cincinnati College of Medicine
Cincinnati, Ohio
Present Address:
Oak Ridge Research Institute
Oak Ridge, Tennessee

RICHARD L. JACKSON
Division of Lipoprotein Research
Department of Pharmacology and Cell
Biophysics
University of Cincinnati College of Medicine
Cincinnati, Ohio

J. DAVID JOHNSON
Department of Pharmacology and Cell Biophysics
University of Cincinnati College of Medicine
Cincinnati, Ohio
Present Address:
Department of Physiological Chemistry
Ohio State University Medical Center
Columbus, Ohio

LARRY R. JONES
Krannert Institute of Cardiology
Department of Medicine and Department of Pharmacology and Toxicology
Indiana University School of Medicine
Indianapolis, Indiana

ALLAN S. MANALAN
Department of Medicine and Department of Pharmacology and Toxicology
Indiana University School of Medicine, Krannert Institute of Cardiology, and The Veterans Administration Medical Center
Indianapolis, Indiana
Present address:
Cardiovascular Institute
Department of Medicine
Michael Reese Hospital and Medical Center
Chicago, Illinois

MOHAMMED A. MATLIB
Department of Pharmacology and Cell Biophysics
University of Cincinnati College of Medicine
Cincinnati, Ohio

P. M. MATTHEWS
Department of Biochemistry
University of Oxford
Oxford, England
Present address:
Department of Pharmacology
Stanford University School of Medicine
Stanford, California

R. W. MILLARD
Department of Pharmacology and Cell Biophysics
University of Cincinnati College of Medicine
Cincinnati, Ohio

JUN NAKAMURA
Department of Pharmacology and Cell Biophysics
University of Cincinnati College of Medicine
Cincinnati, Ohio
Present Address:
Tanabe Pharmaceutical Company
Higashi-Ku, Osaka, Japan

EDWARD D. PAGANI
Department of Physiology
University of Cincinnati College of Medicine
Cincinnati, Ohio
Present Address:
Department of Anesthesia Research
Brigham and Women's Hospital
Boston, Massachusetts

JAMES D. POTTER
Department of Pharmacology and Cell Biophysics
University of Cincinnati College of Medicine
Cincinnati, Ohio
Present Address:
Department of Pharmacology
University of Miami School of Medicine
Miami, Florida

G. K. RADDA
Department of Biochemistry
University of Oxford
Oxford, England

STEVEN ROBERTSON
Department of Pharmacology and Cell Biophysics
University of Cincinnati College of Medicine
Cincinnati, Ohio
Present Address:
Miles Laboratory
Human Research Division
Elkhart, Indiana

DENISE E. ROBINSON
Department of Pharmacology and Cell Biophysics
University of Cincinnati College of Medicine
Cincinnati, Ohio
Present Address:
Department of Pharmacology
Georgetown University
Washington, D.C.

WILLIAM ROUSLIN
Department of Pharmacology and Cell Biophysics
University of Cincinnati College of Medicine
Cincinnati, Ohio

ARNOLD SCHWARTZ
Department of Pharmacology and Cell Biophysics
University of Cincinnati College of Medicine
Cincinnati, Ohio

R. JOHN SOLARO
Departments of Physiology and Pharmacology and Cell Biophysics
University of Cincinnati College of Medicine
Cincinnati, Ohio

PAL L. VAGHY
Department of Pharmacology and Cell Biophysics
University of Cincinnati College of Medicine
Cincinnati, Ohio

TAITZER WANG
Department of Pharmacology and Cell Biophysics
University of Cincinnati College of Medicine
Cincinnati, Ohio

AUGUST M. WATANABE
Department of Medicine and Department of Pharmacology and Toxicology
Indiana University School of Medicine, Krannert Institute of Cardiology, and The Veterans Administration Medical Center
Indianapolis, Indiana

LAURA A. WITTENAUER
Department of Pharmacology and Cell Biophysics
University of Cincinnati College of Medicine
Cincinnati, Ohio
Present Address:
Department of Physiological Chemistry
Ohio State University Medical Center
Columbus, Ohio

Preface

It is a pleasure to introduce Volume 5 in the Methods in Pharmacology series. In 1971, Volume 1 of this series was published while I was Head of the Division of Myocardial Biology in the Department of Pharmacology at Baylor College of Medicine in Houston, Texas. I dedicated that first volume to Sir Henry Hallet Dale, who died on July 23, 1968. In the Preface I pointed out that many of the pharmacological advancements that occurred during the last century were direct descendants from the classic paper published in 1910 by Professor Dale and his colleague, Dr. Barger. In this paper, the concept of "specific receptor sites" was introduced by the statement that "the relationship of the recepted mechanism to the base [i.e., drug base] may well be one of solid solution of adsorption and, therefore, more analogous to that of an enzyme to its substrate. . . ." I also pointed out at that time that the search for drug receptors continues and that fundamental knowledge of the nature of receptors and drug–receptor interaction will eventually lead to a rational approach to drug design. Since 1971, the study of receptors and their interaction with specific chemical substances has continued at an accelerated pace and this is due, in particular, to the introduction of new and exciting methodologies. The death last year of Professor Raymond P. Ahlquist, who pioneered the introduction of specific adrenergic receptors, represents the close of yet another era.

In the first volume, we discussed ways in which one could study the effects of local anesthetics and methodologies involved in myocardial metabolism, how to set up and study isolated atrial preparations, and how to relate those findings to intact cardiac muscle. We provided recipes for the study of hypertension, methods for evaluating antiarrhythmic drugs, and methods for isolating mitochondria, sarcoplasmic reticulum, the Na,K-ATPase, and contractile proteins. We discussed in some detail how to analyze high energy phosphate compounds and even how to use microelectrodes in muscle. It is of interest, in particular, that Dr. James J. Fischer (in Chapter 14) discussed how nuclear magnetic resonance might be applied to pharmacology. At that time, very little was known about the newer instruments and, in particular, about phosphorous nuclear magnetic resonance spectroscopy as applied to problems in cardiovascular disease.

It was time to reconsider the techniques available to pharmacology and attempt to highlight those areas that have developed since the publication of Volume 1, some 13 years ago. The present volume provides alterations in the recipes for the various organelle systems, as well as for contractile proteins, so that the preparations that are available for study will be much purer and much better characterized. In addition, the extremely important area of radioligand-binding techniques is discussed in considerable detail, as are biophysical techniques used to study chemically induced changes in membranes and in proteins. We have also tried to provide up-to-date information on various isolated and intact organ systems, in order for the investigator who is interested in this area to be able to quantitate effects of drugs on these components. Of considerable interest is an updated chapter on nuclear magnetic resonance spectroscopy from the laboratory of Professor George Radda. Here the reader will see the tremendous advances that have been made in this important "noninvasive" technique to study the mechanism of action of drugs.

I hope that these "recipes" will assist the student and young scientist, as well as the mature investigator, in fulfilling the hopes and dreams of the search for information on the mechanism of action of drugs.

Arnold Schwartz

Cincinnati, Ohio

Contents

Chapter 1

Isolation of Canine Cardiac Sarcolemmal Vesicles

Larry R. Jones and Henry R. Besch, Jr.

Krannert Institute of Cardiology
Department of Medicine
and Department of Pharmacology and Toxicology
Indiana University School of Medicine
Indianapolis, Indiana

I. INTRODUCTION

Isolation and characterization of sarcolemmal membrane fragments from the heart has been a goal of several research laboratories for some time (Wollenberger and Will, 1978). This is because of the fundamental importance of the sarcolemma in maintaining the electrophysiological and contractile properties of the heart by regulating transmembrane fluxes of the inotropically active cations Na^+, K^+, and Ca^{2+} between intracellular and extracellular compartments. Both purity and morphological form of the isolated membranes are equally important considerations in any isolation scheme for cardiac sarcolemma (Besch *et al.*, 1976). In analogy to results first observed with cardiac sarcoplasmic reticulum membrane preparations, it seems highly advantageous to isolate sarcolemmal membrane fragments from the heart in the form of tightly sealed vesicles so that not only enzymic activity but also active and passive transport of ions can be measured in the same membrane preparation.

Recently, we have successfully isolated highly purified, tightly sealed sarcolemmal membrane fragments from canine myocardium, which exhibit such properties (Jones *et al.*, 1979, 1980). These preparations exhibit high specific activities of enzymes thought to be importantly involved in the regulation of cardiac contractility such as Na^+,K^+-ATPase, adenylate cyclase, cAMP-dependent protein kinase, and Ca^{2+}–calmodulin-dependent protein kinase (Jones *et al.*,

1979, 1980, 1981). In addition, other investigators recently have shown that these preparations are also suitable for characterization of the functional properties of cardiac sarcolemma in that they exhibit a $Na^+ : Ca^{2+}$ exchange mechanism (Reeves and Sutko, 1979), an active transport of Na^+ catalyzed by the Na^+,K^+-ATPase (Pitts, 1979), and an active transport of Ca^{2+} mediated by a sarcolemmal Ca^{2+} pump (Caroni and Carafoli, 1980).

This report describes in detail our isolation procedure for canine cardiac sarcolemmal vesicles. In addition, we also describe our standard ATPase assay, which is used for monitoring the purity of the membrane fractions. The Na^+,K^+-ATPase is the positive enzymic marker for the sarcolemmal membranes, whereas the very active Ca^{2+},K^+-ATPase of sarcoplasmic reticulum vesicles is the negative enzymic marker used to assess sarcoplasmic reticulum contamination. Azide-sensitive ATPase activity conveniently can be used to estimate the mitochondrial contamination that is present in either membrane fraction. Because the sarcolemmal membrane fraction is vesicular and the vesicles are tightly sealed, much latent Na^+,K^+-ATPase enzymic activity is present in the preparation. Several agents useful for unmasking this activity are also described because it is necessary to unmask the latent activities inherent in the vesicular form in order to insure that enzymic turnover provides a valid assessment of enzymic content. It should be pointed out that the technique of unmasking activities after the fractions have been harvested applies equally well to mixed microsomes as to purified sarcolemmal vesicles. The unmasking technique as applied to cardiac microsomes eliminates the need for the more time-consuming and laborious treatments with preparative media containing various chaotropic agents that have previously been thought necessary for obtaining cardiac Na^+,K^+-ATPase of high activity.

II. ISOLATION OF CANINE CARDIAC SARCOLEMMAL VESICLES

The general strategy behind the isolation of purified cardiac sarcolemmal vesicles is to obtain a microsomal fraction from the heart that is enriched in sarcolemmal vesicles and deficient in sarcoplasmic reticulum vesicles and then to further purify the sarcolemmal vesicles from the crude microsomes by means of sucrose density gradient centrifugation. We used a Ca^{2+}–oxalate loading step in the original procedure to increase the density of the sarcoplasmic reticulum vesicles selectively and thus facilitate their separation from crude cardiac microsomes (Jones *et al.*, 1979). In subsequent experiments, however, it was shown that this latter maneuver was unnecessary (Jones *et al.*, 1980). The initial brief homogenizations and low-speed centrifugations that are incorporated in the procedure (Jones *et al.*, 1979) selectively extract most of the sarcoplasmic reticulum membrane fragments from the bulk of the particulate material. Sarcolemmal vesicles are then formed from this remaining particulate material by subsequent vigorous homogenizations.

A. Solutions

1. Medium I (1.5 Liters)

0.75 *M* NaCl.
10 m*M* histidine (free base).

The pH of histidine (free base) dissolved in H_2O is about 7.5. Therefore, it is not necessary to adjust the pH of preparative media containing histidine.

2. Medium II (1.5 Liters)

10 m*M* $NaHCO_3$.
5 m*M* histidine (free base).

3. Medium III (50 ml)

0.6 *M* sucrose.

The 0.6 *M* sucrose is dissolved in a solution containing 300 m*M* NaCl, 100 m*M* tris base, and 50 m*M* tetrasodium pyrophosphate (pH adjusted to 7.1 by addition of concentrated HCl). The purpose of the salts incorporated into medium III is to reduce nonspecific aggregation of membranes (Heller and Harary, 1977).

4. Medium IV (100 ml)

0.25 *M* sucrose.
10 m*M* histidine (free base).

B. Procedure

1. Homogenization of Tissue and Removal of Sarcoplasmic Reticulum

All preparative procedures are performed at 4°C. The left ventricles from two large dogs are well trimmed with scissors by removing the main coronary arteries, pericardium, endocardium, and fat; 180 to 200 g of trimmed ventricle is then minced by passing the tissue through a meat grinder. The ground tissue is divided into six equal portions, and each portion is added to a Beckman JA-14 centrifuge tube containing 100 ml of medium I. Each portion is homogenized directly in the centrifuge tube one time for 5 sec with a Polytron PT-20 (Brinkman Instruments, Inc.) set at half-maximal speed. The homogenates are centrifuged at 10,000 rpm (14,000 $\times$ *g* max) for 20 min in a Beckman JA-14 rotor. The supernatants containing the fragmented sarcoplasmic reticulum are discarded, and each pellet is resuspended in 100 ml of medium I by shaking. The suspensions are homogenized and centrifuged a second time as described above. The supernatants are discarded, and the pellets are now resuspended in 100 ml of medium II. The suspensions are then homogenized and centrifuged a third time as described above. The supernatants are discarded, and each pellet is resuspended in 100 ml of medium II.

2. *Isolation of Microsomes Enriched in Sarcolemmal Vesicles*

The membrane suspensions are next homogenized three times for 30 sec with the Polytron PT-20 set a half-maximal speed. This longer time of homogenization causes formation of sealed sarcolemmal vesicles. The suspensions are centrifuged at 10,000 rpm for 20 min in the JA-14 rotor to remove nuclei, cell debris, and mitochondria. The supernatants are divided between a Beckman JA-20 rotor (eight tubes of about 35 ml each) and a type 30 rotor (12 tubes of about 25 ml each), and the microsomes are sedimented at 19,000 rpm (44,000 × *g* max) for 30 min. The supernatants are discarded, and microsomal pellets are combined by resuspending them to a total volume of 60 ml with medium IV. Twenty milliliters of the resuspended microsomes are added to each of three Beckman 30 rotor tubes, and the suspensions are centrifuged at 12,000 rpm (17,000 × *g* max) for 20 min. The purpose of this step is to selectively sediment remaining mitochondrial fragments from the microsomes. The supernatants are poured into three clean type 30 rotor tubes, and the membrane suspensions are centrifuged at 30,000 rpm (106,000 × *g* max) for 30 min. This yields a firm brown pellet with a white rim of membrane material. The white membrane material, consisting of sarcolemmal-enriched microsomes, is collected from each of the three 30 rotor tubes by aspiration with a syringe. The volume of this material is approximately 15 ml.

3. *Density Gradient Centrifugation of Sarcolemmal Vesicles*

Ten milliliters of medium III are added to three Beckman 30 rotor centrifuge tubes. Approximately 5 ml of the sarcolemmal-enriched microsomes are layered over the medium III in each centrifuge tube. The tubes are centrifuged at 40,000 rpm (170,000 × *g* max) for 90 min in a Beckman 42.1 fixed-angle rotor. The white membrane material at the interface of medium III is collected from the three tubes by aspiration with a syringe and diluted with four volumes of ice-cold water into three clean type 30 rotor tubes. The membrane material is sedimented at 40,000 rpm for 30 min in the 42.1 rotor to yield the purified cardiac sarcolemmal vesicles. The sarcolemmal vesicles are resuspended in a total volume of approximately 1 to 2 ml of medium IV, distributed into 100-μl aliquots in small tubes, and stored frozen at −20°C. Protein concentration is determined by the method of Lowry *et al.* (1951). The final yield of membrane material is about 6 mg per 100 g of heart. The time required to prepare the membranes is about 8 hr.

For comparative purposes in this report, ATPase activities in sarcolemmal vesicles are compared to ATPase activities in sarcoplasmic reticulum vesicles and mitochondria also isolated from canine heart. The sarcoplasmic reticulum fraction used is our E fraction, which has been purified by density gradient centrifugation after Ca^{2+}–oxalate loading (Jones *et al.*, 1979). Crude mitochondria were prepared by sedimenting a postnuclear fraction at 6,000 × *g* for 10 min. The mitochondria were then further purified by centrifugation through 1.2 *M* sucrose.

III. ASSAY OF ATPase ACTIVITIES

Purity of membrane fractions is conveniently monitored by measuring ATPase activities. ATPase activities are ideal enzymic markers for cardiac membranes because they are measured reliably and quickly with minimal effort for large numbers of samples and because they are selectively activated and inhibited by different agents in sarcolemma, sarcoplasmic reticulum, and mitochondria. ATPase activity is determined by a colorimetric method that measures the hydrolysis of inorganic phosphate from ATP (Harris and Popat, 1954).

A. Solutions

1. Na^+, K^+-ATPase Assay Medium

Aliquots of 0.9 ml of a medium containing 50 m*M* histidine (free base), 3 m*M* $MgCl_2$, 111 m*M* NaCl, 11 m*M* KCl, 3.33 m*M* phosphoenolpyruvate, 75 μg pyruvate kinase, 11 m*M* NaN_3, and 1.1 m*M* ethylene glycol bis(β-amino ethyl ether)-N,N,N′,N′-tetracetic acid (EGTA) are added to test tubes. Reaction tubes are set up that contain this medium plus or without 1.11 m*M* ouabain. Typically, duplicate or triplicate reaction tubes plus and without ouabain are processed for each membrane sample. Phosphoenolpyruvate and pyruvate kinase are included to regenerate ATP from ADP produced during the reactions.

2. Ca^{2+},K^+-ATPase Assay Medium

Aliquots of 0.9 ml of a medium containing 50 m*M* histidine (free base), 3 m*M* $MgCl_2$, 111 m*M* KCl, 3.33 m*M* phosphoenolpyruvate, 75 μg pyruvate kinase, 3 μg A23187, and 1.11 m*M* EGTA are added to test tubes. Reaction tubes are set up that contain this medium plus or without 0.67 m*M* $CaCl_2$. A23187, a calicum-specific ionophore, is added to prevent Ca^{2+} build-up inside sarcoplasmic reticulum vesicles during the assay (Jones *et al.*, 1977, 1978a).

3. Azide-Sensitive ATPase Assay Medium

Aliquots of 0.9 ml of a medium containing 50 m*M* histidine (free base), 3 m*M* $MgCl_2$, 111 m*M* KCl, 3.33 m*M* phosphoenolpyruvate, 75 μg pyruvate kinase, 1.11 m*M* ouabain, and 1.11 m*M* EGTA are added to test tubes. Reaction tubes are set up that contain this medium plus or without 11 m*M* NaN_3.

4. ATP Blanks

Aliquots of 0.9 ml of a medium containing 50 m*M* histidine (free base), 3 m*M* $MgCl_2$, 111 m*M* KCl, 3.33 m*M* phosphoenolpyruvate, and 75 μg of pyruvate kinase are added to test tubes. These reaction tubes do not receive membrane protein and are included to control for the small amount of inorganic phosphate that is detected that is not generated by ATPase activity. EGTA, A23187, and other additives indicated above do not alter the background level of absorbance that is detected with the use of these blank samples.

5. *Phosphate Standard*

Aliquots of 0.9 ml of 50 m*M* histidine and 3 m*M* $MgCl_2$ are added to reaction tubes; 0.1 ml of 5 mM sodium phosphate is also included, which brings the final volume to 1 ml. These samples do not receive ATP or membrane protein.

6. *ATP Start Solution*

ATP (Tris salt), 30 m*M*, is dissolved in 50 m*M* histidine (free base) and 3 m*M* $MgCl_2$ at the time of assay.

7. *Stop Solution for Detection of Inorganic Phosphate*

Inorganic phosphate is determined by the method of Harris and Popat (1954). Three concentrated stock solutions are made (A, B, and C), which are stable indefinitely when stored at 4° in the dark. These solutions are the following:

1. Solution A: 15 g of sodium bisulfite and 5 g of *p*-methylaminophenol sulfate in 500 ml of water.
2. Solution B: 12.5 g of molybdic acid (ammonium salt) in 500 ml of water.
3. Solution C: 68 ml of concentrated H_2SO_4 diluted to 500 ml with water.

For determination of inorganic phosphate, 1 volume each of stock solutions A, B, and C are mixed with four volumes of water, and 2.5 ml of the resultant stop solution is then added to the ATPase assay tubes to detect inorganic phosphate as described below.

B. Procedure

1. *Preincubation of Membranes*

The stock sarcolemmal, mitochondrial, and sarcoplasmic reticulum fractions at a protein concentration of 6 to 8 mg per ml are prediluted 1:10, and 10 to 20 μl of the diluted membranes are added to 0.9 ml of solutions 1, 2, and 3 for assay of each of the ATPase activities in each of the subfractions. Sarcolemmal membranes must first be treated with a suitable unmasking agent during the predilution to allow detection of all of their Na^+,K^+-ATPase activity, as described in the next section. After addition of membrane protein, all reaction tubes are preincubated at 37°C for 10 min.

2. *Starting the Reactions*

Reactions are initiated at 37°C by adding 0.1 ml of solution 6 (ATP start solution) to 0.9 ml of reaction samples 1, 2, 3, and 4. Solution 5, the phosphate standard, does not receive ATP. After addition of ATP, the pH of the reaction mixtures will be approximately 6.8–7.0 without prior adjustment. The reactions are conducted for 15 to 30 min at 37°C.

Table I. ATPase Activities of Purified Cardiac Membrane Fractions[a]

Activity measured	Fraction	Total ATPase activity a	Total ATPase activity b	Specific ATPase activity a − b
		(−) Ou	(+) Ou	
Na^+,K^+-ATPase	SL	149.0	8.6	140.4
	SR	6.5	3.9	2.6
	Mito.	3.1	1.6	1.5
		(+) Ca	(−) Ca	
Ca^{2+},K^+-ATPase	SL	38.7	35.7	3.0
	SR	222.7	4.6	218.1
	Mito.	138.5	144.0	0.0
Azide-sensitive		(−) N_3	(+) N_3	
ATPase	SL	33.7	17.0	16.7
	SR	4.6	5.9	0.0
	Mito.	141.1	1.6	139.5

[a] All values are expressed as micromoles of inorganic phosphate liberated per milligram protein per hour. Sarcolemmal (SL), sarcoplasmic reticular (SR), and mitochondrial (Mito.) activities were determined as described in the text in the presence and absence of ouabain (Ou), calcium (Ca), and sodium azide (N_3). For assay of Na^+,K^+-ATPase, the membranes were first pretreated with the optimal concentration of sodium dodecyl sulfate as depicted in Figure 1. All assays were performed at the same time on the same preparations of membranes.

3. *Stopping the Reactions*

Reactions are terminated by adding 2.5 ml of stop solution (solution 7) to solutions 1, 2, 3, 4, and 5. The stop solution also contains the reagents required for colorimetric determination of inorganic phosphate. After 15 min at room temperature, absorbances are read at a wavelength of 660 nm. The spectrophotometer is blanked with water containing 2.5 ml of stop solution. The phosphate standards should have an absorbance of approximately 0.5. The absorbance read for the ATP blanks (solution 4) should be subtracted from the absorbances read for the reaction tubes that contain membranes if basal ATPase activities of the membranes are to be accurately assessed. The assay for inorganic phosphate is linear to an absorbance of 1.0.

C. Comments

ATPase activities determined for the subcellular fractions are given in Table I. The Na^+,K^+-ATPase activity unmasked by the detergent sodium dodecyl sulfate is defined as that activity inhibited by 1 m*M* ouabain (Jones *et al.*, 1978b). It is evident that Na^+,K^+-ATPase is highly enriched in sarcolemmal vesicles.

The Ca^{2+},K^+-ATPase, defined as that activity dependent on micromolar Ca^{2+} (Jones *et al.*, 1978a,b), is highly enriched in the sarcoplasmic reticulum fraction (Table I). Assuming that this latter fraction is completely purified, an upper limit of sarcoplasmic reticulum contamination in the sarcolemmal fraction is set at 1–2%. The question of whether or not the residual Ca^{2+},K^+-ATPase activity detected in the sarcolemmal fraction represents a low level of sarcoplasmic reticulum contamination or is a manifestation of the activity of the sarcolemmal Ca^{2+} pump will require further investigation before a definitive answer can be obtained (Caroni and Carafoli, 1980; Jones *et al.*, 1980).

Azide-sensitive ATPase, defined as that activity inhibited by 10 m*M* sodium azide, is most enriched in the mitochondrial fraction (Table I). Assuming that this fraction is completely pure, we can estimate an upper limit of mitochondrial contamination in the sarcolemmal fraction of 12%. However, no serious attempt was made to isolate completely pure mitochondria in these studies. Results obtained with the ATPase activities do suggest, however, that the mitochondrial fraction is minimally contaminated with sarcolemma and sarcoplasmic reticulum. The results depicted in Table I clearly establish the validity of using specific ATPase activities as indicators of the purity of cardiac membrane preparations.

IV. UNMASKING AGENTS FOR REVEALING LATENT Na^+,K^+-ATPase ACTIVITIES

Most of the cardiac sarcolemmal vesicles isolated by our procedure are tightly sealed, and as a result most of their enzymic activity is latent. Before Na^+,K^+-ATPase activity can be used as a reliable enzymic marker for sarcolemmal vesicles, therefore, the vesicles must be made leaky. Two effective agents that we have utilized for this purpose are the anionic detergent sodium dodecyl sulfate and the channel-forming peptide ionophore alamethicin (Besch *et al.*, 1977; Jones *et al.*, 1980). Recently Lad and White (1979) have identified two other polypeptide amphiphiles, gramicidin S and melittin, that appear to be effective in unmasking latent activities in membrane vesicles. The protocol below compares the effect of these four agents on the latent Na^+,K^+-ATPase activity of purified cardiac sarcolemmal vesicles.

A. Solutions

1. Sodium Dodecyl Sulfate

A stock solution of sodium dodecyl sulfate is made to 1 mg per ml in 30 m*M* imidazole buffer (pH 7.0). Ultrapure sodium dodecyl sulfate is obtained from Bio-Rad.

2. Gramicidin S

A stock solution of gramicidin S is made to 25 mg per ml in 50% ethanol. Gramicidin S is obtained from Sigma.

3. Melittin

A stock solution of melittin is dissolved in 0.25 *M* sucrose and 10 m*M* histidine (free base) at a concentration of 2 mg per ml. Melittin is obtained from Sigma.

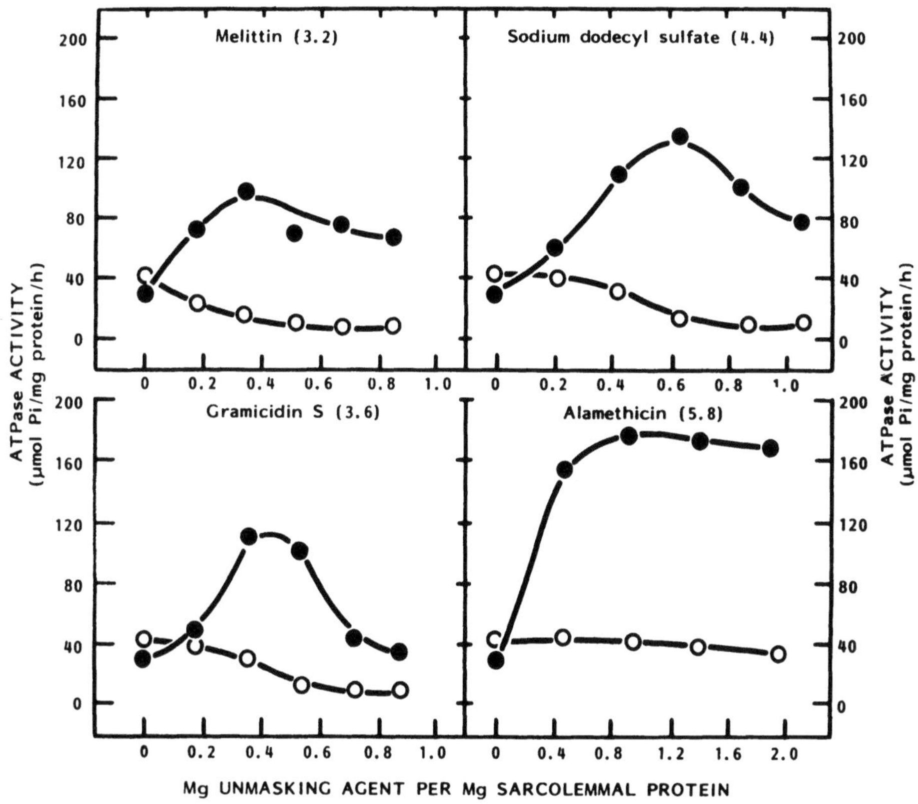

Figure 1. Effect of unmasking agents on the Na^+,K^+-ATPase activity of cardiac sarcolemmal vesicles. Membranes were pretreated with unmasking agents, and their Na^+,K^+-ATPase activities were determined exactly as described in the text. All data points were obtained in the same assay on the same population of sarcolemmal vesicles. Ouabain-inhibitable Na^+,K^+-ATPase activities are indicated by the filled circles. and ouabain-insensitive (basal) ATPase activities are indicated by the open circles (see Table I). Numbers in parentheses indicate the maximum factors of activation of Na^+,K^+-ATPase activities produced by each unmasking agent.

4. *Alamethicin*

A stock solution of alamethicin is dissolved in absolute ethanol at a concentration of 50 mg per ml. Alamethicin was generously supplied by Dr. Joseph Grady of the Upjohn Co.

B. Procedure

The Na^+,K^+-ATPase assays are conducted exactly as described in the previous section. The sarcolemmal fraction (protein concentration 7.1 mg per ml in the specific assay depicted in Figure 1) is prediluted 1:10 in 0.25 *M* sucrose and 10 m*M* histidine that contains increasing concentrations of the amphipathic agents listed above. The concentrations of these unmasking agents in the diluted membrane suspensions are varied as follows: sodium dodecyl sulfate, 0.15 to 0.75 mg per ml; gramicidin S, 0.13 to 0.63 mg per ml; melittin, 0.12 to 0.60 mg per ml; alamethicin, 0.33 to 1.67 mg per ml. The concentration of sarcolemmal protein in these diluted suspensions is kept constant at 0.71 mg per ml. After 20 min at room temperature, 10 μl of pretreated membrane sample is added to each reaction tube, and Na^+,K^+-ATPase activity is then measured by monitoring the ouabain-inhibitable ATPase activity.

C. Comments

Figure 1 demonstrates that each of the four unmasking agents reveals considerable latent Na^+,K^+-ATPase activity in sarcolemmal vesicles. Alamethicin is most effective, giving a 5.8-fold activation, whereas melittin is the least effective, giving only a 3.2-fold activation. Maximal Na^+,K^+-ATPase activities measured in the presence of melittin, gramicidin S, sodium dodecyl sulfate, and alamethicin are 96.5, 109, 133, and 176 μmoles of inorganic phosphate per milligram of protein per hour, respectively. Except for alamethicin, higher concentrations of all of the amphiphiles inhibit both Na^+,K^+-ATPase activity and ouabain-insensitive or basal ATPase activity.

The data in Figure 1 suggest that alamethicin is an ideal unmasking agent for revealing latent Na^+,K^+-ATPase activity in cardiac sarcolemmal vesicles. Alamethicin also increases β-adrenergic receptor-coupled adenylate cyclase activity of sarcolemmal vesicles severalfold as well as cAMP-dependent protein kinase activity (Jones *et al.*, 1980, 1981). Unfortunately, alamethicin is not readily obtainable at the present time, but it is our hope that this interesting ionophore will soon become commercially available. For routine monitoring of purity of cardiac sarcolemmal vesicles, we now employ the detergent sodium dodecyl sulfate, which is the second most effective agent for revealing latent Na^+,K^+-ATPase activity that we have yet identified. Other enzymic activities of cardiac sarcolemmal vesicles are inactivated and/or solubilized by this detergent, however, which makes it unsuitable as a "multipurpose" membrane enzyme-unmasking agent.

V. CONCLUDING REMARKS

The procedures detailed above describe a simple method for preparing highly purified sarcolemmal vesicles from the heart and for monitoring their purity by assay of ATPase activity. The specific activity of Na^+,K^+-ATPase in the sarcolemmal fraction is enriched 40- to 60-fold over that of crude myocardial homogenates (Jones *et al.*, 1980), and this specific activity is so far the highest reported for a cardiac sarcolemmal preparation (Jones *et al.*, 1981). Because the membranes are isolated in a tightly sealed vesicular form, they are suitable not only for enzymic studies but also for studies designed to characterize the physiological properties of sarcolemma such as the regulation of active and passive transport of cations and the generation of transmembrane potentials.

Several caveats should be mentioned, however, with regard to the use of such sarcolemmal vesicles in enzymic and physiological studies. The first is that although the preparation is highly enriched in sarcolemmal vesicles, it is by no means 100% pure. Therefore, any new activities or properties identified in the preparation should be confirmed carefully by both positive and negative marker analysis.

Secondly, the yield of sarcolemmal membranes obtained from the heart is probably 5% or less based on the recovery of Na^+,K^+-ATPase activity from the original myocardial homogenate (unpublished observations). We do not know at this time if the purified vesicles represent a true random sample of the plasma membrane of heart cells or whether they arise from a localized or subspecialized region of the cardiac plasma membrane such as transverse tubules.

The third caveat is that the orientation of the vesicles is probably mixed, although right-side-out sarcolemmal vesicles do account for most of the membrane material (Jones *et al.*, 1980). This sidedness heterogeneity raises important implications for both physiological and enzymic studies, which attempt to characterize the properties of the vesicles. For example, $Na^+:Ca^{2+}$ exchange by the vesicles is usually measured by first passively loading the entire population of vesicles with Na^+ (Reeves and Sutko, 1979). Therefore, both right-side-out and inside-out vesicles are expected to contribute to the $Na^+:Ca^{2+}$-exchange measured when the entire population of Na^+-loaded vesicles is diluted into a second medium devoid of Na^+ and containing radioactive Ca^{2+}. Active transport of Ca^{2+} by sarcolemmal vesicles, on the other hand, may well be contributed by only the inside-out vesicles in the preparation (Caroni and Carofoli, 1980), which probably represent 25% or less of the total vesicle population (Jones *et al.*, 1980).

Problems of interpretation of data also pertain for measurement of enzymic activities. For example, β-adrenergic agonists should bind to only right-side-out vesicles in intact preparations, but resultant stimulation of adenylate cyclase activity in these vesicles should not be detectable because ATP is prevented access to the interior of the vesicles. The low percentage of inside-out vesicles, on the other hand, should contribute most of the adenylate cyclase activity in the intact preparations, but stimulation of their activity by β-adrenergic agonists might not occur because of diffusion limitation of the β agonists.

Because of the caveats mentioned above, we believe that further refinements in purification techniques for sarcolemmal vesicles will be directed toward the isolation of the vesicles in higher yield, the separation of right-side-out from inside-out vesicles, and the identification of suitable unmasking agents that reveal all latent activities uniformly.

ACKNOWLEDGMENTS

This work was supported in part by Grants HL-06308, HL-23704, and GM 07756 from the National Institutes of Health; by the American Heart Association, Indiana Affiliate; by the Herman C. Krannert Fund; and by the Showalter Residuary Trust.

REFERENCES

Besch, H. R., Jr., Jones, L. R., and Watanabe, A. M. 1976. Intact vesicles of canine cardiac sarcolemma. Evidence from vectorial properties of Na^+,K^+-ATPase. *Circ. Res., 39:*586–595.

Besch, H. R., Jr., Jones, L. R., Fleming, J. W., and Watanabe, A. M. 1977. Parallel unmasking of latent adenylate cyclase and (Na^+,K^+)-ATPase activities in cardiac sarcolemmal vesicles. A new use of the channel forming ionophore alamethicin. *J. Biol. Chem., 252:*7905–7908.

Caroni, P., and Carafoli, E. 1980. An ATP-dependent Ca^{2+}-pumping system in dog heart sarcolemma. *Nature, 283:*765–767.

Harris, W. D., and Popat, P. 1954. Determination of the phosphorus content of lipids. *J. Am. Oil Chem. Soc., 31:*124–127.

Heller, M., and Harary, I. 1977. Plasma membranes from cardiac cells in culture. Enzymatic radioiodination, evaluation of preparations and properties of the sarcolemma. *Biochim. Biophys. Acta, 467:*29–43.

Jones, L. R., Besch, H. R., and Watanabe, A. M. 1977. Monovalent cation stimulation of Ca^{2+} uptake by cardiac membrane vesicles. Correlation with stimulation of Ca^{2+}-ATPase activity. *J. Biol. Chem., 252:*3315–3323.

Jones, L. R., Besch, H. R., Jr., and Watanabe, A. M. 1978a. Regulation of the calcium pump of cardiac sarcoplasmic reticulum. Interactive roles of potassium and ATP on the phosphoprotein intermediate of the (K^+,Ca^{2+})-ATPase. *J. Biol. Chem., 253:*1643–1653.

Jones, L. R., Phan, S. H., and Besch, H. R., Jr. 1978b. Gel electrophoretic and density gradient analysis of the (K^+,Ca^{2+})-ATPase and the (Na^+,K^+)-ATPase activities of cardiac membrane vesicles. *Biochem. Biophys. Acta, 514:*294–309.

Jones, L. R., Besch, H. R., Jr., Fleming, J. W., McConnaughey, M. M., and Watanabe, A. M. 1979. Separation of vesicles of cardiac sarcolemma from vesicles of cardiac sarcoplasmic reticulum. Comparative biochemical analysis of component activities. *J. Biol. Chem., 254:*530–539.

Jones, L. R., Maddock, S. W., and Besch, H. R., Jr. 1980. Unmasking effect of alamethicin on the Na^+,K^+-ATPase, β-adrenergic receptor coupled adenylate cyclase, and cAMP-dependent protein kinase activities of cardiac sarcolemmal vesicles. *J. Biol. Chem., 255:*9971–9980.

Jones, L. R., Maddock, S. W., and Hathaway, D. R. 1981. Membrane localization of myocardial type II cyclic AMP-dependent protein kinase activity. *Biochim. Biophys. Acta, 641:*242–253.

Lad, P. J., and White, A. A. 1979. Effect of alamethicin, gramicidin S and melittin upon the particulate guanylate cyclase from rat lung. *Biochim. Biophys. Acta, 570:*198–09.

Lowry, O. H., Rosebrough, N. J., Farr, A. L., and Randall, R. J. 1951. Protein measurement with the folin phenol reagents. *J. Biol. Chem., 193:*265–275.

Pitts, B. J. R. 1979. Stoichimetry of sodium-calcium exchange in cardiac sarcolemmal vesicles. Coupling to the sodium pump. *J. Biol. Chem., 254:*6232–6235.

Reeves, J. P., and Sutko, J. L. 1979. Sodium-calcium ion exchange in cardiac membrane vesicles. *Proc. Natl. Acad. Sci. U.S.A., 76:*590–594.

Wollenberger, A., and Will H. 1978. Protein kinase-catalyzed membrane phophorylation and its possible relationship to the role of calcium in the adrenergic regulation of cardiac contraction. *Life Sci., 22:*1159–1178.

Chapter **2**

Isolation of Sarcolemmal Membranes from Smooth Muscle

Mohammed A. Matlib

Department of Pharmacology and Cell Biophysics
University of Cincinnati College of Medicine
Cincinnati, Ohio

I. INTRODUCTION

Smooth muscle tone is dependent on cytoplasmic free Ca^{2+} concentration, which is regulated by Ca^{2+} influx and efflux across the sarcolemma and across the membranes of intracellular Ca^{2+}-transporting organelles. These Ca^{2+} transport processes may be altered by changes in ionic composition, hormonal stimulation, pharmacological treatments, and by disease conditions. The movements of Ca^{2+} in smooth muscle tissues can be studied by measuring the influx and efflux of $^{45}Ca^{2+}$ under different experimental conditions, but the interpretation of these data is difficult because of the limited knowledge of compartmentalization of cellular Ca^{2+}. Another approach is to isolate membrane vesicles in purified form and to study Ca^{2+} transport *in vitro* to gain an insight into its function *in vivo*. Since the number of smooth muscle cells is small, and they are usually surrounded by nonmuscle cells, it is difficult to isolate substantial amounts of purified subcellular membranes from smooth muscle tissues. In this chapter, a procedure is described that has been found useful in our laboratory for the isolation of reasonable amounts of sarcolemmal membranes from rat myometrium, pig coronary arteries, and dog and rat mesenteric arteries.

II. MATERIALS

A. Chemicals

ATP, 5′-AMP, NADH, NADPH, cytochrome *c*, succinate, atropine, ouabain, morpholinopropanesulfonic acid, and bovine serum albumin (fatty acid-free) were obtained from Sigma Chemical Co., St. Louis. [^{3}H]Ouabain, [^{3}H]quinuclidinyl benzilate, [^{14}C]tyramine, and [^{3}H]wheat germ agglutinin were obtained from New England Nuclear, Boston. [^{3}H]Oxytocin was prepared in the laboratories of Dr. Luis A. Branda, Department of Biochemistry, McMaster University, Hamilton, Ontario, Canada. [^{3}H]Nimodipine was custom synthesized by New England Nuclear for Dr. Alexander Scriabine of Miles Institute of Preclinical Pharmacology, New Haven, Connecticut. All other chemicals were of the purest grade available commercially.

B. Solutions

Five to ten liters of 0.9% NaCl solution. Five hundred ml of freshly prepared isolation medium containing 250 m*M* sucrose, 0.05% bovine serum albumin, and 10 m*M* morpholinopropanesulfonic acid buffer (pH 7.4 at 4°C). All other solutions for enzyme and markers are prepared fresh when required.

C. Instruments

A Polytron® homogenizer, glass–Teflon® homogenizer, refrigerated low- and high-speed centrifuges, spectrophotometer, Millipore™ filtration apparatus, and liquid scintillation counter are required.

D. Tissues

Ten pig or beef hearts may be obtained from a slaughterhouse, should be placed in iced saline and immediately transported to the laboratory. Two mongrel dogs may be anesthetized with pentobarbital (30 mg/kg), and their hearts should be excised. The abdomens are opened, and the entire mesenteric beds are removed and placed in iced saline. Thirty rats (~300 g) may be sacrificed by decapitation with a guillotine. The abdomens are opened, and the mesenteric beds are removed and placed in ice-cold isolation medium.

III. METHODS

A. Separation of Smooth Muscle Cells from Nonmuscle Cells

This process depends on the type of tissue used and is usually carried out at 0–4°C. A cold surface is created on an inverted 500-ml glass beaker by adding a few milliliters of 0.9% NaCl solution to the beaker and packing it with ice. The top of the inverted glass beaker is covered with filter paper moistened with isolation medium. In the case of rat uterine smooth muscle, the uterus is placed on this cold surface and slit open with scissors, and the endometrium and other nonmuscle cells are removed by scraping with a sharp plastic edge made by cutting a white tip of a 5-ml digital pipette (Gilson Pipetman). The remaining myometrium containing smooth muscle cells is then used for the isolation of subcellular membranes.

Right, left, and left-descending coronary arteries of pig or beef hearts are dissected and placed on top of the inverted beaker as described above. The myocardium and fatty tissues are trimmed off, and the vessels are split open. The inside of each vessel is scraped gently to remove blood cells and the endothelial layer. The medial layer containing smooth muscle cells is then scraped from the adventitial layer and placed in ice-cold isolation medium.

In the case of rat mesenteric arteries, the entire mesenteric vasculature is dissected, cooled in ice-cold isolation medium and then placed on top of the inverted glass beaker with veins facing upward. Fat, some mesenteric veins, and other nonmuscle cells are removed by scraping while holding the superior mesenteric artery and vein with a pair of forceps. After removal of the gross fat and lymph nodes, the mesenteries near the superior mesenteric vein are cut free so that the vein can be pulled away from the tissue with a pair of forceps, leaving only the arteries still embedded in the mesentery. The arteries are then gently pulled away from the mesenteric bed on the filter paper and scraped to remove remaining fat and veins. The tissue containing smooth muscle cells from mesenteric beds of several animals is pooled, blotted, and weighed. A procedure to collect rat mesenteric arteries has been described in detail by Kwan *et al.* (1979).

The dog mesenteric beds were spread on a clean surface in a cold room, the superior mesenteric artery was located, and the branches were pulled away with a pair of forceps and placed in ice-cold isolation medium.

B. Preparation of Membrane Fractions

The procedure is similar to the one described previously for rat myometrium (Matlib *et al.*, 1979). The cleaned tissue is minced with scissors. The minced tissue (~2 g) is placed in an ice-cold centrifuge tube and suspended in 5 ml of a solution containing 250 m*M* sucrose, 10 m*M* morpholinopropanesulfonic acid (MOPS) buffer, and 0.05% bovine serum albumin (BSA), pH 7.4, at 4°C. The centrifuge tube is placed in a plastic bottle containing saline and ice. The tissue is then homogenized with a Polytron® (PT 10/35, Brinkman Instruments) twice for 10 sec each at a speed setting of 8 and then twice for 10 sec at a setting of 6.5. After each Polytron® burst, the homogenate is cooled for 2 min before the next burst. The homogenate is diluted (1 g tissue: 10 ml medium), placed in a glass–Teflon® homogenizer, and homogenized by making six passes. The homogenate is then transferred to centrifuge tubes and centrifuged at 1000 × *g* for 10 min to remove nuclei, contractile proteins, and unbroken cells. The supernatant is filtered through two layers of cheesecloth and centrifuged at 10,000 × *g* for 10 min. The resulting supernatant is then centrifuged at 112,000 × *g* for 30 min in a Beckman

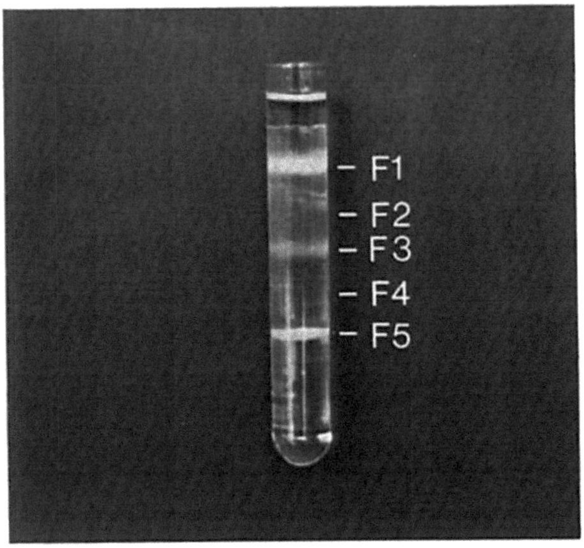

Figure 1. Distribution of membrane bands in discontinuous sucrose density gradient after centrifugation of microsomes of rat myometrium. F1, F3, and F5 are concentrated, and F2 and F4 are diffuse membrane bands.

ultracentrifuge. The pellet, designated as microsomes, is suspended in about 5 ml of the isolation medium.

Fractionation of the microsomes is carried out in a discontinuous sucrose density gradient. The discontinuous gradient is composed of 4 ml of 50% sucrose (w/w), 3 ml of 35% sucrose, and 3 ml of 30% sucrose layered in that order in a 9.5 × 1.5 cm cellulose nitrate tube. The microsomal fraction, in a volume of 3 ml sucrose–MOPS solution containing 7–9 mg protein, is layered on top of the tubes containing the discontinuous sucrose gradient. These are then centrifuged at 112,000 × *g* for 2 hr in a swinging-bucket rotor (Beckman SW40). After centrifugation, three distinct and two diffuse bands are observed (Figure 1). The distinct band at the interface between 8.5% of the loading sucrose–MOPS solution and 30% sucrose is designated as F1, the diffuse band in 30% sucrose as F2, the distinct band at the interface between 30% and 35% sucrose as F3, the diffuse band in 35% sucrose as F4, and, finally, the distinct band at the interface between 35% and 50% sucrose as F5 fraction. Individual fractions are carefully removed with Pasteur pipettes, diluted with distilled water to a sucrose concentration of 8.5% and centrifuged at 102,000 × *g* for 30 min. The resultant pellets are resuspended in a small volume of sucrose–MOPS solution.

C. Electron Microscopy

Pellets of isolated membranes are fixed for 2 hr in 2% glutaraldehyde in 75 m*M* sodium cacodylate buffer (pH 7.4) containing 4.5% sucrose. Fixed pellets are rinsed for 1 hr in the above buffer, postfixed in 2% osmium tetroxide in 50 m*M* cacodylate buffer (pH 7.4), stained *en bloc* for 1 hr with saturated uranyl acetate, dehydrated in graded alcohols, and embedded in Spurr resin. Silver to gray sections are cut with a microtome, suspended on copper grids, stained with lead citrate, and examined in a Philips 301 electron microscope at 60 kV. An electron micrograph of the F1 fraction is shown in Figure 2. This fraction is characterized by sealed and homogeneous membrane vesicles. The other membrane fractions are heterogeneous and probably originate from different sources (electron micrographs not shown).

D. Assays for Membrane Markers

The following enzymes and markers can be employed to determine the distribution and enrichment of membranes in different fractions during the preparation. Unless otherwise mentioned, enzyme assays are carried out after 2–5 min of preincubation at either 30°C or 37°C, depending on the enzyme under study.

5′-Nucleotidase activity is assayed according to Song and Bodansky (1967) by measuring inorganic phosphate liberated from 5′-AMP at 37° during 15 min of incubation in a solution (1 ml) containing 100 m*M* tris-HCl, pH 7.5, 10 m*M* $MgCl_2$, 5 mM 5′-AMP, and 20–50 μg protein. The reaction is started with 5′-AMP after preincubation of the membranes for 5 min at 37°. After 15 min of incubation, the reaction is stopped by adding 1 ml 10% trichloroacetic acid. The precipitate is removed by centrifugation at 3000 rpm for 20 min. Inorganic phosphate in the supernatant is measured according to Bonting *et al.* (1961). Where the enzyme activity is very low, as with pig coronary arteries, a more sensitive assay for inorganic phosphate described by Ames and Dubin (1960) is used.

Total Mg^{2+}*-ATPase* activity is assayed by measuring the liberation of inorganic phosphate from ATP after 5 min incubation at 37°. The assay medium contains 100 m*M* tris-HCl, 5 m*M* $MgCl_2$, 5 m*M* ATP, pH 7.5, and 20–50 μg protein. Inorganic phosphate in the supernatant is determined according to Bonting *et al.* (1961).

Succinate–cytochrome c reductase activity is measured at 30°C according to King (1967) in a solution (1 ml) containing 100 m*M* potassium phosphate buffer pH 7.5, 1 m*M* KCN, 10 μ*M* cytochrome *c*, and 10 m*M* succinate. The reduction of cytochrome *c* is followed in a spectrophotometer set at 550 nm.

NADPH- and NADH–cytochrome c reductase activities are measured according to the method of Sottocasa *et al.* (1967) by following the reduction of cytochrome *c* at 550 nm by NADPH or NADH in the same solution as the one used in the succinate–cytochrome *c* reductase assay except that succinate is replaced with 0.15 m*M* NADPH or NADH. Rotenone (10 μ*M*) is added when required to determine the rotenone-sensitive NADH–cytochrome *c* reductase activity. An extinction coefficient of 19.2 cm^{-1} mM^{-1} for reduced cytochrome *c* is used for the calculations.

Monoamine oxidase activity is determined in 100 m*M* sodium phosphate buffer (pH 7.5) by the radiochemical method of Otsuka and Kobayashi (1964) as modified by Grosso and Gawienowski (1976), using [^{14}C]tyramine as a substrate.

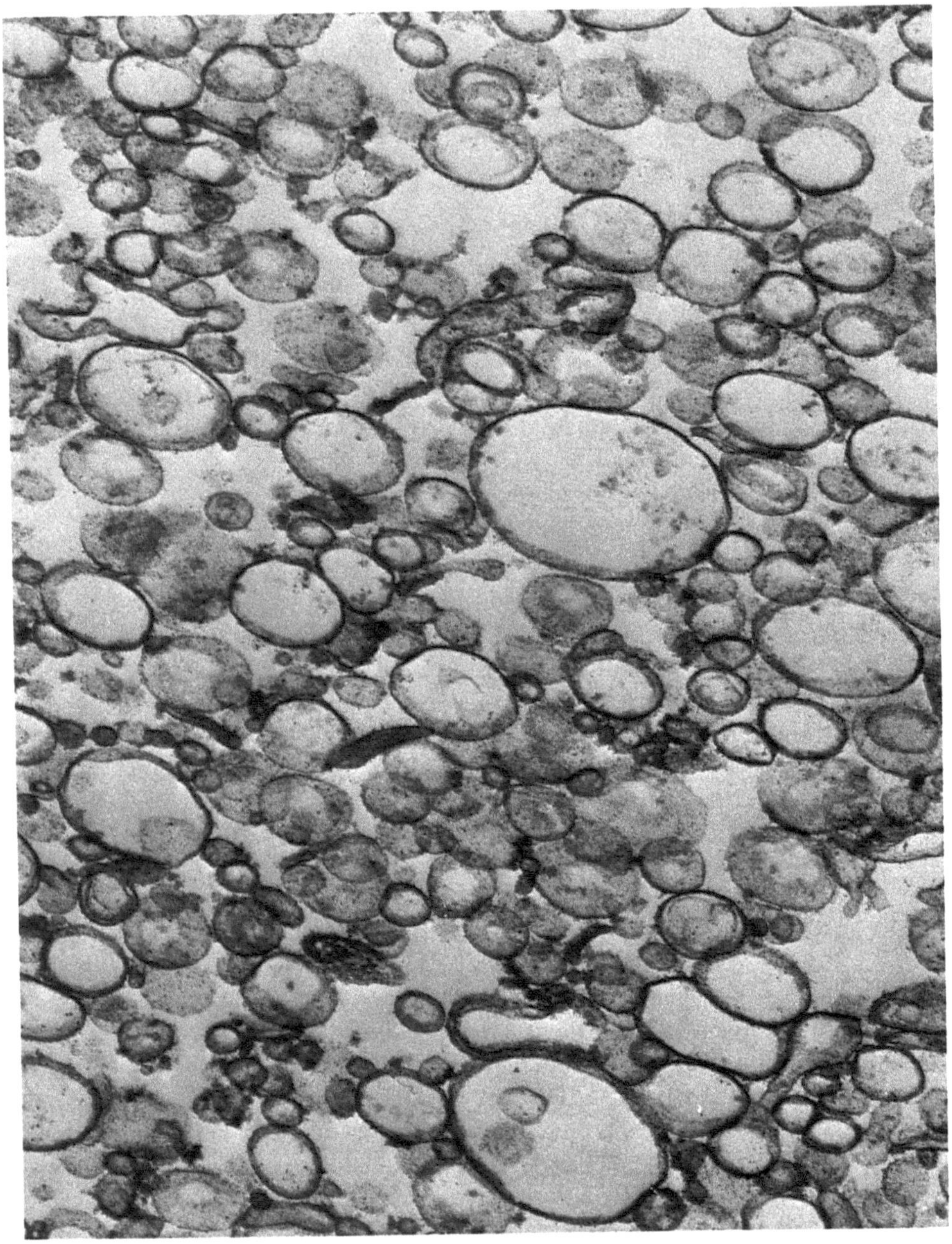

Figure 2. Electron micrograph of the sarcolemmal membranes of rat myometrium concentrated in the F1 fraction. Magnification × 150,000.

E. Ligand Binding Assays

[^{3}H]Ouabain binding is carried out in a 3-ml solution containing 50 m*M* tris-HCl (pH 7.4), 5 m*M* Mg-Pi, and 10^{-7} *M* [^{3}H]ouabain. The binding is initiated by adding 60–120 μg protein after 10 min of preincubation of the solution at 37°C. After 30 min of incubation, a 0.9-ml aliquot is filtered through 0.45-μm GF/F filter (Whatman) and washed three times with 5 ml cold 50 m*M* tris-HCl (pH 7.4). The filters are then counted for radioactivity in 10 ml of Scinti-Verse® E scintillation fluid (Fisher Scientific Co., U.S.A.). The nonspecific binding is defined as binding of [^{3}H]ouabain in the presence of 5.5×10^{-3} *M* unlabeled ouabain. The nonspecific binding is subtracted from total binding before the specific binding in the membranes is determined.

[^{3}H]Quinuclidinyl benzilate ([^{3}H]QNB) binding is carried out at 37°C in a 5-ml solution containing 50 m*M* tris-HCl (pH 7.4), 10 m*M* $MgCl_2$, and 2×10^{-10} *M* [^{3}H]QNB. The solution is incubated in the presence of 100–200 μg protein for 1 hr, filtered through 0.45-μm GF/F filter, and washed three times with 5 ml cold 50 m*M* tris-HCl (pH 7.4). The nonspecific binding is defined as binding of [^{3}H]QNB in the presence of 10^{-6} *M* atropine.

[^{3}H]Nimodipine binding is carried out in a 1-ml solution containing 50 m*M* tris-HCl (pH 7.4) and 2×10^{-10} *M* [^{3}H]nimodipine. The solution is preincubated at 37°C for 5 min and then 10–50 μg membrane protein is added. After 30 min of incubation, the binding is stopped by filtration as described above. The filter papers are washed once with 20 ml and twice with 10 ml cold distilled water. The nonspecific binding is determined in the presence of 10^{-6} *M* unlabeled nimodipine.

[^{3}H]Wheat germ agglutinin ([^{3}H]WGA) and *[^{3}H]oxytocin* bindings to membranes are carried out as described previously (Crankshaw *et al.*, 1978; Matlib *et al.*, 1979).

IV. DATA PRESENTATION

Described below are two examples of characterization of membranes isolated from rat myometrium and dog mesenteric arteries.

The data in Figures 3 through 7 are presented according to the format of deDuve *et al.* (1955). In this format, the specific activity of the constituents in the postnuclear supernatant (1000 × *g* supernatant) is set as unity; the height of each block represents the specific activity of a fraction relative to that of the postnuclear supernatant. The recovery of protein in that fraction is indicated on the abscissa. Therefore, the surface area of each block (relative specific activity times protein) is the percentage of the constituent recovered in the corresponding fraction. The absolute activities of markers in fractions of rat myometrium were obtained from data presented in a previous publication (Matlib *et al.*, 1979).

Figure 3 shows the distribution of wheat germ agglutinin ([^{3}H]WGA) and [^{3}H]oxytocin binding and 5′-nucleotidase activity in different fractions obtained after differential centrifugation of postnuclear supernatant of rat myometrium. All of these markers were enriched in the microsomal fraction, although some remained in the soluble supernatant. When the microsomal fraction was subjected

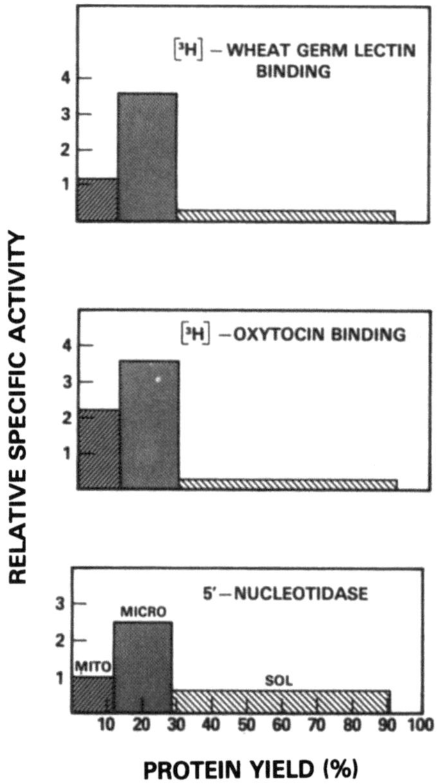

Figure 3. Distribution of specific binding of [^{3}H]wheat germ agglutinin (lectin) and [^{3}H]oxytocin and 5′-nucleotidase activity in mitochondria (MITO), microsomes (MICRO), and soluble supernatant (SOL) of rat myometrium.

to discontinuous sucrose density gradient centrifugation, these markers were found to be concentrated in the F1 fraction (Figure 4). This fraction was designated as enriched sarcolemmal membranes, since these three markers are considered located in sarcolemmal membranes (Crankshaw *et al.*, 1978; Chang *et al.*, 1975; Janis *et al.*, 1977). Succinate–cytochrome *c* reductase and rotenone-sensitive NADH-cytochrome *c* reductase located in the mitochondrial inner membrane (Greenawalt and Schnaitman, 1968) were concentrated in the mitochondrial fraction (Figure 5). These enzyme activities were decreased in F1 fraction and increased in F4 fraction in the sucrose density gradient (Figure 6). Monoamine oxidase activity located in the mitochondrial outer membrane (Schnaitman *et al.*, 1967) was found to be distributed almost equally in all the fractions. This enzyme appears not to be suitable as a marker for the smooth muscle mitochondrial outer membranes, probably because of the very low activity compared to that of liver and brain. There is no known marker for endoplasmic reticulum or sarcoplasmic reticulum in smooth muscle. NADPH–cytochrome *c* reductase or rotenone-insensitive (RI)-NADH–cytochrome *c* reductase activities were employed as possible markers for this organelle. In rat myometrium, these enzyme activities were found to be enriched in the F4 fraction (Figure 7). It is apparent from these marker studies that F1 fraction was enriched with sarcolemmal membranes. The other fractions were found to contain membranes of heterogeneous origin.

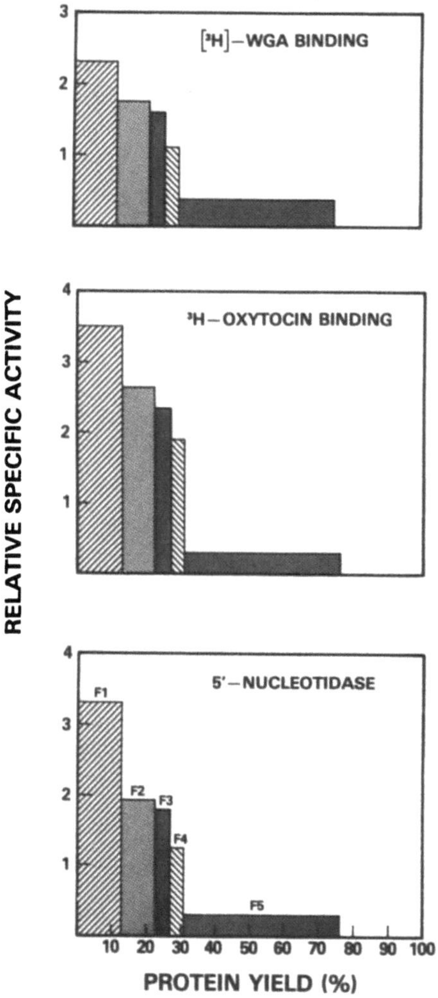

Figure 4. Distribution of specific binding of [^{3}H]wheat germ agglutinin ([^{3}H]WGA) and [^{3}H]oxytocin, and 5'-nucleotidase activities in membrane fractions separated after centrifugation of microsomes of rat myometrium in a discontinuous sucrose density gradient.

Table I. Distribution of Sarcolemmal Markers in Membrane Fractions of Dog Mesenteric Arteries

Fractions	5'-Nucleotidase activity (nmoles/mg protein per hr)	[^{3}H]Ouabain binding (pmoles/mg protein)	[^{3}H]QNB binding (fmoles/mg protein)	[^{3}H]Nimodipine binding (fmoles/mg protein)
Homogenate	505 ± 79	1.02 ± 0.26	11.2 ± 5.5	6.77 ± 3.17
Mitochondria	484 ± 45	0.79 ± 0.23	1.1 ± 0.8	—
Microsomes	836 ± 114	1.30 ± 0.17	33.7 ± 8.4	20.93 ± 6.96
F1	5956 ± 890	12.27 ± 1.26	141.7 ± 27.8	50.70 ± 9.78
F3	2721 ± 351	4.37 ± 0.24	92.5	24.30
F5	486 ± 67	0.66 ± 0.20	40.8 ± 22.3	12.90 ± 7.01

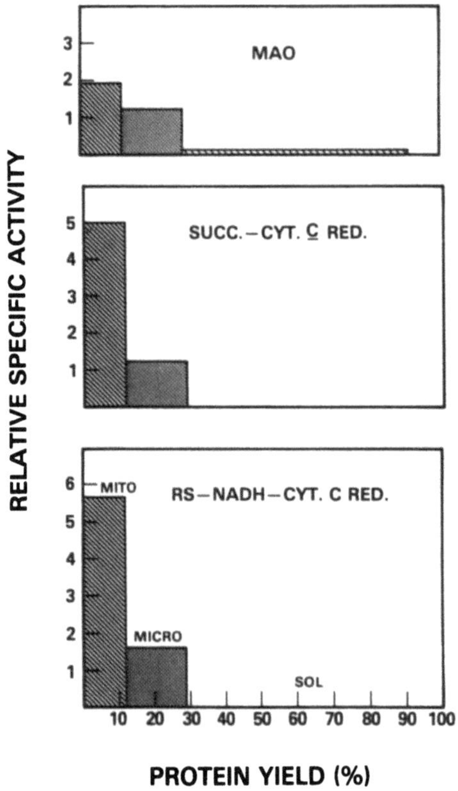

Figure 5. Distribution of monoamine oxidase (MAO), succinate–cytochrome *c* reductase (SUCC.-CYT C RED.), and rotenone-sensitive NADH–cytochrome *c* reductase (RS-NADH-CYT C RED.) activities in mitochondria (MITO), microsomes (MICRO), and soluble supernatant (SOL) of rat myometrium.

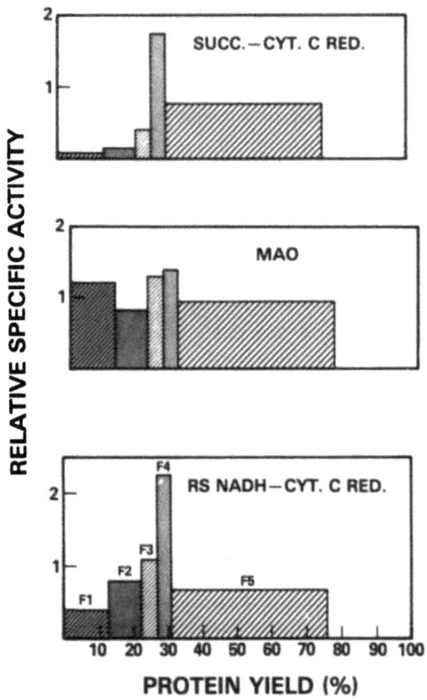

Figure 6. Distribution of monoamine oxidase (MAO), succinate–cytochrome *c* reductase (SUCC.-CYT C RED.), and rotenone-sensitive NADH–cytochrome *c* reductase (RS-NADH-CYT C RED.) activities in membrane fractions of rat myometrium separated after centrifugation of microsomes in a discontinuous sucrose density gradient.

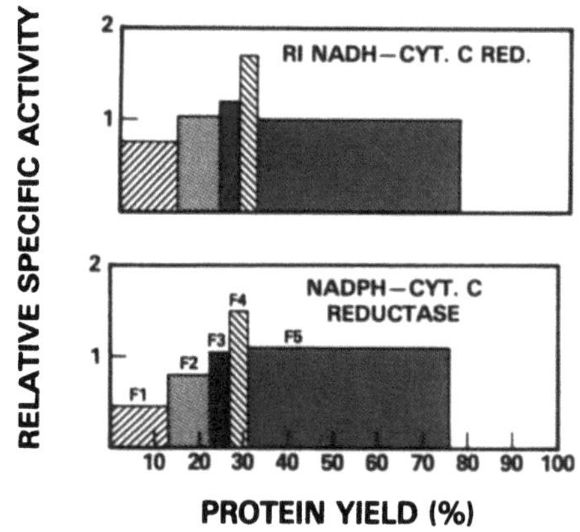

Figure 7. Distribution of NADPH–cytochrome *c* reductase activity in membranes separated after centrifugation of microsomes of rat myometrium in a discontinuous sucrose density gradient.

The same procedure was employed to fractionate membranes of dog mesenteric arteries. The data presented in Table I indicate that the F1 fraction was enriched with 5′-nucleotidase activity. This fraction was also enriched with [^{3}H]ouabain (inhibitor of Na^+,K^+-ATPase), [^{3}H]QNB (antagonist of muscarinergic receptor), and [^{3}H]nimodipine (inhibitor of slow inward calcium channels) binding. Since 5′-nucleotidase activity was found to be a specific marker for sarcolemmal membrane in smooth muscle (Chang *et al.*, 1975; Janis *et al.*, 1977; Crankshaw *et al.*, 1978; Matlib *et al.*, 1979; Kwan *et al.*, 1979), it was concluded that sarcolemmal membranes of dog mesenteric arteries are also the site of [^{3}H]ouabain, [^{3}H]QNB, and [^{3}H]nimodipine binding. This membrane fraction is therefore suitable for studies on ion transport and characterization of certain hormone and drug receptors.

ACKNOWLEDGMENTS

Part of this work was carried out in the laboratories of Dr. Edwin E. Daniel at the Department of Neurosciences, McMaster University, Hamilton, Ontario, Canada. The author thanks Ms. Janet Simons for typing the manuscript.

REFERENCES

Ames, B. N., and Dubin, D. T. 1960. The role of polyamines in the neutralization of bacteriophage deoxyribonucleic acid. *J. Biol. Chem., 235*:769–775.

Bonting, S. L., Simon, K. A., and Hawkins, N. A. 1961. Studies on sodium–potassium-activated adenosine triphosphatase. 1. Quantitative distribution in several tissues of the cat. *Arch. Biochem. Biophys., 95*:416–423.

Chang, K.-J., Bennet, V., and Cautrecassas, P. 1975. Membrane receptors as general markers for plasma membrane isolation procedures. *J. Biol. Chem. 250*:488–500.

Crankshaw, D. J., Branda, L. A., Matlib, M. A., and Daniel, E. E., 1978, Localization of the oxytocin receptor in the plasma membrane of rat myometrium, *Eur. J. Biochem., 86*:481–486.

deDuve, C., Pressman, B. C., Gianetto, R., Wattiaux, R., and Appelmans, F. 1955. Tissue fractionation studies. 6. Intracellular distribution patterns of enzymes in rat-liver tissue. *Biochem., J., 60:*604–617.

Greenawalt, J. W., and Schnaitman, C. 1968. Enzymatic properties of the inner and outer membranes of rat liver mitochondria. *J. Cell Biol., 38:*158–175.

Grosso, D. S., and Gawienowski, A. M. 1976. Inhibition of mitochondrial monoamine oxidase of the rat uterus and liver by clorgyline, pargyline and hermine. *Biochem. Pharmacol., 25:*957–961.

Janis, R. A., Crankshaw, D. J., and Daniel, E. E. 1977. Control of intracellular Ca^{2+} activity in rat myometrium. *Am. J. Physiol., 232:*C50–C58.

King, T. E. 1967. Preparation of succinate–cytochrome *c* reductase and cytochrome *b–c*, particle, and reconstitution of succinate–cytochrome *c* reductase. In: *Methods in Enzymology*, Volume 10, pp. 216–217. Ed. by Estabrook, R. W., and Pullman, M. E. Academic Press, New York.

Kwan, C.-Y., Garfield, R., and Daniel, E. E. 1979. An improved procedure for the isolation of plasma membranes from rat mesenteric arteries. *J. Mol. Cell. Cardiol., 11:*639–659.

Matlib, M. A., Crankshaw, J., Garfield, R. E., Crankshaw, D. J., Kwan, C-Y., Branda, L. A., and Daniel, E. E. 1979. Characterization of membrane fractions and isolation of purified plasma membranes from rat myometrium. *J. Biol. Chem., 254:*1834–1840.

Otsuka, S., and Kobayashi, Y. 1964. A radioisotopic assay for monoamine oxidase determinations in human plasma. *Biochem. Pharmacol., 13:*995–1006.

Schnaitman, C., Erwin, V. G., and Greenawalt, J. W. 1967. The submitochondrial localization of monoamine oxidase. *J. Cell Biol., 32:*719–735.

Song, C. S., and Bodansky, O. 1967. Subcellular localization and properties of 5′-nucleotidase in rat liver. *J. Biol. Chem., 242:*694–699.

Sottocasa, G. L., Kuylenstierna, B., Ernster, L., and Bergstrand, A. 1967. An electron transport system associated with outer membrane of liver mitochondria. *J. Cell Biol., 32:*415–438.

Chapter 3

Isolation of Cardiac Muscle Mitochondria: An Update

Mohammed A. Matlib, William Rouslin, Pal L. Vaghy, and Arnold Schwartz

Department of Pharmacology and Cell Biophysics
University of Cincinnati College of Medicine
Cincinnati, Ohio

I. INTRODUCTION

In cardiac muscle cells, mitochondria occupy about 40% of the total volume (Page and McCallister, 1973) and provide about 90% of the ATP required under normal aerobic conditions (Neely and Morgan, 1974). In addition to being the major source of ATP, mitochondria contain distinct Ca^{2+} influx and efflux systems (Carafoli, 1979), the role of which in cell function is still incompletely understood. The structure and function of mitochondria are known to be damaged in such disease conditions as myocardial ischemia (Jennings and Ganote, 1974; Rouslin, 1983; Rouslin and Millard, 1980, 1981; Sordahl and Stewart, 1980; Wood *et al.*, 1979; Nagao *et al.*, 1980) and heart failure (Lindenmayer *et al.*, 1968, 1970, 1971; Lochner *et al.*, 1968; Meerson *et al.*, 1964; Rouslin *et al.*, 1979; Schwartz and Lee, 1962; Wollenberger *et al.*, 1963). A major thrust of research in this area has been the elucidation of mechanisms and factors responsible for mitochondrial damage and the design of pharmacological interventions to prevent cellular injury. In most of these studies, it is necessary to study the structure and function of mitochondria *in vitro* after isolation and purification.

Procedures for the isolation of mitochondria from various tissues have been described in detail in Volume 1 of this series (Sordahl *et al.*, 1971). In the past, the major concern was the isolation of intact and functionally active mitochondria. However, a more recent concern in this area has been the yield of mitochondria.

By increasing the number of mitochondria that can be isolated from normal and diseased tissues, it is hoped that more "representative" organelle populations reflecting diverse situations *in situ* may be obtained. In this chapter, procedures for the isolation of cardiac muscle mitochondria are described that are now used routinely in this and other laboratories.

II. ISOLATION PROCEDURES

A. Isolation of Mitochondria by Polytron® Treatment

Mitochondria may be prepared essentially according to the method of Sordahl *et al.* (1971) as modified in this laboratory (Rouslin, 1983). All steps are carried out at ice-bucket temperatures. Briefly, myocardial samples are drained and then minced finely. Approximately 10 volumes of ice-cold isolation medium containing 180 m*M* KCl, 10 m*M* EGTA [ethyleneglycol-bis(β-aminoethylether)-N,N′-tetra-acetic acid]-tris, pH 7.4, 0.5% bovine serum albumin (Sigma fraction V), and 10 m*M* HEPES (N-2-hydroxyethylpiperazine-N′-2-ethanesulfonic acid)–KOH buffer, final medium pH of 7.4, (KEAH medium) are added to the tissue mince. This is homogenized as gently as possible by several rapid passes with a Polytron® type PT 10/35 tissue homogenizer (Brinkman Instruments) set at a low speed just sufficient to homogenize fully the tissue mince fragments in the 12 sec total employed. The homogenates are then centrifuged at 450 *g* for 10 min.

The low-speed supernatants are decanted through two layers of cheesecloth and centrifuged at 10,000 *g* for 10 min. The tops of the 10,000-*g* pellets are rinsed carefully to remove any light or fluffy material, and the mitochondrial pellets are then suspended in the KEAH isolation medium using glass homogenizers with loose-fitting Teflon® pestles at as high a final protein concentration as is practicable (*ca.* 40 mg/ml). This procedure, involving a minimum of handling of the subcellular fraction, has been applied successfully by us to the isolation of cardiac muscle mitochondria from dogs (Rouslin, 1983; Rouslin and Millard, 1980), pigs (Rouslin and Millard, 1981), and rabbits (Rouslin *et al.*, 1979). The yield is 7 to 8 mg/g wet wt. or *ca.* 15–20% of the total mitochondrial population.

1. *Assays of Polytron®-Prepared Mitochondria*

State 3 rates are measured polarographically at 30°C using a Gilson model K-IC Oxygraph equipped with a Clark oxygen electrode. Approximately 1.5 mg of mitochondrial protein are used per assay and the assay medium contains 0.25 *M* sucrose, 10 m*M* HEPES–KOH, pH 7.4, 2.5 m*M* phosphate, 536 nmoles ADP, and either 6.25 m*M* glutamate plus 6.25 m*M* malate or 6.25 m*M* succinate plus 1 μg rotenone/ml.

NADH–coenzyme Q reductase or electron transfer complex I is assayed spectrophotometrically by measuring the rotenone-sensitive initial rate of oxidation of NADH at 340 nm at a full-scale sensitivity of 0.1 O.D. unit (Rouslin and Millard, 1980). The 1.5-ml reaction mixture contains 120 μmoles of tris-HCl buffer,

Table I. Activities of Control Canine Heart Mitochondria Prepared Using the Polytron® Procedure[a]

State 3 Qo_2 (natoms O_2/min per mg)	
Glutamate + malate (n = 10)	184 ± 7
Succinate + rotenone (n = 6)	125 ± 9
Enzyme activity (μmoles/min per mg)	
Complex I (NADH–CoQ reductase) (n = 7)	0.100 ± 0.007
Complex II (succinate–CoQ reductase) (n = 5)	0.044 ± 0.005
Complex III (QH_2–c reductase) (n = 5)	3.36 ± 0.29
Complex IV (cytochrome c oxidase) (n = 4)	5.03 ± 0.41
Complex V (oligomycin-sensitive ATPase) (n = 6)	1.41 ± 0.12

[a] From Rouslin (1983).

pH 8.0, 5.0 μmoles of NaN_3, 40 μg of oxidized coenzyme Q_2, and 100 μl of mitochondria that have been diluted to 2.0 mg/ml and sonicated a total of 45 sec. The reaction is begun by the addition of 1.5 μmoles of NADH.

Succinate–coenzyme Q reductase or electron transfer complex II is assayed spectrophotometrically by measuring the rate of reduction of 2,6-dichloroindophenol at 600 nm. The 3.0-ml reaction mixture contains 300 μmoles of potassium phosphate buffer, pH 7.4, 0.3 μmole of EDTA, 0.1% (v/v) Triton X-100, 3 μg of rotenone, 6 μmoles of NaN_3, 50 μl of 0.1% (w/v) 2,6-dichloroindophenol, and 100 μl of mitochondria diluted to 4 mg/ml and swollen for 20 min at 30° in 0.1 M potassium phosphate, pH 7.4. After allowing for the depletion of endogenous substrates, the reaction is begun by the addition of 0.1 ml of 0.5 M succinate–KOH, pH 7.4.

Reduced coenzyme Q–cytochrome c reductase or electron transfer complex III and cytochrome c oxidase (complex IV) are assayed spectrophotometrically at 550 nm by determining the first-order rate constants for the reduction or oxidation, respectively, of oxidized or reduced cytochrome c as described earlier (Rouslin, 1975). The mitochondria used for these assays are swollen for 20 min at 30° in 0.1 M potassium phosphate, pH 7.4.

Mitochondrial ATPase or complex V is assayed by a modification of the method of Tzagoloff *et al.* (1968). The 1.0-ml reaction mixture contains 50 μmoles tris-HCl, pH 7.8, 10 μmoles $MgCl_2$, and 50 μl sonicated mitochondria. The reaction is started by the addition of 10 μmoles ATP-tris, run for 5 min at 30°C, and stopped by the addition of 1 ml 10% trichloroacetic acid. After protein removal, inorganic phosphate is determined (against a zero-time blank) according to the method of Bonting *et al.* (1961). Protein is determined by the method of Lowry *et al.* (1951). Table I shows mitochondrial functional and enzymatic activities measured using the above-described assay procedures.

Table II. Respiration and Oxidative Phosphorylation in Isolated Rabbit Heart Mitochondria in Sucrose and KCl Medium by the Glass–Teflon® Homogenization Procedure[a]

Assay medium	N	State 3	State 4	RCI	ADP:O	OPR
Sucrose	4	312.5 ± 19.1[b]	26.8 ± 1.4[b]	11.8 ± 0.5	2.92 ± 0.05	911 ± 53[b]
KCl	4	583.4 ± 52.8	53.8 ± 3.5	11.1 ± 1.2	2.87 ± 0.03	1675 ± 164

[a] These mitochondria were isolated by the glass–Teflon® homogenization procedure. The assay media contained 250 mM sucrose, 1 mM pyruvate, and 5 mM potassium phosphate buffer (pH 7) or 150 mM KCl, 1 mM pyruvate, and 2 mM potassium phosphate buffer (pH 7) at 37°C. The experiments were started by the addition of 1 mg of mitochondrial protein to 1.5 ml of test medium. State 3 respiration was induced by the addition of 500 nmoles ADP. Statistical significances were calculated by Student's t-test. States 3 and 4 are expressed in nanoatoms oxygen consumed by 1 mg of mitochondrial protein per min. OPR is the oxidative phosphorylation rate expressed as nmoles ATP synthesized by 1 mg of mitochondrial protein per min. RCI is the respiratory control index (the ratio of state 3 to state 4 oxygen consumption).

[b] Values are significantly different between sucrose and KCl medium ($P < 0.05$).

B. Isolation of Mitochondria by Glass–Teflon® Homogenization

1. *Isolation of Mitochondria*

The method is the same as that described in a previous publication (Vaghy *et al.*, 1981). Male and female albino rabbits weighing 2–3 kg may be employed. The chest is opened after cervical dislocation, and the heart is quickly removed and immediately placed in ice-cold physiological saline solution to wash it free of blood. The heart is then transferred to an ice-cold medium containing 180 mM KCl, 10 mM EGTA, and 0.5% bovine serum albumin (BSA, fraction V, Sigma Chemical Co., St. Louis, MO), pH 7.4, at 4°C (KEA medium). All subsequent steps are carried out in a cold room at 4°C.

The ventricular tissue is cut free of fat, large vessels and atria; the weight is determined. Approximately 1.5 to 2.0 g of tissue is minced and then homogenized in 10 ml of KEA medium with the aid of an electrically driven Teflon® pestle at 2500 rpm in a glass homogenizing vessel immersed in iced saline solution. Three times three passes are made with a 30-sec rest period after each three passes. Then, 25 ml of KEA medium is added to the homogenate, which is homogenized again as described above. The homogenate is centrifuged at 500 g for 10 min using a Beckman J-21C type centrifuge fitted with a JA-20 rotor. The supernatant fraction is then filtered through two layers of cheesecloth into centrifuge tubes and is centrifuged at 8000 g for 10 min. The resultant pellet is washed by resuspension and centrifugation at 8000 g for 10 min. The washing procedure is repeated, and the final mitochondrial pellet is resuspended in a small volume of KEA medium to make a mitochondrial protein concentration of 20–30 mg per ml.

This isolation method results in a yield of 20–22 mg mitochondria protein/g wet tissue representing about 40% of the total based on citrate synthase activity distribution (Scheme 1). Mitochondria isolated by this procedure are qualitatively similar to those isolated by the Polytron® method (Sordahl *et al.*, 1971). The

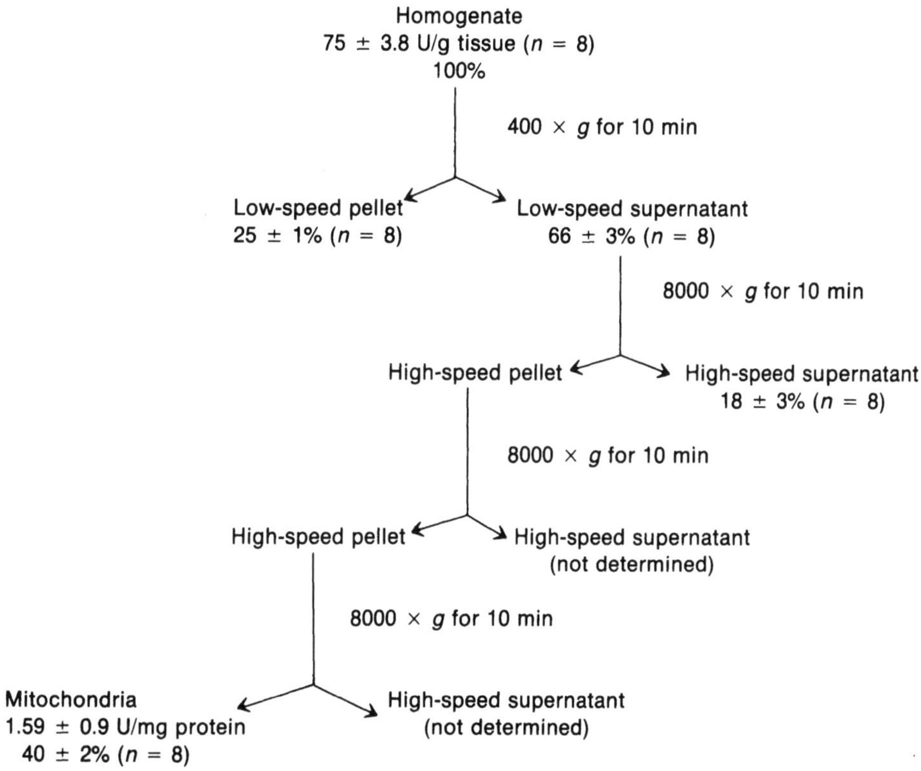

Scheme 1. Distribution of the citrate synthase activity in various fractions of rabbit heart.

protein concentration of the final mitochondrial suspension is determined by the method of Lowry *et al.* (1951) with bovine serum albumin as a standard. The procedure just described has been applied successfully by us for the isolation of cardiac muscle mitochondria from dog, pig, and rat. However, the yield and respiratory properties of mitochondria vary with species.

2. *Measurement of Oxidative Phosphorylation*

The oxygen consumption of mitochondria is determined polarographically with the aid of a Clark oxygen electrode fitted to an Oxygraph model K-IC (Gilson Medical Electronics). The assays are carried out at 37°C using 1 mg mitochondrial protein in 1.5 ml assay medium. The compositions of the various assay media are indicated in the legend of the table. State 3 and state 4 respiration and the RCI and the ADP:O ratio are calculated according to Estabrook (1967). State 4 respiration is determined after the added ADP is phosphorylated. The rate of respiration is expressed in nanoatoms oxygen consumed by 1 mg mitochondrial protein per min. The oxidative phosphorylation rate (OPR) is calculated according to Edoute *et al.* (1979) and is expressed as nmoles ATP synthesized by 1 mg mitochondrial protein per minute. Table II shows the characteristics of mitochondria isolated from rabbit heart by glass–Teflon® homogenization.

3. Measurement of Citrate Synthase Activity

Citrate synthase activity is determined spectrophotometrically at 30°C according to the method of Srere (1969). All the samples are sonicated four times, 10 sec each, separated by 30-sec cooling intervals. The assay medium contains 0.1 *M* tris-HCl (pH 8.5), 0.1 m*M* 5-dithiobis-2-nitrobenzoic acid (DTNB), 250 μ*M* acetyl CoA, 500 μ*M* oxaloacetic acid, and a 10-μl aliquot of sonicated sample of either mitochondria or homogenate in a total volume of 1 ml. The reaction is started with oxaloacetate. The rate of DTNB reduction before the oxaloacetate addition, which occurs through deacylase activity, is subtracted from the rate after oxaloacetate addition. One unit of enzyme is defined as 1 μmole oxaloacetate utilized/min per mg protein.

4. Electron Microscopy

One milligram of isolated mitochondria is suspended in 1.5 ml ice-cold isolation medium and centrifuged in an Eppendorf microfuge model 5412 for 2 min at maximum speed. The supernatant is removed, and 1.5 ml ice-cold 2% glutaraldehyde in 0.1 *M* cacodylate buffer (pH 7.4) is added on top of the pellet for fixation for 2–3 hr. The pellet is postfixed in 1% osmium tetroxide for 1 hr, dehydrated in graded ethanol and propylene oxide, and embedded in Spurr medium. Thin sections of the embedded mitochondrial pellet are cut in a microtome, stained in uranyl acetate and lead citrate, and examined in a Zeiss 9S electron microscope. Figure 1 is a representative micrograph of mitochondria isolated from rabbit heart by glass Teflon homogenization.

5. Uptake and Na^+-Induced Ca^{2+} Release from Isolated Heart Mitochondria

In addition to oxidative phosphorylation, mitochondria in general contain an energy-dependent Ca^{2+} uptake system. Mitochondria of excitable tissues also contain a Na^+-induced Ca^{2+} release system. These properties of mitochondria can be studied *in vitro* spectrophotometrically with Ca^{2+}-sensitive dyes or with a Ca^{2+}-sensitive electrode or by radiochemical technique using $^{45}Ca^{2+}$. The spectrophotometric technique of Scarpa *et al.* (1978) using arsenazo III is employed in the present study. The assay is carried out in a dual-beam dual-wavelength spectrophotometer (Aminco or Hitachi–Perkin Elmer) at 675–685 nm (Scarpa *et al.*, 1978). The assay medium (3 ml) contains 120 m*M* KCl, 10 m*M* MOPS, 5 m*M* K-glutamate, 5 m*M* K-malate, 50 μ*M* arsenazo III, 2 mg mitochondrial protein, pH 7.0, at 37°C. The mixture is continuously stirred with a built-in magnetic stirrer in the spectrophotometer. Usually, the reaction is started with the addition of known amount of $CaCl_2$. After the completion of the uptake of Ca^{2+}, 1 μ*M* ruthenium red is added to prevent the reuptake of Ca^{2+}. The release of Ca^{2+} can then be induced with Na^+ or other agents. When the effect of a drug or inhibitor is tested, it is added before the addition of $CaCl_2$. Figure 2 depicts a typical experiment on the effect of diltiazem, a calcium-channel-blocking drug, on Ca^{2+} uptake and Na^+-induced Ca^{2+} release.

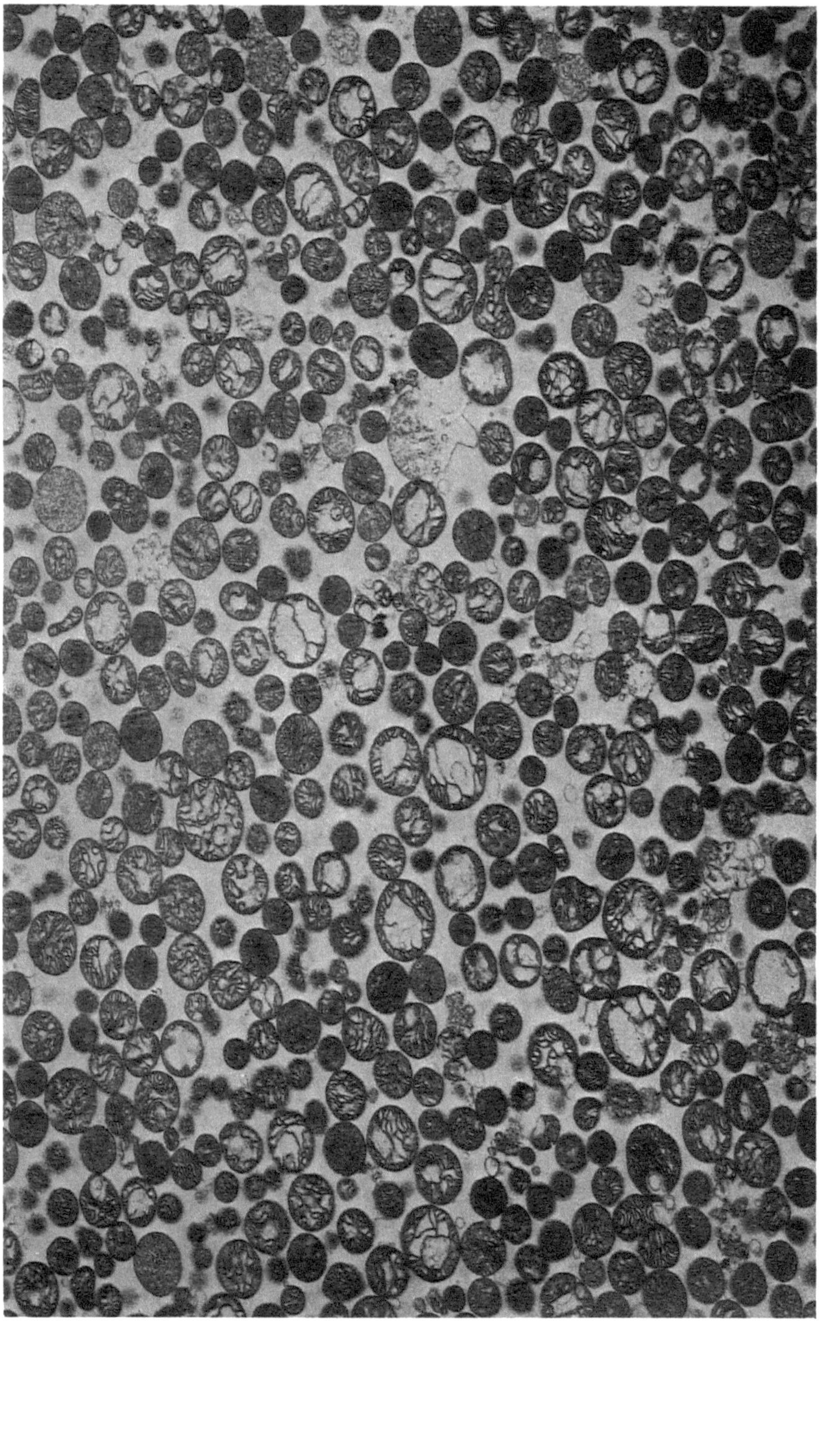

Figure 1. Electron micrograph of mitochondria isolated from rabbit heart by glass–Teflon® homogenization technique.

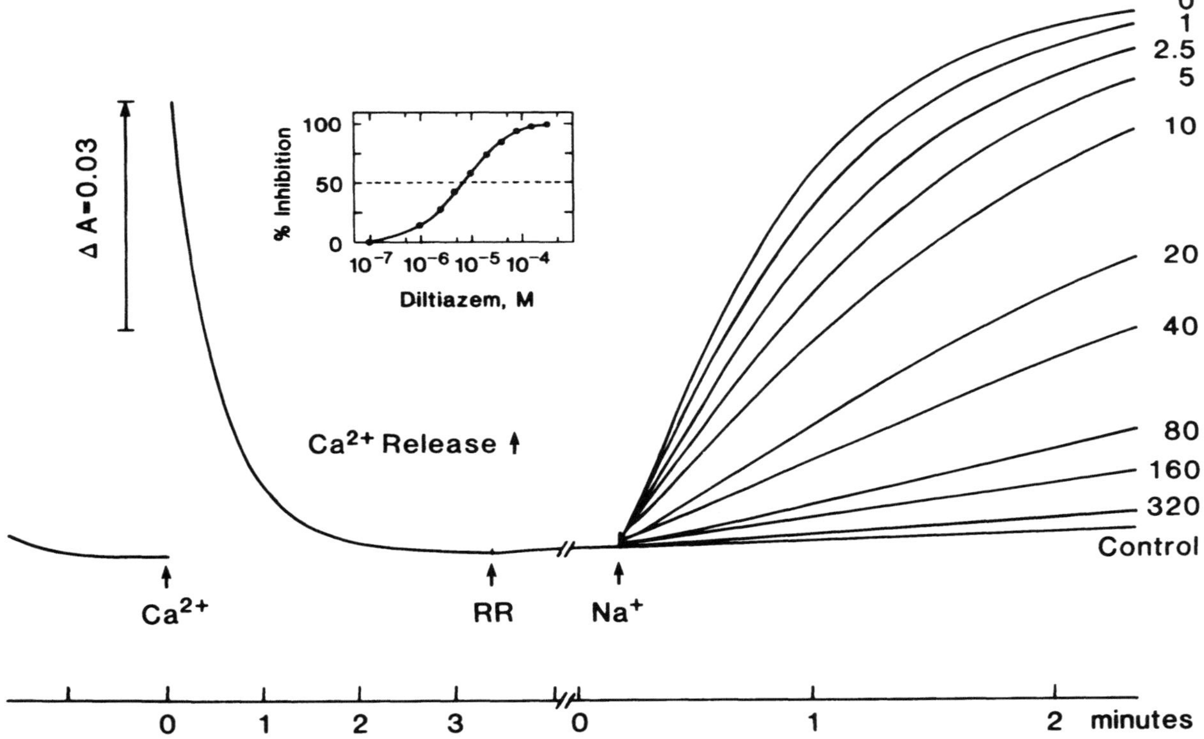

Figure 2. Effect of diltiazem on the respiration-dependent Ca^{2+} uptake and on Na^{+}-induced Ca^{2+} release from mitochondria of rabbit heart isolated by the glass–Teflon® homogenization procedure. Where indicated by arrows, 40 nmoles $CaCl_2$ (Ca^{2+}), 1 μM ruthenium red (RR), and 10 m*M* NaCl (Na^{+}) were added. In control experiments, NaCl was not added. Diltiazem, when present, was added to the assay medium 1 min before adding mitochondria. The numbers indicate the diltiazem concentrations (μM). The time scale has been changed to monitor Na^{+}-induced Ca^{2+} release. The insert shows the percent inhibition of the rate of Na^{+}-induced Ca^{2+} release by different concentrations of diltiazem. This figure was taken from a previous publication (Vaghy *et al.*, 1982) for illustration.

C. Isolation of Mitochondria by Nagarse Treatment

The following procedure for preparation of rat heart mitochondria was described by Vercesi *et al.* (1978). The hearts are quickly excised following decapitation of rats, chilled, opened, and thoroughly washed with ice-cold 0.25 *M* sucrose. They are finely minced with chilled sharp scissors into about 1 ml per heart of a cold medium of 0.25 *M* sucrose, 0.5 m*M* EGTA, and 3.0 m*M* HEPES buffer, pH 7.2; fine mincing of the hearts is a critical step. The minced heart suspension is then diluted to 10 ml per heart with cold medium to which 0.1 mg of nagarse (Enzyme Development Corp., New York, NY) per milliliter has been added. After 15 min of incubation at 0°C with occasional stirring, the suspending medium is decanted and discarded. The finely minced tissue is washed once with 10 ml of cold 0.25 *M* sucrose to remove excess nagarse and then resuspended in 10 ml of cold 0.25 *M* sucrose per heart.

The now soft and easily dispersed minced heart tissue is homogenized by hand in a glass Dounce or Ten Broeck homogenizer. Three to six gentle strokes of a previously chilled, loose-fitting pestle are employed to yield a uniform but somewhat coarse homogenate. To complete the homogenization, a tighter pestle is then used for three or four additional strokes, also gentle; exposure of the homogenate to vigorous shearing force or to suction is deleterious. The resulting homogenate is diluted with cold 0.25 M sucrose to 20 ml per heart and centrifuged at 600 × *g* for 5 min in the SS-34 rotor (radius, 4.25 inches) of a Sorvall RCB-2 refrigerated centrifuge. The supernatant medium is carefully removed by decantation (leaving behind a mobile fluffy layer) and centrifuged for 10 min at 10,000 × *g* to sediment the mitochondria. The resulting pellet is suspended in 10 ml of cold 0.15 M sucrose per heart and recentrifuged for 10 min at 12,000 × *g*. Suspension in 0.25 M sucrose (5 ml per heart) and centrifugation are repeated once more; the upper light layer of sediment is then decanted from the final pellet as cleanly as possible and discarded. The red–brown lower layer is resuspended in 0.5 ml of 0.25 M sucrose per heart, and the concentration adjusted to give 20 mg of mitochondrial protein per ml. The entire procedure is carried out at 0°C. Ordinarily four rat hearts are carried through the procedure, yielding about 15 to 18 mg of mitochondrial protein per gram wet weight of heart. The respiratory control ratio with succinate as substrate usually exceeds 4.0.

D. Isolation of "Two Populations" of Mitochondria

Palmer *et al.* (1977) described a procedure for the isolation of "subsarcolemmal" and "interfibrillar" mitochondria from cardiac muscle. The authors claim that this procedure produces a separation of mitochondria located beneath the sarcolemma from those located between the myofibrils. However, the degree of the separation of these two subpopulations produced by this procedure is arguable (Matlib *et al.*, 1981). The procedure, as described by Palmer *et al.* (1977), is as follows.

For each experiment, three to five rats (250–300 g) are decapitated and bled for 10 to 20 sec. Their hearts are removed and immediately placed in cold buffer

A (220 m*M* mannitol, 70 m*M* sucrose, 5 m*M* MOPS, pH 7.4). Basically, the procedure of Sordahl *et al.* (1971) is used for preparation of Polytron® mitochondria. After removal of extraventricular tissue, the hearts are rinsed five to ten times, blotted dry, and weighed. The tissue is finely minced and brought to a final concentration of 10 g of tissue/100 ml of buffer A plus 2 m*M* EGTA and 0.2% bovine serum albumin. The tissue suspension is homogenized with a Polytron® tissue processor (Brinkmann Instruments) for exactly 2.4 sec at a rheostat setting of 6.5. The time from decapitation to initial homogenization should not exceed 15 min.

The Polytron® homogenate is centrifuged in a Sorvall RC-5 (SS-34 head). In order to insure complete recovery of Polytron® mitochondria from the Polytron® homogenate, the original Polytron® pellet is resuspended to the original volume by use of a Potter–Elvehjem homogenizer in buffer A (plus 2 mM EGTA and 0.2% albumin) and recentrifuged at 500 × *g* for 10 min. The resultant supernatants are combined and centrifuged at 3000 × *g* for 10 min to obtain the mitochondrial fraction, which is then washed twice. The final Polytron® mitochondrial pellet is resuspended in buffer A (0.5 m*M* EGTA) to give a final protein concentration of approximately 25 mg/ml and designated as "subsarcolemmal population." All supernatants from these washes are combined to yield the total Polytron® supernatant.

The nagarse mitochondrial fraction is derived from nagarse treatment of the washed Polytron® pellet obtained after 500 × *g*. The pellet is resuspended in buffer B (100 m*M* KCl, 50 m*M* MOPS, pH 7.4) plus 2 m*M* EGTA and 0.2% albumin, and nagarse mitochondria are prepared according to the procedure of Chance and Hagihara (1960) as modified by Tomec and Hoppel (1975). Nagarse is added to a final concentration of 5 mg/g wet weight of tissue, and the homogenate is immediately homogenized with a Potter–Elvehjem homogenizer, diluted twofold with buffer B, and immediately centrifuged at 5000 × *g* for 5 min.

The high-speed pellet remaining after the nagarse treatment is resuspended in the original volume of buffer B and sedimented at low speed to yield the nuclear pellet. In order to quantitate recovery of mitochondria from this pellet, it is washed twice in buffer B (2 m*M* EGTA; 0.2% albumin), and the supernatants are added back to the original nuclear supernatant. These are centrifuged at 3000 × *g* for 10 min. The resulting pellet is washed twice and then resuspended in buffer B (0.5 m*M* EGTA) to a final concentration of 25 mg/ml. This procedure yields about 10 mg mitochondrial protein/g tissue by Polytron® treatment and about 20 mg protein/g tissue by subsequent nagarse treatment. Based on recoveries of five mitochondrial marker enzymes, these yields represent 60–85% of the mitochondria in the cell. These mitochondria are designated "interfibrillar population."

E. Isolation of Mitochondria by Combined Polytron and Nagarse Treatment

Sordahl and Stewart (1980) described a procedure combining Polytron® and nagarse treatments and were able to isolate about 60% of the total mitochondrial population in the normal and ischemic canine myocardial samples. The procedure described by Sordahl and Stewart (1980) is essentially a modification of previously published procedures (Palmer *et al.*, 1977; Sordahl *et al.*, 1971).

Briefly, heart tissue (1–2 g) is minced into very small pieces with scissors. One-gram portions of tissue are put into individual size C glass homogenizers (A. H. Thomas, Co.), and 20 ml of 0.25 *M* sucrose, 5 m*M* tris-HCl, 10 m*M* EGTA medium, pH 7.2, are added (5% wt/vol homogenate). The tissue is homogenized with a Polytron® PT-20 tissue processor (Brinkmann Instruments) at a setting of 4.6 for 4 sec. The homogenate is then centrifuged at 27,000 *g* for 10 min. The supernatant, which contains no cytochrome *c* oxidase activity, is discarded, the single-gram pellets are combined, and 1 mg nagarse (Enzyme Development Corp.) per gram starting tissue is added (nagarse solution is made up by adding 10 mg nagarse enzyme to 10 ml of the sucrose–tris–EGTA medium plus 100 μl 1.0 *M* tris base). The suspension is thoroughly mixed with a vortex mixer and allowed to incubate at 4°C for 8 min. It has been determined that optimally functional and intact mitochondria are obtained with this length of incubation time.

After incubation, a solution of 0.18 *M* KCl, 5 m*M* tris-HCl, 10 m*M* EGTA, 0.5% bovine serum albumin (fraction V, Sigma), pH 7.2, is added to obtain a 5% wt./volume homogenate. This suspension is homogenized by making one pass with a motor-driven Teflon® pestle and then centrifuged at 500 *g* for 5 min. Half of the supernatant is poured through one layer of cheesecloth and saved. The other half of the supernatant and the pellet are suspended and centrifuged at 12,000 *g* for 10 min. The mitochondria are "washed" once and resuspended in 0.18 *M* KCl, 5 m*M* tris-HCl, 0.5% bovine serum albumin medium, pH 7.2, at a final concentration of approximately 30 mg/ml. Protein determinations are made by a biuret method (Jacobs *et al.*, 1956). This procedure yields about 27 mg mitochondrial protein/g tissue.

ACKNOWLEDGMENTS

This work was supported in part by grants from NIH (HL 22619 IV-B, V-A, and Cores 1 and 2). The authors thank Ms. Janet Simons for typing the manuscript and Ms. Gwen Kraft for drawing Figure 1. The electron micrograph was provided by Dr. M. Ashraf.

REFERENCES

Bonting, S. L., Simon, K. A., and Hawkins, N. A. 1961. Studies on sodium–potassium-activated adenosine triphosphatase. 1. Quantitative distribution in several tissues of the cat. *Arch. Biochem. Biophys.*, *95*:416–423.

Carafoli, E. 1979. The calcium cycle. *FEBS Lett.*, *104*:1.

Chance, B., and Hagihara, B. 1960. Initiation of succinate oxidation in aged pigeon heart mitochondria. *Biochem. Biophys. Res. Commun.*, *3*:1–5.

Edoute, Y., Kotze, J. C. N., and Lochner, A. 1979. Oxidative phosphorylation rate: An index for evaluation of mitochondrial function in myocardial ischemia. *J. Mol. Cell. Cardiol.*, *11*:831–833.

Estabrook, R. W. 1967. Mitochondrial respiratory control and the polarographic measurement of ADP:O ratios. In: *Methods in Enzymology*, Volume 10, pp. 41–47. Ed. by Estabrook, R. W., and Pullman, M. E. Academic Press, New York.

Jacobs, E. E., Jacob, M., Sanadi, D. R., and Bradley, L. B. 1956. Uncoupling of oxidative phosphorylation by cadmium ion. *J. Biol. Chem., 223*:147–156.

Jennings, R. B., and Ganote, C. E. 1974. Structural changes in myocardium during acute ischemia. *Circ. Res., 34/35*(Suppl. III):156–172.

Lindenmayer, G. E., Sordahl, L. A., and Schwartz, A. 1968. Reevaluation of oxidative phosphorylation in cardiac mitochondria from normal animals and animals in heart failure. *Circ. Res., 23*:439–450.

Lindenmayer, G. E., Harigaya, S., Bajusz, E., and Schwartz, A. 1970, Oxidative phosphorylation and calcium transport of mitochondria isolated from cardiomyopathic hamster hearts, *J. Mol. Cell. Cardiol., 1*:249.

Lindenmayer, G. E., Sordahl, L. A., Harigaya, S., Allen, J. C., Besch, H. R., and Schwartz, A. 1971, Some biochemical studies on subcellular systems isolated from fresh recipient human cardiac tissue obtained during transplantation, *Am. J. Cardiol., 27*:277.

Lochner, A., Opie, L. H., and Brink, A. J. 1968. A defective oxidative phosphorylation in hereditary myocardiopathy in Syrian hamster. *Cardiovasc. Res., 2*:297–307.

Lowry, O. H., Rosebrough, N. J., Farr, A. L., and Randall, R. J. 1951. Protein measurement with the phenol reagent. *J. Biol. Chem., 193*:265–275.

Matlib, M. A., Rebman, D., Ashraf, M., Rouslin, W., and Schwartz, A. 1981. Differential activities of putative subsarcolemmal and interfibrillar mitochondria from cardiac muscle. *J. Mol. Cell. Cardiol., 13*:163–170.

Meerson, F. Z., Zaletayeva, T. A., Lagutchev, S. S., and Pshennikova, M. G. 1964. Structure and mass of mitochondria in the process of compensatory hyperfunction and hypertrophy of the heart. *Exp. Cell Res., 36*:568–578.

Nagao, T., Matlib, M. A., Franklin, D., Millard, R. W., and Schwartz, A. 1980. Effects of diltiazem, a calcium antagonist, on regional myocardial function and mitochondria after brief coronary occlusion. *J. Mol. Cell. Cardiol., 12*:29–43.

Neely, J. R., and Morgan, H. E. 1974. Relationship between carbohydrate and lipid metabolism and the energy balance of heart muscle. *Annu. Rev. Physiol., 36*:413–459.

Page, E., and McCallister, L. P. 1973. Quantitative electron microscopic description of heart muscle cells. *Am. J. Cardiol., 31*:172–181.

Palmer, J. W., Tandler, B., and Hoppel, C. L. 1977. Biochemical properties of subsarcolemmal and interfibrillar mitochondria isolated from rat cardiac muscle. *J. Biol. Chem., 252*:8731–8739.

Rouslin, W. 1975. Oxygen dependence of promitochondrial and cytoplasmic protein synthesis in the formation of electron transfer complexes III and IV in adapting bakers' yeast. *Arch. Biochem. Biophys., 168*:685–692.

Rouslin, W. 1983. Mitochondrial complexes I, II, III, IV, and V in myocardial ischemia and autolysis. *Am. J. Physiol., 244*:H743–H748.

Rouslin, W., Cubicciotti, R. S., Edward, W. D., Matlib, M. A., Wilson, D. R., Hamrell, B. B., and Schwartz, A. 1979. Phosphorylative respiratory activity of mitochondria isolated from the left and right ventricles of rabbit hearts following partial pulmonary trunk occlusion. *J. Mol. Cell. Cardiol., 11*:91–99.

Rouslin, W., and Millard, R. W. 1980. Canine myocardial ischemia: Defect in mitochondrial electron transfer complex I. *J. Mol. Cell. Cardiol., 12*:639–645.

Rouslin, W., and Millard, R. W. 1981. Mitochondrial inner membrane enzyme defects in porcine myocardial ischemia. *Am. J. Physiol., 240*:H308–H313.

Scarpa, A., Brinley, F. J., Jr., and Dubyak, G. 1978. Antipyrylazo III, a "middle range" Ca^{2+} metallochromic indicator. *Biochemistry, 17*:1378–1386.

Schwartz, A., and Lee, K. S. 1962. Study of heart mitochondria and glycolytic metabolism in experimentally induced cardiac failure. *Circ. Res., 10*:321–332.

Sordahl, L. A., Johnson, C., Blailock, Z. R., and Schwartz, A. 1971. The mitochondrion. In: *Methods in Pharmacology*, Volume 1, pp. 247–286. Ed. by Schwartz, A. Appleton-Century-Crofts, New York.

Sordahl, L. A., and Stewart, M. L. 1980. Mechanisms(s) of altered mitochondrial calcium transport in acutely ischemic canine hearts. *Circ. Res., 47:*814–820.

Srere, P. A. 1969. Citrate synthase. In: *Methods in Enzymology*, Volume 13, pp. 3–11. Ed. by Lowenstein, J. M. Academic Press, New York.

Tomec, R., and Hoppel, C. 1975. Carnitine palmitoyltransferase in bovine fetal heart mitochondria. *Arch. Biochem. Biophys., 170:*716–723.

Tzagoloff, A., Byington, K. H., and MacLennan, D. H. 1968. Studies on the mitochondrial adenosine triphosphatase system. *J. Biol. Chem., 243:*2405–2412.

Vaghy, P. L., Matlib, M. A., Szekeres, L., and Schwartz, A. 1981. Protective effects of verapamil and diltiazem against inorganic phosphate induced impairment of oxidative phosphorylation of isolated heart mitochondria. *Biochem. Pharmacol., 30:*2603–2610.

Vaghy, P. L., Johnson, J. D., Matlib, M. A., Wang, T., and Schwartz, A. 1982. Selective inhibition of Na^+-induced Ca^{2+} release from heart mitochondria by diltiazem and certain other Ca^{2+} antagonist drugs. *J. Biol. Chem., 257:*6000–6002.

Vercesi, A., Reynafarjee, B., and Lehninger, A. L. 1978. Stoichiometry of H^+ ejection and Ca^{2+} uptake coupled to electron transport in rat heart mitochondria. *J. Biol. Chem., 253:*6379–6385.

Wollenberger, A., Kleitke, B., and Raabe, G. 1963. Some metabolic characteristics of mitochondria from chronically overloaded, hypertrophied hearts. *Exp. Mol. Pathol., 2:*251–260.

Wood, J. H., Hanley, H. G., Entman, M. L., Hartley, C. J., Swain, J. A., Busch, U., Chang, C. H., Lewis, R. M., Morgan, W. J., and Schwartz, A. 1979. Biochemical and morphological correlates of acute experimental myocardial ischemia in the dog. *Circ. Res., 44:*52–61.

Chapter 4

Cardiac Sarcoplasmic Reticulum

Purification of Ca^{2+}-ATPase

Taitzer Wang, Jun Nakamura, and Arnold Schwartz

Department of Pharmacology and Cell Biophysics
University of Cincinnati College of Medicine
Cincinnati, Ohio

I. INTRODUCTION

The sarcoplasmic reticulum is a membranous subcellular system in muscle cells. Its principal physiological function is to pump cytoplasmic calcium ions into the SR lumen and, as a consequence of decreased Ca^{2+} concentration, cause muscle relaxation (Ebashi *et al.*, 1969; MacLennan and Holland, 1975; Tada *et al.*, 1978; Hasselbach, 1979; DeMeis and Inesi, 1982; Ikemoto, 1982). The SR, or part of it, as a major Ca^{2+} pool inside the muscle cells, may also release Ca^{2+} to the cytoplasm and consequently bring about muscle contraction (Endo, 1977; Winegrad, 1982; Fabiato, 1983). Ca^{2+} release from SR has not been studied as thoroughly as its function as a "relaxing factor." To date, our knowledge of the SR and its physiological function is largely based on the results obtained from studies of skeletal muscle. The SR in cardiac muscle cells possess similar properties, and recent studies of this particular "suborganelle" in cardiac muscles are beginning to reveal some properties of its own. Among these, the most important is the finding that the cardiac SR Ca^{2+}-ATPase protein may be regulated by phospholamban, a 22,000-dalton protein present in SR (Adams and Schwartz, 1980; Tada *et al.*, 1982). Phosphorylation of phospholamban by cAMP-dependent and/or Ca^{2+}- and calmodulin-dependent protein kinase enhances the Ca^{2+}-ATPase and Ca^{2+}-transport activities of the cardiac SR.

Present address for Jun Nakamura: Tantabe Pharmaceutical Company, Higshi-Ku, Osaka, Japan.

Isolated cardiac SR (microsomes) are composed of proteins and lipids (Ebashi *et al.*, 1969; MacLennan and Holland, 1975; Tada *et al.*, 1978; Hasselbach, 1979; DeMeis and Inesi, 1982; Ikemoto, 1982; Levitsky *et al.*, 1982). A number of proteins are always observed when the SR microsomes are subjected to SDS treatment followed by electrophoresis. It is not certain whether all of these proteins are an essential part of the Ca^{2+} pump system or some of them are contaminating proteins derived from sarcolemmal and mitochondrial fragments. Among the proteins, the best characterized is the Ca^{2+}-ATPase protein, which has a molecular weight of approximately 100,000 (Levitsky *et al.*, 1976; Van Winkle *et al.*, 1978; Bidlack *et al.*, 1982; Nakamura *et al.*, 1983). The 55,000-dalton protein in cardiac SR has been characterized as calsequestrin (Campbell *et al.*, 1983), which is similar to the skeletal calsequestrin of 63,000 molecular weight found in the terminal cisternae, where large amounts of Ca^{2+} are stored. Two glycoproteins of 53,000 and 130,000 molecular weight are similar to those (53,000 and 160,000 dalton) observed in skeletal SR (Campbell *et al.*, 1983). The regulatory 22,000-dalton protein in cardiac SR as described above is not present in the fast-twitch skeletal SR (Kirchberger and Tada, 1976; Adams and Schwartz, 1980; Tada *et al.*, 1982).

In this chapter, we describe procedures for isolation of SR microsomes from the dog cardiac muscle (Sumida *et al.*, 1978; Wang *et al.*, 1979) and the purification of the 100,000-dalton Ca^{2+}-ATPase from the SR microsomes (Nakamura *et al.*, 1983).

II. PREPARATION OF DOG CARDIAC SR MICROSOMES

A. Removal of Heart from Anesthesized Dog

1. Equipment

One 600-ml beaker, ice bucket, 20-ml syringe, needle (20 × 1″), scalpel, Bard–Parker surgical blade (No. 21 or 22) and knife handle, hair clipper, a pair of curved-on-flat operating scissors, and several pairs of plastic gloves are required.

2. Solutions

Sodium pentobarbital (1 grain/ml, Veterinary Laboratory, Inc., Lenexa, KS) and 500 ml of saline solution (0.9% NaCl, prepared by dissolving 9.0 g of NaCl in 1000 ml of distilled H_2O and stored in 4°C cold room before use) are used.

3. Procedure

Fill the 600-ml beaker with 500 ml of cold saline solution. Keep the solution cold in an ice bucket filled with crushed ice.

Administer about 15 ml of sodium pentobarbital intravenously (1 ml per 5 lb body weight) to the dog. After the dog is completely anesthetized, open the chest and remove the heart. The heart should be kept in the cold saline solution and homogenized within 15 min.

B. Homogenization and Centrifugation

1. Equipment

One Sorvall Omni mixer assembly (Ivan Sorvall, Inc., Newtown, CT) with a 420-ml cup, knife, cutting board, ice bucket, Beckman J14 centrifuge, Beckman L5-50 ultracentrifuge, J14 rotor and four 250-ml centrifuge tubes, rotor 35K and ten 65-ml centrifuge tubes (all centrifuge tubes and caps are weight-matched), two pairs of curved-on-flat operating scissors, four 600-ml beakers, a 100-ml and a 10-ml glass–Teflon® homogenizer, a stopwatch, cheesecloth, and some paper towels are used.

2. Solutions

Tris Maleate, 30 mM, pH 7.1. The final concentration is 30 m*M* tris and 15 m*M* maleate. The solution is prepared by dissolving the required amount of Trizma base in a maleic anhydride solution in water. Store in the cold room.

KCl-Tris Buffer. A buffer solution of 0.6 *M* KCl-20 m*M* tris maleate, pH 6.8, is prepared and stored in a refrigerator.

Sucrose. A solution of 2 *M* sucrose is stored in a refrigerator.

3. Procedure

Squeeze the heart a few times in the cold saline solution to remove the remaining blood and replace the heart into the crushed ice before carrying out the homogenization in a cold room.

In the cold room, cut the heart open, remove the atria, and clean the ventricles of fat. Weigh the cleaned ventricles. The total weight of the heart may range from 100 to 180 g.

Cut the ventricular muscle into small pieces and place them in a 600-ml beaker. Avoid using more than 130 g of tissue. Chop up the tissue in the beaker with two pairs of sharp scissors held together. This chopping of tissues usually takes 1 to 2 min. Transfer the chopped tissues to the 420-ml Omni mixer cup and fill the cup to the top with the cold 30 m*M* tris maleate (pH 7.1). Run the Omni mixer at the maximum speed continuously for 40 sec with the cup immersed in crushed ice to prevent temperature elevation.

Pour the contents into a 600-ml beaker and rinse the Omni mixer cup with about 30 ml of the 30 m*M* tris maleate buffer solution. Combine and make up to a total of 500 ml. Pour the contents into two 250-ml centrifuge tubes and balance them by eye. Centrifuge at 8000 rpm for 10 min (Beckman J14 centrifuge).

Filter the supernatant through three to four layers of cheesecloth into a beaker to remove fat and other large debris. Centrifuge the filtrate (a total of about 300 ml) in two 250-ml centrifuge tubes at 10,000 rpm for 20 min (Beckman J14 centrifuge).

Filter the supernatant through three to four layers of cheesecloth. Care should be exerted to avoid contaminating the filtrate with the fat or denatured protein formed as loose white particles on the walls of the centrifuge tubes.

Equally divide the filtrate into six of the 65-ml centrifuge tubes and centrifuge at 35,000 rpm for 30 min (Beckman L5-50 ultracentrifuge). The resultant pellets are soft, and often there are some unwanted white particles remaining on the walls of the tubes. Discard most of the supernatant carefully. Loosen by shaking the tubes gently in the remaining supernatant and transfer the soft pellets to a 100-ml glass–Teflon® homogenizer. Homogenize with 60 ml of 20 m*M* tris maleate containing 0.6 *M* KCl. Equally divide the homogenate into four 65-ml centrifuge tubes and add the same buffer solution to near the top of each tube. Shake the tubes a few times. Each pair of the four tubes is balanced by eye.

Centrifuge the suspensions in the four tubes at 35,000 rpm for 45 min (Beckman L5-50 ultracentrifuge). The resultant pellets are soft but can be separated from the supernatant. The pellets may first be homogenized in 2.0 ml of 0.6 *M* KCl-20 m*M* tris maleate buffer, pH 6.8. Total yield is 50–70 mg; specific Ca^{2+}-ATPase activity is 40–50 μmoles Pi/mg per hr. After determining the protein by the Biuret method, add 0.5 ml of 2 *M* sucrose (based on a final volume of 4.5 ml), quick freeze with liquid N_2 or dry ice–ethyl alcohol, and store the preparation in a −80°C freezer. It is important that the final suspensions contain 0.2 *M* sucrose.

C. Determination of SR Protein by the Biuret Method

1. Equipment

A UV–visible spectrophotometer, ten disposable glass test tubes (12 × 75 mm), a hotplate, a 100-ml beaker, some boiling chips, and four small marbles are used.

2. Solutions

Standard BSA protein solution (bovine serum albumin, Sigma, 20 mg/ml), 1 *N* NaOH, and biuret reagent (0.75 g $CuSO_4 \cdot 5H_2O$, 3.0 g K,Na-tartrate, 15 g NaOH, and 0.5 g NaI in 500 ml final H_2O solution) are used.

3. Procedure

Duplicate samples of 0, 25, and 50 μl of BSA solution and SR suspension are made up to 100 μl with water in ten test tubes, and each is mixed with 0.5 ml of 1 *N* NaOH. The SR mixture is heated at 100°C (with test tubes covered with marbles) for five minutes to solubilize the protein until clear. After cooling, 2 ml of biuret reagent is added with mixing to develop the color. The same amount of the biuret reagent is used for the BSA mixture. After 10 min, the solutions are read at 540 nm. The SR protein concentration is determined against the standard BSA.

D. Assay of SR Ca^{2+}-ATPase Specific Activity

1. Equipment

A UV–visible spectrophotometer, eleven test tubes (12 × 75 mm), a test tube rack, a shaker bath, an ice bucket, and a stopwatch are required.

2. *Solutions*

The SR suspension (tenfold diluted), standard phosphate solutions (1, 3, 5, 7, and 9 m*M*), working buffer solution (pH 7.0, 45.5 m*M* L-histidine, 9.1 m*M* $MgCl_2$, 182 m*M* KCl, 182 μ*M* EGTA, and 9.1 m*M* NaN_3), ammonium molybdate–ferrous sulfate solution (prepared fresh by dissolving 0.35 g $FeSO_4 \cdot 7H_2O$ in 7 ml of 1.25% ammonium molybdate in 1 *N* H_2SO_4), and 10% trichloroacetic acid (TCA, w/v) are used.

3. *Procedure*

Duplicate samples of 0, 0, and 100 μl of 1 m*M* $CaCl_2$ are made up to 0.375 ml with water in six test tubes followed by addition of 0.55 ml of working buffer. The mixture is equilibrated in a shaker bath at 37°C for 5 min, and 25 μl of tenfold-diluted SR suspension is added. For easy control of reaction time, the additions of enzyme and later of TCA and ATP solutions are done at 15-sec intervals. After incubation of the enzyme for 6 min, 1 ml of 10% TCA is added (to denature the enzyme) to two tubes that contain no Ca^{2+}, and 50 μl of 100 m*M* ATP is added to the remaining four tubes, two of which contain Ca^{2+}. The incubation is allowed for another 6 min, at the end of which 50 μl ATP is added to the two TCA-containing tubes for background, and 1 ml of TCA is added to the other four to stop the enzymatic reaction. To develop the color, 1 ml of ammonium molybdate–$FeSO_4$ solution is added, and after 15 min at room temperature the solution is read at 700 nm.

The determination of standard phosphate at 700 nm is similarly done by mixing 100 μl of each of the standard phosphate solutions with 0.325 ml of water, 0.55 ml of working buffer, and 25 μl of SR suspension followed by addition of TCA and ammonium molybdate–$FeSO_4$ solutions.

The amount of phosphate ion formed in the enzymatic reaction is determined against the phosphate standard and is used for calculation of the specific activity of the SR.

III. PURIFICATION OF DOG CARDIAC SR

A. Solubilization of SR Microsomes

1. *Equipment*

A magnetic stirrer, a stirring bar, a 100-ml beaker, a Pasteur pipette, and ice containers are used.

2. *Solutions*

Solutions of 2 *M* KCl, 2 *M* sucrose, 1 *M* tris-HCl (pH 8.5), 1 *M* tris maleate (pH 7.1), 0.5 *M* $CaCl_2$, 10 m*M* dithiothreitol (prepared fresh by dissolving 13 mg in 8.5 ml of H_2O), 100 m*M* ATP, and 10% Triton X-100 (w/v) and the SR microsome suspension (fresh or frozen) are utilized.

3. *Procedure*

Prepare 32.4 ml of buffer solution by mixing 15 ml of 2 *M* KCl, 7.7 ml of 2 *M* sucrose, 6 ml of 1 *M* tris-HCl (pH 8.5), 2.4 ml of 0.5 *M* $CaCl_2$, and 1.3 ml of H_2O. Divide the solution into two equal parts (16.2 ml each) and keep the solution cold on ice.

Stir 16.2 ml of the buffer solution in a 100-ml beaker cooled on ice and add 3 ml of 10 m*M* DTT, 1.5 ml of 100 m*M* ATP, and 2.8 ml of H_2O. Add 6.5 ml of 17.9 mg/ml SR suspension (total SR protein 116 mg) to make up a final total of 30 ml. It is important to keep the SR concentration 3–4 mg/ml constantly stirred in this suspension.

Keep the mixture and sucrose concentration 0.3 *M* and add dropwise, slowly, a total of 0.58 ml of the 10% Triton X-100 (58 mg) by means of a Pasteur pipette. The addition usually takes 1 to 2 min. After addition of the Triton X-100, the mixture is stirred gently for 5 min. The resultant mixture becomes less cloudy than the original SR mixture.

B. Centrifugation

1. *Equipment*

An ultracentrifuge (Beckman L5-50), rotor Ti-50, 20 centrifugation tubes ($\frac{3}{4}$ × 3″, weight-matched), and a 10-ml glass–Teflon® homogenizer are required.

2. *Procedure*

Fill five centrifuge tubes each with about 6 ml of the SR-Triton X-100 mixture and the sixth tube with water. Balance by eye each pair of the six tubes. Centrifuge at 40,000 rpm (124,000 × *g*) for 1 hr. The resultant pellets are densely packed, but the supernatant is somewhat cloudy.

Transfer the supernatant to another set of six tubes (the sixth tube filled with H_2O), balance (by eye) the tubes, and centrifuge at 45,000 rpm (165,000 × *g*) for 1 hr.

Transfer the supernatant to a 100-ml beaker placed on ice. Keep the solution cold and stirred while diluting it by slowly adding 30 ml of a buffer mixture consisting of 16.2 ml of the original buffer, 3 ml of the 10 m*M* DTT, 0.65 ml of 2 *M* sucrose, and 10.15 ml of H_2O. The slow addition usually takes 5 min and the resultant solution is kept under stirring for another 5 min.

Transfer the diluted mixture to eight tubes, balance each pair of the tubes by eye, and centrifuge at 40,000 rpm (113,000 × *g*) for 1 hr. The resultant pellet is soft and light brown (purified Ca^{2+}-ATPase) (see Figure 1). Discard the supernatant very carefully. Add 4–5 drops of the final buffer (see below) to each tube, gently shake the tube, and transfer by means of a Pasteur pipette to a 10-ml homogenizer. Rinse the tubes with several drops of the final buffer. The total suspension should be around 1 ml. Total yield is 4 to 6 mg; specific Ca^{2+}-ATPase activity is 470–750 μmoles ADP/mg per hr.

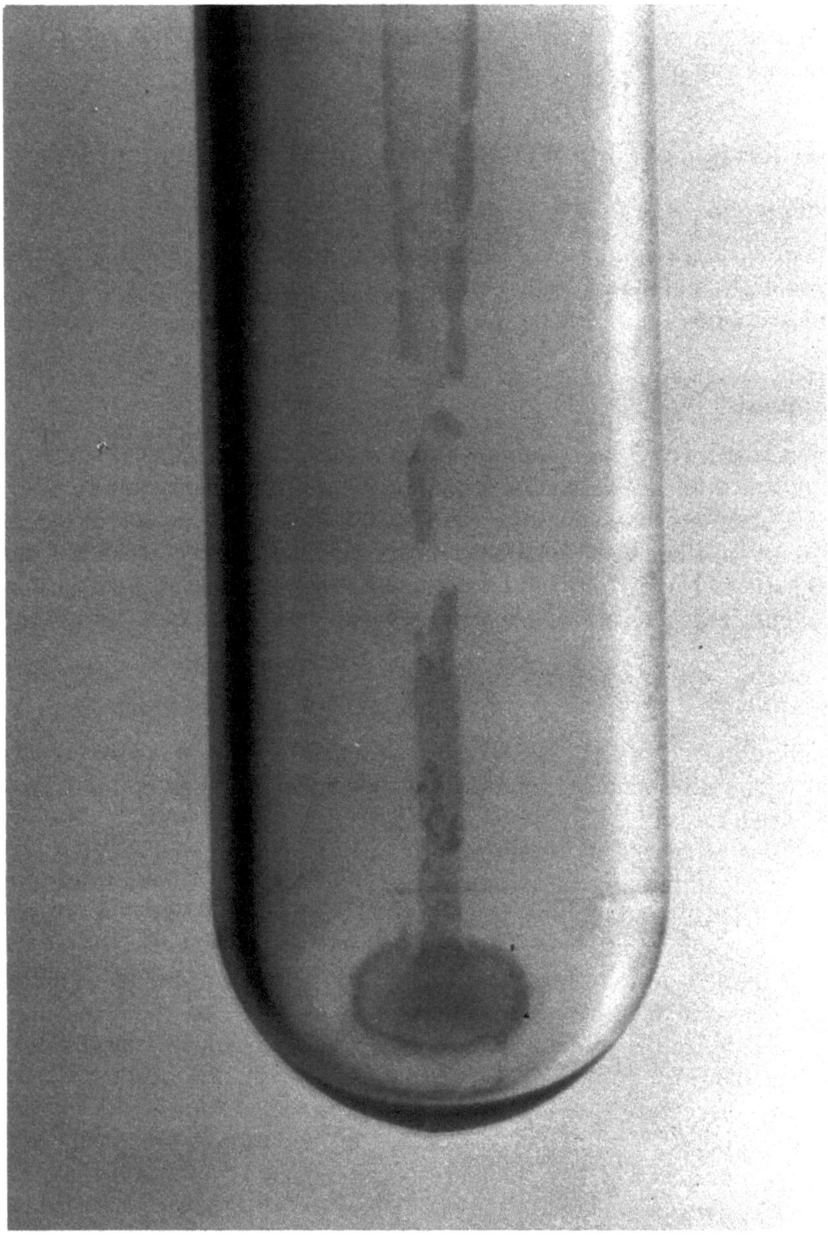

Figure 1. Final pellet of the purified dog cardiac SR Ca^{2+}-ATPase in the Ti-50 centrifugation tube. The light brown, soft pellet is surrounded by denatured protein residues.

This final product may be washed again in two centrifuge tubes each with 5 to 7 ml of the final buffer. This washing results in no significant loss of protein. The final buffer is prepared by mixing 3.75 ml of 2 *M* KCl, 2.25 ml of 2 *M* sucrose, 0.3 ml of 1 *M* tris maleate (pH 7.1), 0.03 ml of 0.5 *M* $CaCl_2$, 2.25 ml of 10 m*M* DTT, and 6.42 ml of H_2O.

C. Determination of Ca^{2+}-ATPase Protein by Modified Lowry Method

1. Equipment

The procedure requires a UV–visible spectrophotometer, tabletop centrifuge (Beckman TJ-6), hotplate, 250-ml beaker, boiling chips, marbles, Kimwipe™ tissue, and test tubes (13 × 100 mm).

2. Solutions

Standard BSA protein solution (bovine serum albumin, Sigma, 0.50 mg/ml, freshly diluted from a 20 mg/ml solution), Ca^{2+}-ATPase suspension (tenfold diluted), 1% sodium deoxycholate (NaDOC), 10% trichloroacetic acid (TCA), 1 *N* NaOH, 0.02% alkaline Cu^{2+} solution (1 part of 2% $CuSO_4$, 1 part of Na,K-tartrate, and 100 parts of Na_2CO_3, mixed fresh), and 1 *N* phenol reagent (freshly diluted from commercially available 2 *N* phenol reagent, Fisher Scientific) are used.

3. Procedure

Duplicate samples of 0, 20, 40, 60, and 80 μl of Ca^{2+}-ATPase suspension and 0.50 mg/ml BSA standard solution are made up to 100 ml with water. To each tube is added 100 μl of 1% NaDOC with mixing to insure solubilization of the Ca^{2+}-ATPase protein. This is followed by addition of 1 ml of 10% TCA to precipitate the denatured protein. Another 1 ml of 10% TCA is used to rinse off the protein particles formed on the internal wall of the test tubes. The tubes are then centrifuged at 3000 rpm for 10 min, and the supernatant is carefully decanted. Kimwipe® tissue is used to remove the last drops of the supernatant at the tip of the tube while it is in an inverted position.

To resolubilize the protein, 0.5 ml of 1 *N* NaOH is added, and the mixture is heated at 100°C for 2 min with the test tubes covered with marbles. Vortexing is sometimes necessary to bring all the protein particles into the hot NaOH solution. After cooling, 2 ml of 0.02% alkaline Cu^{2+} solution is added with mixing, and 10 min later 0.5 ml of 1 *N* phenol reagent is added to develop the color. The solutions are allowed to stand for 30 min before the absorbances are read at 750 nm. The amount of Ca^{2+}-ATPase protein is determined against the BSA standard.

D. Assay of Ca^{2+}-ATPase Specific Activity

The same procedure for the assay of SR Ca^{2+}-ATPase described in Section II.D can be used for the purified Ca^{2+}-ATPase.

ACKNOWLEDGMENTS

We thank Ms L.-I. Tsai for her excellent technical assistance in developing these procedures. Supported by NIH PO1 22619-06 (IVA-1).

REFERENCES

Adams, R. J., and Schwartz, A. 1980. Comparative mechanisms for contraction of cardiac and skeletal muscle. *Chest, 78:*123–139.

Bidlack, J. M., Ambudkar, I. S., and Shamoo, A. E. 1982. Purification of phospholamban, a 22,000-dalton protein from cardiac sarcoplasmic reticulum that is specifically phosphorylated by cyclic AMP-dependant protein kinase. *J. Biol. Chem., 257:*4501–4506.

Campbell, K. P., MacLennan, D. H., Jorgensen, A. O., and Mintzer, M. C. 1983. Purification and characterization of calsequestrin from canine cardiac sarcoplasmic reticulum and identification of the 53,000 dalton glycoprotein. *J. Biol. Chem., 258:*1197–1204.

DeMeis, L., and Inesi, G. 1982. The transport of calcium by sarcoplasmic reticulum and various microsomal preparations. In: *Membrane Transport of Calcium*, pp. 141–186. Ed. by Carafoli, E. Academic Press, New York, London.

Ebashi, S., Endo, M., and Ohtsuki, T. 1969. Control of muscle contraction. *Q. Rev. Biophys., 2:*351–386.

Endo, M. 1977. Calcium release from the sarcoplasmic reticulum. *Physiol. Rev., 57:*71–108.

Fabiato, A. 1983. Calcium-induced release of calcium from the cardiac sarcoplasmic reticulum. *Am. J. Physiol., 245:*C1–C14.

Hasselbach, W. 1979. The sarcoplasmic calcium pump. A model of energy transduction in biological membranes. *Top. Curr. Chem., 78:*1–56.

Ikemoto, N. 1982. Structure and function of the calcium pump protein of sarcoplasmic reticulum. *Annu. Rev. Physiol., 44:*297–317.

Kirchberger, M. A., and Tada, M. 1976. Effects of adenosine 3′ : 5′-monophosphate-dependent protein kinase on sarcoplasmic reticulum isolated from cardiac and slow and fast contracting skeletal muscles. *J. Biol. Chem., 251:*725–729.

Levitsky, D. O., Aliev, M. K., Kuzmin, A. V., Levchenko, T. S., Smirnov, V. N., and Chazov, E. I. 1976. Isolation of calcium pump system and purification of calcium-ion-dependent ATPase from heart muscle. *Biochim. Biophys. Acta, 443:*468–484.

Levitsky, D. O., Benevolensky, D. S., Levchenko, T. S., and Kuzmin, A. V. 1982. The cardiac relaxing system. Its nature, calcium ion capacity, and influence of hydrogen and magnesium ions on initial velocity of calcium binding. In: *Advances in Myocardiology*, Volume 3, pp. 393–405. Ed. by Chazov, E., Smirnov, V., and Dhalla, N. S. Plenum Press, New York, London.

MacLennan, D. H., and Holland, P. C. 1975. Calcium transport in sarcoplasmic reticulum. *Annu. Rev. Biophys. Bioeng., 4:*377–404.

Nakamura, J., Wang, T., Tsai, L. I., and Schwartz, A. 1983. Properties and characterization of a highly purified sarcoplasmic reticulum Ca^{2+}-ATPase from dog cardiac and rabbit skeletal muscle. *J. Biol. Chem., 258:*5079–5083.

Sumida, M., Wang, T., Mandel, F., Froehlich, J. P., and Schwartz, A. 1978. Transient kinetics of Ca^{2+} transport of sarcoplasmic reticulum. *J. Biol. Chem., 253:*8772–8777.

Tada, M., Yamamoto, T., and Tonomura, Y. 1978. Molecular mechanism of active calcium transport by sarcoplasmic reticulum. *Physiol. Rev., 58:*1–79.

Tada, M., Yamada, M., Kadoma, M., Inui, M., and Ohmori, F. 1982. Calcium transport by cardiac sarcoplasmic reticulum and phosphorylation of phospholamban. *Mol. Cell. Biochem., 46:*73–95.

Van Winkle, W. B., Pitts, B. J., and Entman, M. L. 1978. Rapid purification of canine cardiac sarcoplasmic reticulum Ca^{2+}-ATPase. *J. Biol. Chem., 253:*8671–8673.

Wang, T., Tsai, L. I., Solaro, R. J., Grassi de Gende, A. O., and Schwartz A. 1979. Effects of potassium on vanadate inhibition of sarcoplasmic reticulum Ca^{2+}-ATPase from dog cardiac and rabbit skeletal muscle. *Biochem. Biophys. Res. Commun., 91:*356–361.

Winegrad, S. 1982. Calcium release from the sarcoplasmic reticulum. *Annu. Rev. Physiol., 44:*451–462.

Chapter 5

Methods for Measuring Functional Properties of Sarcoplasmic Reticulum and Myofibrils in Small Samples of Myocardium

Edward D. Pagani* and R. John Solaro*†

Departments of *Physiology and †Pharmacology and Cell Biophysics
University of Cincinnati College of Medicine
Cincinnati, Ohio

I. INTRODUCTION

We describe here methods developed to study properties of sarcoplasmic reticulum (SR) and myofibrils in the same sample of heart muscle. We wanted to do this because regulation of SR and myofibrils appears to be coordinated in both short-term and long-term regulation of the heart. In short-term regulation of beating hearts, both SR and myofibrillar proteins are phosphorylated by activation of cAMP-dependent protein kinases (Solaro *et al.*, 1976, 1980; E. G. Kranias and R. J. Solaro, unpublished observations). These phosphorylations alter cardiac function by increasing the velocity of Ca^{2+} transport by the SR (Katz, 1979) and by decreasing the Ca^{2+} sensitivity of myofibrillar activation (Solaro *et al.*, 1976; Holroyde *et al.*, 1979), and these changes are likely to be responsible for the decreased contraction–relaxation cycle time of hearts responding to sympathetic nerve stimulation. During relatively long-term stress, such as exercise (Pagani and Solaro, 1981), pressure overload, or thyrotoxicosis (Alpert *et al.*, 1979), kinetic properties of SR and myofibrils change in a way that suggests that these chronic signals might also induce coordinated changes in the SR and the con-

Present Address for Edward D. Pagani: Department of Anesthesia Research, Brigham and Women's Hospital Boston, Massachusetts.

tractoregulatory protein complex. For example, hearts of hyperthyroid rabbits show increased rates of contraction and relaxation, and this is undoubtedly a manifestation of increased velocity of Ca^{2+} transport by the SR and the increased rate of myofibrillar cross-bridge cycling. It is also clear that some pharmacological agents, general and local anesthetics, for example, affect both SR and myofibrillar function and thus may affect coordination between these organelles.

In our own work in the area of coordinated control of SR and myofibrils in chronically stressed rats and rabbits (Martin *et al.*, 1981; Pagani and Solaro, 1981), we find it important to assess the functional properties of these organelles in preparations from single hearts rather than in preparations from pooled hearts. We find considerable biological heterogeneity independent of methodological variability, and this indicates that information will be obscured in studies with preparations from pooled hearts. There are, however, methodological problems in preparing and studying SR preparations and myofibrils with the relatively small hearts of rats and rabbits that are commonly used in studies probing questions about chronic changes in cardiac function. The methods we describe here provide one way of overcoming these problems.

II. GENERAL APPROACH

An obstacle in studying SR function in small tissue samples is that the yield of SR vesicles is too small, and many times too impure, to make reliable measurements, particularly if one wants to compare samples from control and stressed hearts. Past studies using dog heart (Solaro and Briggs, 1974, 1977) and fast and slow skeletal muscles (Briggs *et al.*, 1977) indicated that we could overcome this problem by studying Ca^{2+} transport of SR vesicles in the homogenate itself. The strategy we used employs incubation conditions that enhance Ca^{2+} transport by the SR vesicles and diminish non-SR Ca^{2+} transport or binding to trivial levels.

With some modifications shown below, we have applied this idea to studies of rat and rabbit hearts. By using the homogenate preparation to study SR function, we can measure Ca^{2+} transport properties of the SR vesicles quickly after sacrifice in a small sample of heart. We quantitate SR function by using a Millipore® filtration technique and ^{45}Ca to measure the velocity of SR Ca^{2+} transport and the steady-state filling of the SR vesicles with Ca^{2+}; from these data, we compute a rate constant. Only a small portion of the homogenate is needed to make a variety of measurements. We use the rest of the homogenate to prepare cardiac myofibrils essentially as described by Solaro *et al.* (1971). We quantitate myofibrillar function by measuring the relationship between free Ca^{2+} concentration and Mg^{2+}-ATPase activity in miniaturized reactions using P_i and protein assays of relatively high sensitivity. By adjusting the salt and free metal concentrations of the reaction mixtures, we also measure the Ca^{2+}-activated, Mg^{2+}-activated, and K^+-EDTA ATPase activity of myofibrillar myosin.

III. PREPARATION OF CARDIAC HOMOGENATE AND MYOFIBRILS

A. Solutions

1. Homogenizing solution: 25 m*M* imidazole, pH 7.0.
2. Solution A: 60 m*M* KCl, 30 m*M* imidazole, 2.5 m*M* $MgCl_2$, pH 7.0.
3. Solution B: 60 m*M* KCl, 30 m*M* imidazole, pH 7.0.

B. Procedure

We sarcifice rats and rabbits by cervical dislocation, quickly opening the chest and excising the heart. The heart is immediately immersed in ice-cold homogenizing solution and washed free of blood. The atria and remnants of valves and blood vessels are trimmed away, and the ventricles are blotted dry on filter paper and weighed. We then mince the heart with scissors and suspend the pieces in 15 volumes of ice-cold homogenizing solution. All procedures are performed at 0–4°C.

We homogenize the heart in a Teflon®–glass Thomas tissue grinder (Cat. no. A-43277) using a motor-driven pestle at 500 rpm for 20 to 40 pestle passes. (As discussed below, this type of homogenization procedure is critical for reliable and reproducible results.)

A small portion of the homogenate is placed on ice, and measurements of SR Ca^{2+} transport are begun, usually within 20 min of sacrifice.

The rest of the homogenate is diluted to 40 volumes per gram of heart with ice-cold solution A and centrifuged at 10,000 × *g* for 15 min.

The supernatant is discarded, and the pellet is resuspended in about 40 ml of solution A and homogenized in the Thomas Teflon®–glass tissue grinder. This suspension is centrifuged at 4000 × *g* for 10 min.

We repeat the procedure in the previous step a total of three times. However, the solution used the third time contains 1 m*M* EGTA. We then resuspend the pellet in 40 ml of solution A containing 1% Triton X-100 (v/v). This suspension is homogenized and centrifuged at 4000 × *g* for 10 min.

We wash the pellet from the previous step by resuspension in 60 m*M* KCl, 30 m*M* imidazole, pH 7.0 (solution B), homogenize, and centrifuge at 4000 × *g* for 10 min. This is repeated a total of three times.

The final pellet suspension should be milky white. We remove connective tissue by resuspending the pellet in about 1–2 ml of solution B using the Thomas homogenizer. The Teflon® pestle is then used to collect the connective tissue. Connective tissue will adhere to the pestle on each pass, and it can then be washed away. The pestle is passed through the myofibrillar preparation and washed until no connective tissue adheres to the pestle.

The protein concentration of the myofibrillar preparation is immediately determined, and the myofibrils are assayed for ATPase activity on the same day.

IV. MEASUREMENTS OF SR Ca^{2+} TRANSPORT IN CARDIAC HOMOGENATES

A. "Uptake" Solution

	Stock	Final bath
Potassium chloride	117.6 m*M*	100 m*M*
Potassium oxalate	1.176–11.76 m*M*	1–10 m*M*
Imidazole	44.4 m*M*	40 m*M**
Sodium azide	11.76 m*M*	10 m*M*
Magnesium chloride	5.3 m*M*	4.5 m*M*
Sodium ATP	2.94 m*M*	2.5 m*M*
Creatine phosphokinase	2.36 Units/ml	2.0 Units/ml
Creatine phosphate	3.54 m*M*	3.0 m*M*
pH	7.0	7.0

B. ^{45}Ca-EGTA Solution

	Stock		Final bath	
	Ca^{2+}	EGTA	Ca^{2+}	EGTA
"Velocity" solution	0.5 m*M*	0.31 m*M*	25 μ*M*	15.5 μ*M*
"Capacity" solution	3.0 m*M*	2.9 m*M*	150 μ*M*	145 μ*M*
^{45}Ca activity	3.7 μCi/ml		0.185 μCi/ml	

C. Procedure

To insure that the assay solutions are identical from week to week, we prepare a large volume of stock uptake solution (approximately 75 ml). The solution is stored in 1.7-ml aliquots at −20°C. At the time of the assay, an appropriate number of tubes is brought to 37°C in a temperature-controlled water bath.

The homogenate is resuspended by one pass of the Teflon® pestle, and a portion (usually 0.18 ml) is added to a reaction tube with gentle "vortexing" at a known time. We preincubated this reaction mixture for 5 min. This not only insures temperature equilibration but also insures that contaminant extravesicular Ca^{2+} will be transported into the vesicles of the SR. We add 20 μl of base, acid, or homogenization solution to precisely adjust the pH to 7.0.

After the 5-min preincubation, Ca^{2+} transport is initiated by addition of 0.1 ml of ^{45}Ca-EGTA, which yields the final desired concentration of total and free calcium as well as ^{45}Ca (usually about 0.18 μCi/ml bath or about 400,000 cpm/ml).

At appropriate times, a sample (usually 0.5 ml) is removed from the reaction tube and rapidly filtered by suction through a Millipore® filter (HA 0.45 μm).

Radioactivity in an aliquot (usually 0.1 ml) of the filtrate and reaction mixture is then determined using a liquid scintillation spectrometer by standard procedures.

* Includes amount added with homogenate.

The amount of Ca^{2+} removed by the SR vesicles in the reaction mixture during the time of the assay is computed by multiplying the total added Ca^{2+} (given in nmoles/ml) by the fraction of counts taken up (f), where:

$$f = [(\text{cpm/ml})_{\text{total}} - (\text{cpm/ml})_{\text{filtrate}}]/(\text{cpm/ml})_{\text{total}}$$

Uptake is expressed per gram of heart by dividing this product by grams wet heart/ml reaction mixture. The velocity of transport is given by the slope of a line (generated by sequential samples) relating time to Ca^{2+} uptake or by the total amount of Ca^{2+} removed at a single point in time provided it has been shown that the uptake is linear at that time. At a given free Ca^{2+} concentration, the units for the velocity measurements are expressed as nmoles Ca^{2+}/g heart per min. The capacity for Ca^{2+} uptake or steady-state filling of the SR vesicles with Ca^{2+} is given by the Ca^{2+} uptake at the plateau of the relationship between time and Ca^{2+} uptake and has the units of nmoles Ca^{2+}/g wet heart. It is reasonable to interpret the capacity measurement as a reflection of the total volume of SR vesicles in a particular sample, which appears to be independent of vesicle geometry. We find that the measured SR capacity for Ca^{2+} is the same for one sample when divided in half and treated as two separate samples. Therefore, when both the velocity and capacity for Ca^{2+} transport are measured under identical conditions, a catalytic rate constant for Ca^{2+} transport can be computed. The rate constant is calculated by dividing the maximum velocity of Ca^{2+} transport by the capacity and has the units of t^{-1}.

V. MEASUREMENT OF MYOFIBRILLAR AND MYOSIN ATPase ACTIVITY

A. Assay Solutions

1. Protein Determination

The following solutions are used (modified from Lowry *et al.*, 1951):

A. 2% Na_2CO_3 in 0.1 N NaOH.
B. 2% $CuSO_4$.
C. 4% Na or K tartate.
D. 50 parts A + 0.25 parts each of B and C, adding B last.
E. Phenol Reagent diluted 1:1 with deionized H_2O.
F. Stock standard bovine serum albumin (0.5 mg/ml).

2. P_i Determination

The following are required (modified from King, 1938):

G. 10% trichloroacetic acid.
H. 8.75% perchloric acid.
I. 5% ammonium molybdate.

J. A.N.S. solution (25 ml, dissolve 3 g $NaHSO_3$ and 0.6 g Na_2SO_3 in H_2O. Add 0.005 g 1-amino-2-naphthol-4-sulfonic acid; filter).
K. Stock standard KH_2PO_4 (1 m*M*).

B. Incubation Solutions

1. Myofibrillar Actomyosin ATPase (Ca^{2+}-Stimulated Mg-ATPase)

	Stock	Final
Potassium chloride	60 m*M*	60 m*M**
Imidazole	30 m*M*	30 m*M**
Magnesium chloride	10 m*M*	7.5 m*M*
Sodium ATP	6.67 m*M*	5.0 m*M*
$CaCl_2$	1.33 m*M*	1.0 m*M*
EGTA	0–1.37 m*M*	0–1.03 m*M*
pH	7.0	7.0

2. Myofibrillar Myosin ATPase

	Stock	Final
Potassium chloride	580 m*M*	450 m*M**
Imidazole	43 m*M*	40 m*M**
$CaCl_2$ or EDTA (for assay of Ca- or K-EDTA-stimulated ATPase, respectively)	13.3 m*M*	10 m*M*
Sodium ATP	6.66 m*M*	5 m*M*
pH	7.5	7.5

C. Procedure

Determine myofibrillar protein concentration. We add 0 to 50 μg BSA to standard tubes and bring to a volume of 100 μl with solution A.

Standard tubes are prepared by adding 0–50 μg BSA. The volume is made to 100 μl with solution A. Triplicate unknown tubes are prepared by adding 100-μl samples of a 1:20 dilution of myofibrils in solution D. To these tubes, 1.0 ml of solution D is added with vortexing. The tubes stand for 15 min to insure that the protein is dissolved. To begin the color reaction, 100 μl of solution E is added to each tube, followed by "vortexing." After 30 min, absorbance at 770 nm is measured. We obtain an absorbance of about 0.0135 units/μg protein.

Tubes containing the myofibrillar ATPase reaction solutions can be prepared and stored frozen (0.75-ml aliquots) as described for the homogenate experiment.

* Note that myofibrils are suspended in 60 m*M* KCl, 30 m*M* imidazole.

At the time of the assay, tubes are brought to 37°C in a temperature-controlled water bath. An amount of myofibrillar solution B is added to the reaction mixture so that with the addition of the myofibrillar protein the final bath volume is 1.0 ml.

Myofibrillar protein (final 0.25 mg/ml bath) is added to the reaction solution to start the reaction.

At various times, the reaction is stopped by the addition of 1.0 ml ice-cold 10% tricholoroacetic acid (TCA) with immediate "vortexing." The tubes are placed on ice for 10 min and then centrifuged to pellet the precipitated protein; after centrifuging, the tubes must be kept on ice. A blank tube is made by adding protein to a reaction tube already containing 1.0 ml of TCA. A 0.1-ml sample of the supernatant is assayed for P_i.

Phosphate is determined in 1.0-ml assay tubes. A 0.1-ml supernatant sample is added to a tube containing 0.8 ml of 8.75% perchloric acid (PCA). Immediately following the addition of the sample, 70 μl of 5% w/v ammonium molybdate (AM) and 30 μl of A.N.S. solution are added to the tube with vortexing at room temperature. The tubes are brought to room temperature, and after 10 min, the absorbance is read at 660 nm. A standard P_i curve is generated by adding 0–100 nmoles of KH_2PO_4 from the 1 m*M* stock standard to tubes containing 0.8 ml of 8.75% PCA, bringing them to a final volume of 0.9 ml, and then assaying as described for the supernatant sample. In our laboratory, we obtain 0.0036 absorbance units/nmole P_i.

VI. RESULTS AND DISCUSSION

A. Homogenate Studies

We show some typical results in this section and discuss the verification of the methods described above. Our assertion in the homogenate studies is that the incubation conditions restrict Ca^{2+} transport to the SR vesicles in the homogenate. Estimates of the magnitude of the potential Ca^{2+} binding and transport properties of components in a canine cardiac homogenate under similar conditions show that Ca^{2+} transport by SR vesicles in the homogenate is virtually all that we are measuring (Solaro and Briggs, 1977). Compared to oxalate-enhanced Ca^{2+} transport, the binding or transport of Ca^{2+} by myofibrils, mitochondria, and sarcolemma (SL) is trivial under the incubation conditions. Yet, although it is clear that 10 m*M* azide will inhibit cardiac mitochondrial Ca^{2+} transport essentially to zero (Solaro and Briggs, 1974) and that myofibrillar Ca^{2+} binding is very low (Solaro and Shiner, 1976) compared to oxalate-enhanced SR Ca^{2+} uptake, it might still be debated whether SL Ca^{2+} transport can be eliminated by our incubation conditions. The reason for this is that preparation of a pure cardiac SL fraction has not been achieved, and it is not certain that the SL preparations have the same specific activity as SL vesicles in the homogenate. We therefore further tested our assertion that homogenate SL Ca^{2+} transport is low relative to oxalate-enhanced SR Ca^{2+} transport by using verapamil. Verapamil has been shown to partially inhibit Ca^{2+} binding to SL membrane at a concentration of 20 μ*M* (Pang,

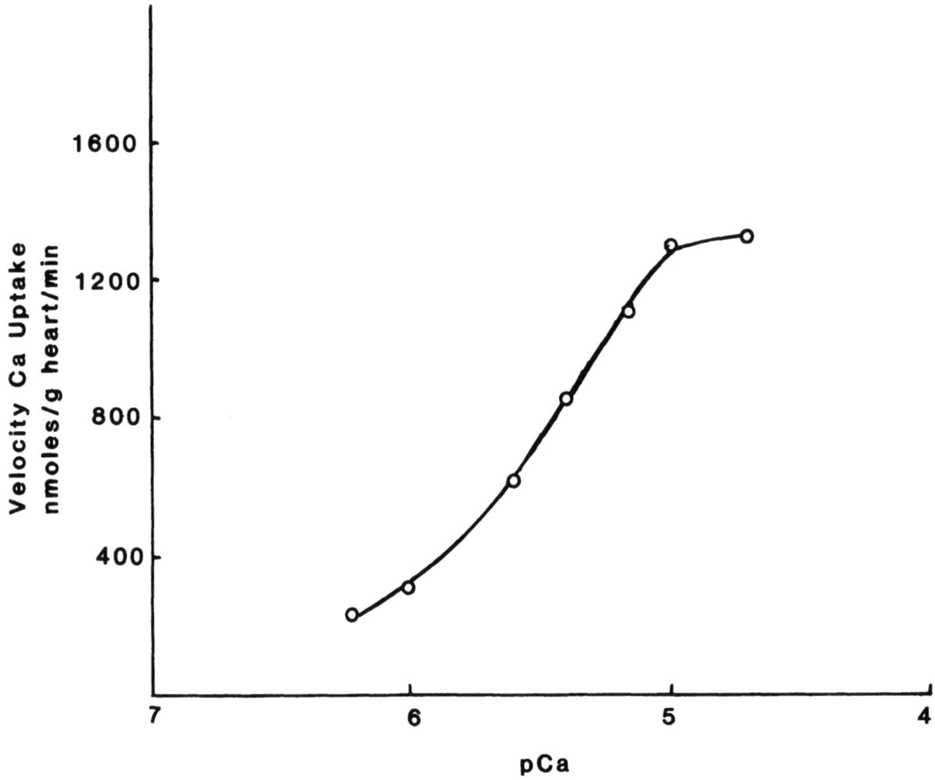

Figure 1. Velocity of Ca^{2+} uptake by SR vesicles in a rat ventricular homogenate as a function of free Ca^{2+} concentration. Measurements were made from a single rat heart (ventricular wet weight 1.0 g). Conditions were as described in the text for SR "uptake" experiments.

1980) and almost completely at 100 μM. When 100 μM verapamil was added to our reaction solution, Ca^{2+} uptake was decreased by less than 5%. This indicates that Ca^{2+} transport into SR vesicles in the homogenate is the main measurement we are making.

We have found that the homogenization procedure affects the stability of the SR vesicles as judged by Ca^{2+} transport. When we used a Sorvall Omnimixer to homogenize rat hearts, the rate of Ca^{2+} transport decayed considerably when measured at various times over a 90-min period. To determine the extent and possible cause of the decay, we prepared homogenates of cardiac and skeletal muscle using the Omnimixer in an identical manner. We prepared a third homogenate by combining equal portions of the skeletal and cardiac homogenates. After 90 min, Ca^{2+} transport of the cardiac homogenate decayed to 12% of the value obtained immediately after homogenization, whereas Ca^{2+} transport in skeletal homogenate decayed to 70% of the maximal value. We then compared the rate of Ca^{2+} transport that we measured in the skeletal–cardiac sample to the predicted rate of calcium transport calculated from the individual rates of Ca^{2+} transport of the cardiac and skeletal homogenates. Again, after 90 min, the measured rate of transport of the combined skeletal–cardiac preparation was signifi-

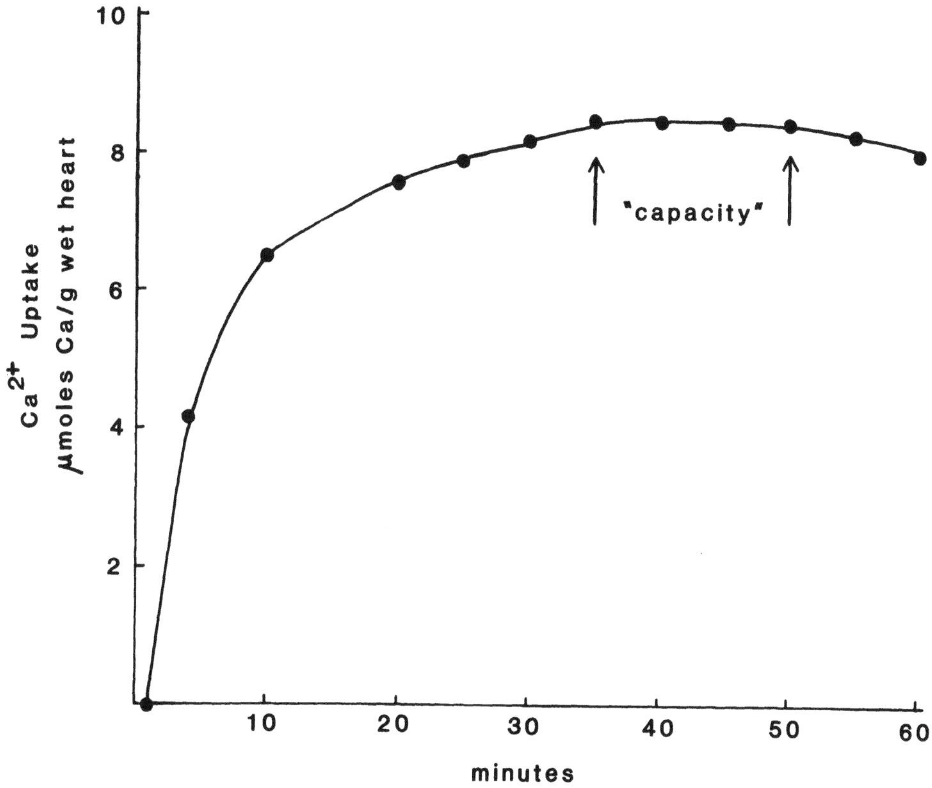

Figure 2. Time course of Ca^{2+} uptake by SR vesicles in a rat ventricular homogenate. Conditions were as described in the text for SR "capacity" experiments.

cantly less than the rate obtained by addition of the individual rates of each. This suggested to us that Omnimixer homogenization released a substance in rat heart that induces decay of Ca^{2+} transport by SR vesicles. We were able to overcome this problem by changing the method of homogenization. When rat cardiac tissue was homogenized using the Thomas homogenizer, described above, we observed a minimal amount of decay in Ca^{2+} transport over the same time period. The addition of phenylmethylsulfonylfluoride (PMSF, a protease inhibitor) to this preparation prevented the decay of Ca^{2+} transport, but because we are able to complete our measurements of SR function within 60 min of homogenization, we did not routinely add PMSF to the homogenates.

In homogenizing the tissue using a Thomas homogenizer, we wanted to know if the number of pestle passes had an effect on SR Ca^{2+} transport. We reasoned that the extent of tissue homogenization could produce conditions between two extremes of functional states. Either little vesiculation of the SR would be achieved because of an inadequate number of pestle passes or the SR would be damaged as a result of an excessive number of pestle passes. To determine an optimal number of pestle passes to give reproducible results, we carried out the following experiments. We minced one heart and divided the tissue in half. We

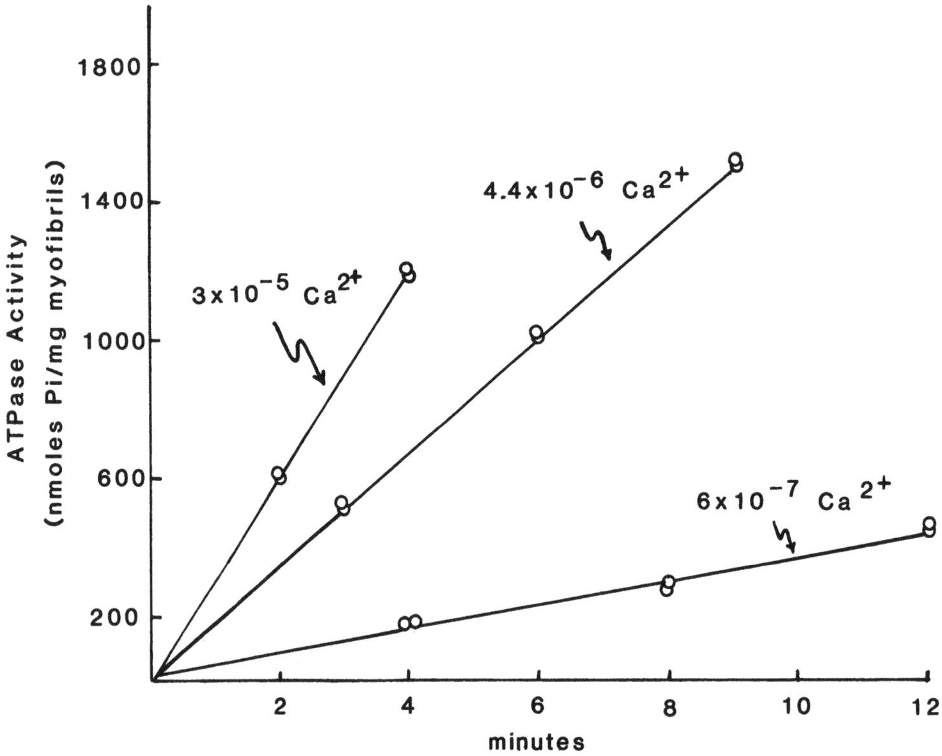

Figure 3. Time course of Ca^{2+}-activated myofibrillar Mg^{2+}-ATPase at three free Ca^{2+} concentrations.

then ground each of the samples to a state that first approached a homogeneous suspension. At this point, we further homogenized a sample of an additional number of pestle passes. Using this system, we obtained identical rates of Ca^{2+} transport when the samples were homogenized with an additional 20 to 40 pestle passes. This number of pestle passes for our system to give reproducible results may vary in another system because of a variety of factors. Therefore, this control experiment should be performed in first setting up a homogenization procedure. Any method of homogenization can be used if the decay of Ca^{2+} transport and optimal homogenization duration are evaluated to insure that the homogenization method produces consistent results. For example, in experiments with dog heart, we found little decay of activity over a 90-min period following Omnimixer homogenization.

In measuring the velocity and capacity of SR Ca^{2+} transport, a number of parameters must be checked to insure that they are not artificially altering Ca^{2+} transport during the assay. These parameters are temperature, pH, ATP concentration, and the final level of extravesicular free Ca^{2+}. We routinely monitor pH and temperature at the beginning and end of our assay by setting up a control bath. The level of ATP is maintained throughout our assay by using an ATP-regenerating system. The level of extravesicular free Ca^{2+} is calculated at the end of each assay. This measurement is made by determining the amount of Ca^{2+}

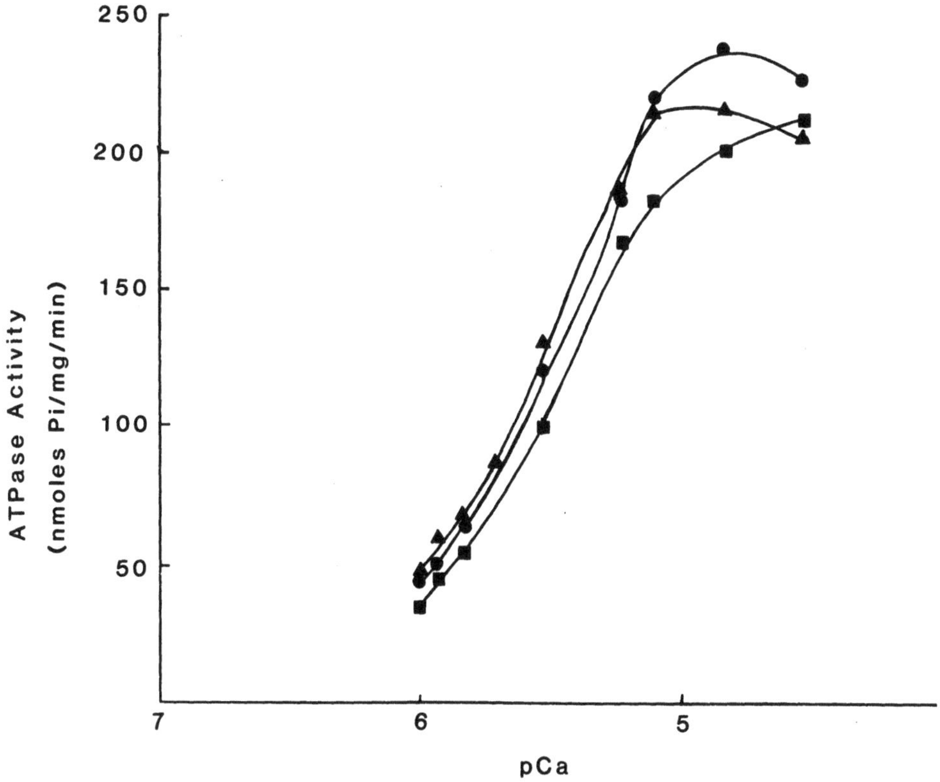

Figure 4. Relationship between free Ca^{2+} concentration and myofibrillar Mg^{2+}-ATPase for preparations from three individual rat hearts.

removed by the SR and subtracting this amount from the initial amount of total calcium in the assay medium to obtain the final extravesicular total calcium and then calculating the amount of extravesicular free Ca^{2+} using the final level of total Ca^{2+} and the initial amount of EGTA. The level of extravesicular free Ca^{2+} should not be reduced to the extent that the velocity of Ca^{2+} transport or Ca^{2+} transport at capacity is affected.

In Figure 1 we show typical results obtained using these methods to measure the relationship between free Ca^{2+} and the velocity of Ca^{2+} transport by SR vesicles in a rat ventricle or homogenate. We find that the v_{max} for Ca^{2+} transport varies from heart to heart, and we attribute this to biological heterogeneity. Likewise, the capacity for Ca^{2+} also varies from heart to heart. We show typical results of a determination for SR Ca^{2+} uptake capacity in Figure 2. When the capacity for Ca^{2+} is reached, the extravesicular free Ca^{2+} concentration (4 μM) is still high enough to support Ca^{2+} transport even though net transport ceases.

B. Myofibrillar ATPase Studies

Data in Figure 3 show the results of a typical experiment in which we measured Ca^{2+}-activated Mg-ATPase activity in myofibrils obtained from one rat heart. We chose the duration of the ATPase assay so that the rate of ATP hydrolysis is linear and the total amount of ATP hydrolyzed is not more than 10% of the total. In Figure 4, we show the relationship between free Ca^{2+} concentration and myofibrillar ATPase activity for preparations from three rats. Data in Figure 4 illustrate the biological variation in the magnitude of the ATPase activity.

We also measured myosin ATPase activity using the myofibrillar preparations and emphasize that the differences in the Ca^{2+}-stimulated myosin ATPase activities among these hearts are not attributable to methodological variability but rather to biological heterogeneity. In other studies, which are not reported here, we have shown that the differences in Ca^{2+}-stimulated myosin ATPAse activity among normal rat and rabbit hearts are related to dissimilar proportions of ventricular myosin isoenzymes (Martin *et al.*, 1981).

In our own work using methods described here, we have been able to make the kind of measurements shown in the figures in single rat and rabbit hearts. With slight modifications and a set of appropriate pilot studies, these methods are very likely to be useful for studies of hearts of other animals or for the study of biopsy material.

ACKNOWLEDGMENTS

Support for work described here came from N.I.H. grants RO1 HL22231, PO1 HL22619 (III B), and a B.R.S.G. grant. Dr. Solaro is the recipient of Research Career Development Award HL00464, and Dr. Pagani was the recipient of a Ryan Fellowship.

REFERENCES

Alpert, N. R., Mulieri, L. A., and Litten, R. Z. 1979. Functional significance of altered myosin adenosine triphosphatase activity in enlarged hearts. *Am. J. Cardiol., 44*:947–953.

Briggs, F. N., Poland, J. L., and Solaro, R. J. 1977. Relative capabilities of sarcoplasmic reticulum in fast and slow mammalian skeletal muscle. *J. Physiol.* (*Lond.*), *266*:587–594.

Holroyde, M. J., Howe, E., and Solaro, R. J. 1979. Modification of calcium requirements for activation of cardiac myofibrillar ATPase by cAMP dependent phosphorylation. *Biochim. Biophys. Acta, 586*:63–69.

Katz, A. M. 1979. Role of contractile proteins and sarcoplasmic reticulum in the response of the heart to catecholamines: An historical review. *Adv. Cyclic Nucleotide Res., 11*:303–343.

King, E. J. 1938. Colorimetric determination of phosphorous. *Biochem. J., 26*:292–297.

Lowry, O. H., Rosenbrough, N. J., Farr, A. L., and Randall, R. J. 1951. Protein measurement with folin phenol reagent. *J. Biol. Chem., 193*:265–275.

Martin, A. F., Pagani, E. D., and Solaro, R. J. 1981. Thyroxine induced redistribution of isoenzymes of rabbit ventricular myosin. *Cir. Res., 50*:117–124.

Pagani, E. D., and Solaro, R. J. 1981. A relation between the calcium uptake properties of sarcoplasmic reticulum and the ATPase of myofibrils in hearts of exercising rats. *Biophys. J., 33*:88a.

Pang, D. C. 1980. Effect of inotropic agents on the calcium binding to isolated cardiac sarcolemma. *Biochim. Biophys. Acta 598*:528–542.

Solaro, R. J., and Briggs, F. N. 1974. Estimating the functional capabilities of sarcoplasmic reticulum in cardiac muscle: Calcium binding. *Circ. Res., 34*:531–540.

Solaro, R. J., and Briggs, F. N. 1977. Calcium oxalate transport as a measure of sarcoplasmic reticulum function. In: *Methodological Surveys in Biochemistry*, Volume 6, *Membranous Elements and Movement of Molecules*, pp. 114–124. Ed. by Reid, E. John Wiley & Sons, Chichester.
Solaro, R. J., and Shiner, J. S. 1976. Modulation of Ca^{++} control of dog and rabbit cardiac myofibrils by Mg^{++}: Comparison with rabbit skeletal myofibrils. *Circ. Res.* *39*:8–14.
Solaro, R. J., Pang, D. C., and Briggs, F. N. 1971. The purification of cardiac myofibrils with Triton X-100. *Biochim. Biophys. Acta*, *245*:259–262.
Solaro, R. J., Moir, A. J. G., and Perry. S. V. 1976. Phosphorylation of troponin I and the inotropic effect of adrenalin in the perfused rabbit heart. *Nature*, *262*:615–617.
Solaro, R. J., Holroyde, M. J., Herzig, J. W., and Peterson, J. 1980. Cardiac relaxation and myofibrillar interactions with phosphate and vanadate. *Eur. J. Cardiol.*, *1*(Suppl. A):21–27.

Chapter **6**

The Regulation of Free Ca^{2+} Ion Concentration by Metal Chelators

Steven Robertson and James D. Potter

Department of Pharmacology and Cell Biophysics
University of Cincinnati College of Medicine
Cincinnati, Ohio

I. INTRODUCTION

The importance of maintaining adequate control of the calcium ion concentration in biological experiments is clearly emphasized by the number of studies in this volume alone that utilize various calcium chelators. Furthermore, most physiological mechanisms regulated by Ca^{2+} are fully activated by the contaminating (10^{-6} *M*) levels of this ion present in typical test solutions. Thus, one of the uses of divalent metal chelators or ion-exchange resins is to reduce the activity of this ion to levels below that required to affect regulation. If the chelator used to alleviate the problem of contaminating metal has an apparent affinity for Ca^{2+} about equal to that of the biological system in question, then it will also serve as a divalent metal buffer, enabling an accurate determination of the Ca^{2+} dependence of that system. This second use of metal chelators is the topic of this chapter. Two metal chelators are compared, and their temperature, pH, and ionic strength dependencies discussed. Finally, methods for calculating the complex equilibria, along with suggestions for solving these calculations by computer, will be presented.

Although many metal chelators have been employed for biological research and more are being developed (Tsien, 1980), two of the most commonly used are

Present address for Steven Robertson: Miles Laboratory, Human Research Division, Elkhart, Indiana.
Present address for James D. Potter: Department of Pharmacology, University of Miami School of Medicine, Miami, Florida.

Table I. Stability Constants and Enthalpy Changes for H^+, K^+, Ca^{2+}, and Mg^{2+} Binding to EGTA and EDTA at 20°C and 0.1M Ionic Strength[a]

	EGTA		EDTA	
Ligand·metal complex	log K (20°C)	ΔH (kcal/mole)	log K 20°C	ΔH (kcal/mole)
K_{HE} = HE/H·E	9.47	−5.48	10.24	−5.67
K_{H_2E} = H_2E/H·HE	8.85	−5.8	6.16	−4.34
K_{H_3E} = H_3E/H·H_2E	2.66	—	2.66	4.34
K_{H_4E} = H_4E/H·H_3E	2.00	—	2.00	0.3
K_{KE} = KE/K·E	—	—	0.8	—
K_{CaE} = CaE/Ca·E	10.97	8.1	10.69	−6.6
K_{CaHE} = CaHE/Ca·HE	5.29	—	3.63	—
K_{MgE} = MgE/Mg·E	5.21	5.0	8.79	3.5
K_{MgHE} = MgHE/Mg·HE	3.36	—	2.58	—

[a] Data from Martell and Smith (1974), Volume 1.

ethyleneglycol-bis(β-aminoethyl ether)-N,N,N',N'-tetraacetic acid (EGTA) and ethylenediaminetetraacetate (EDTA). Both of these aminocarboxylic acids have high affinities for Ca^{2+}. However, because EGTA also has a high selectivity for Ca^{2+} over Mg^{2+}, it has become the buffer of choice for most biological research. For simplicity, we focus our discussion of metal buffers on EGTA. Nevertheless, the specific examples we cite illustrate principles that apply to the use of all the metal buffers.

II. PROPERTIES OF CHELATORS

One unfortunate feature of these compounds is that their nitrogens bind protons with pK_as near the normal working pH range (6–8), rendering their metal-binding properties strongly pH dependent. For example, increasing the pH from 6.5 to 7.5 increases the apparent affinity of EGTA for Ca^{2+} by ~100-fold and increases that for EDTA by ~15-fold. It is therefore apparent that accurate and precise determination and control of the test solution pH is one prerequisite for valid use of these chelators as metal-ion buffers. The importance of continued monitoring of the test solution pH during metal titration is emphasized by the fact that divalent cation binding to these chelators releases protons. Thus, following each addition of Ca^{2+}, some OH^- will be required to maintain pH constant.

Cation binding to these chelators is also temperature and ionic strength dependent. The effects of these two properties are compensated for by selecting stability constants that were obtained under conditions similar to those of the experiment at hand. But, when available, enthalphy changes can be used to adjust the stability constants for different experimental temperatures.

Throughout this chapter we use the stability constants listed in Table I as reported by Martell and Smith (1974) for 20°C and 0.1 M ionic strength. The ΔH

values for various stability constants are also listed in Table I. This will enable both temperature and pH effects to be accounted for in the calculations shown below. For a more complete discussion concerning how changes in ionic strength affect these stability constants, see Fabiato and Fabiato (1979).

There are two basic methodological approaches to experiments involving metal buffers. One is to calculate the free ion concentrations that exist in solution when the total concentrations of each ligand and metal have been specified. For example the $[Ca^{2+}]$ in a solution containing 10 m*M* EGTA and 7.28 m*M* $CaCl_2$ at pH 7.0 and 20°C can be calculated. The other approach is based on a prior knowledge of the desired concentrations of various ligand–metal complexes or free metal-ion concentrations and calculates the total concentration of each ligand and metal required. For example, the concentration of $CaCl_2$ that will produce a $[Ca^{2+}]$ of 10^{-6} *M* in the presence of 10 m*M* EGTA at pH 7.0 and 20°C can be determined. Both of these problems are solved by first writing the following set of simultaneous equations that describe the complex equilibria for a solution containing K_4EGTA and $CaCl_2$ at a specific pH and temperature:

$$E_T = EGTA^{4-} + HEGTA^{3-} + H_2EGTA^{2-} + H_3EGTA^- + H_4EGTA + CaEGTA^{2-} + CaHEGTA^- \quad (1)$$

$$Ca_T = Ca^{2+} + CaEGTA^{2-} + CaHEGTA^- \quad (2)$$

where E_T is total EGTA and Ca_T is total Ca.

Note that although the ions K^+ and Cl^- are important for ionic strength calculations (see Fabiato and Fabiato, 1979), they are not needed to determine $[Ca^{2+}]$. By dropping the charge signs and using the stability constant definitions and abbreviations shown in Table I, each complex can be expressed as a product of free ligand (E), free cation (H or Ca), and the appropriate stability constants as follows:

$$E_T = E + H\cdot E\cdot K_{HE} + H\cdot E\cdot K_{HE}\cdot H\cdot K_{H_2E} + H\cdot E\cdot K_{HE}\cdot H\cdot K_{H_2E}\cdot H\cdot K_{H_3E} + H\cdot E\cdot K_{HE}\cdot H\cdot K_{H_2E}\cdot H\cdot K_{H_3E}\cdot H\cdot K_{H_4E} + Ca\cdot E\cdot K_{CaE} + H\cdot E\cdot K_{HE}\cdot Ca\cdot K_{CaHE} \quad (1')$$

$$Ca_T = Ca + Ca\cdot E\cdot K_{CaE} + H\cdot E\cdot K_{HE}\cdot Ca\cdot K_{CaHE} \quad (2')$$

These two equations can be simplified by combining terms as shown below:

$$E_T = E\cdot(e_H + Ca\cdot e_{Ca}) \quad (3)$$

$$Ca_T = Ca\cdot(1 + E\cdot e_{Ca}) \quad (4)$$

where $e_H = 1 + H\cdot K_{He}\cdot\{1 + H\cdot K_{H_2E}\cdot[1 + H\cdot K_{H_3E}\cdot(1 + H\cdot K_{H_4E})]\}$ and $e_{Ca} = K_{CaE} + H\cdot K_{HE}\cdot K_{CaHE}$.

Table II. Factors That Convert "Concentration" Stability Constants into "Proton" Stability Constants at Various Ionic Strengths[a]

Ionic strength	Increase in log K
0.05	0.09
0.10	0.11
0.15	0.12
0.2	0.13
0.5	0.15
1.0	0.14

[a] Data from Martell and Smith (1974), Volume 1.

The first step in solving either of the two problems posed above is to adjust the log K values if the experimental temperature is not 20°C. The log K_t values for any temperature t can be found using the following equation:

$$\mathrm{d}\log K_t/\mathrm{d}t = \Delta H/\ln(10)\cdot R\cdot(T + 273.2)^2$$

where R is the universal gas constant, 0.001987 kcal/°C per mole, T is the temperature in °C at which ΔH and log K were measured, and t is in °C. Thus, with the log K and ΔH values that are listed in Table I for 20°C, this equation becomes:

$$\log K_t = \log K + \Delta H\cdot(t - 20)/393.3 \tag{5}$$

Note that equilibria involving protons are expressed in terms of concentration; thus, some adjustment must be made to account for the fact that hydrogen ion activity (pH) is usually specified. This can be done either by converting pH values to hydrogen ion concentrations using appropriate hydrogen ion activity coefficients or by converting the concentration constants listed in Table I to Bronsted or mixed constants using Table II (Martell and Smith, 1974). We use the second approach so that, for our example (0.1 ionic strength), all the log K values listed in Table I involving proton reactions will be increased by 0.11.

Following these adjustments, e_{H} and e_{Ca} can be calculated. The values of e_{H} and e_{Ca} are 3.5×10^4 and 9.3×10^{10}, respectively, for the two problems mentioned above. Finally, both problems are solved by substituting eq. 3 into eq. 4, yielding:

$$\mathrm{Ca_T} = \mathrm{Ca}\cdot[1 + \mathrm{E_T}\cdot e_{\mathrm{Ca}}/(e_{\mathrm{H}} + \mathrm{Ca}\cdot e_{\mathrm{Ca}})] \tag{6}$$

or

$$\mathrm{Ca}^2\cdot e_{\mathrm{Ca}} + \mathrm{Ca}\cdot[e_{\mathrm{H}} - e_{\mathrm{Ca}}\cdot(\mathrm{E_T} - \mathrm{Ca_T})] - \mathrm{Ca_T}\cdot e_{\mathrm{H}} = 0 \tag{7}$$

The answer to the first problem we discussed previously, where total EGTA and total Ca are known, is obtained by applying the quadratic formula to eq. 7 as shown below.

$$\mathrm{Ca} = -\beta + (\beta^2 + \mathrm{Ca_T}\cdot e_\mathrm{H}/e_\mathrm{Ca})^{1/2}$$

where $\beta = [e_\mathrm{H} + e_\mathrm{Ca}\cdot(\mathrm{E_T} - \mathrm{Ca_T})]/2e_\mathrm{Ca}$. The second problem, in which total EGTA and free Ca were given, is solved by using eq. 6 directly. Note that these two examples describe the same test solution, since the $[Ca^{2+}]$ in the first is 10^{-6} *M*, whereas $\mathrm{Ca_T}$ in the second is 7.28 m*M*.

III. INTERACTION WITH MAGNESIUM

Many times it is important to know the calcium dependence of a biological parameter in the presence of physiological levels of Mg^{2+}. The analysis of this problem is complicated by the fact that most calcium chelators also bind Mg^{2+}. In spite of this complication, the set of equations describing this situation is similar to eqs. 1 and 2. The equation for $\mathrm{E_T}$ will have the extra terms $\mathrm{MgEGTA^{2-}} + \mathrm{MgHEGTA^{-}}$, and an additional equation for total Mg ($\mathrm{Mg_T}$) will have to be added. Following substitution and collection of terms as described above, the following set of equations can be obtained:

$$\mathrm{E_T} = \mathrm{E}\cdot(e_\mathrm{H} + \mathrm{Ca}\cdot e_\mathrm{Ca} + \mathrm{Mg}\cdot e_\mathrm{Mg}) \tag{8}$$

$$\mathrm{Ca_T} = \mathrm{Ca}\cdot(1 + \mathrm{E}\cdot e_\mathrm{Ca}) \tag{9}$$

$$\mathrm{Mg_T} = \mathrm{Mg}\cdot(1 + \mathrm{E}\cdot e_\mathrm{Mg}) \tag{10}$$

where $e_\mathrm{Mg} = K_\mathrm{MgE} + \mathrm{H}\cdot K_\mathrm{HE}\cdot K_\mathrm{MgHE}$ and e_H and e_Ca are as described for eqs. 3 and 4. Although there are six unknowns in these equations, most experimental protocols specify $\mathrm{E_T}$ and are not concerned with E. Thus, any two of the remaining four variables, $\mathrm{Ca_T}$, Ca, $\mathrm{Mg_T}$, and Mg, must be fixed before a unique solution can be obtained.

The method for solving eqs. 8–10 depends on which two of the four metal unknowns are specified. If both the free metal ion concentrations, Ca and Mg, are given, then E is obtained immediately from eq. 8, enabling direct calculation of $\mathrm{Ca_T}$ and $\mathrm{Mg_T}$ using eqs. 9 and 10. In contrast, if $\mathrm{Ca_T}$ and $\mathrm{Mg_T}$ are fixed, then a third-order expression in E must be solved before Ca and Mg can be found. This illustrates the fact that, independent of the number of ligands and metals present, the mathematical solution of the equations describing the complex equilibria is simplest when all free cation concentrations are specified.

We have calculated the [total Ca]/[total chelator] ratio for both EGTA (Figure 1) and EDTA (Figure 2) when [total chelator] = 2 m*M* in the absence and presence of 1 m*M* free Mg^{2+}. Figure 1 clearly illustrates the high selectivity EGTA has for Ca^{2+} over Mg^{2+}, whereas the curves in Figure 2 emphasize the degree to which

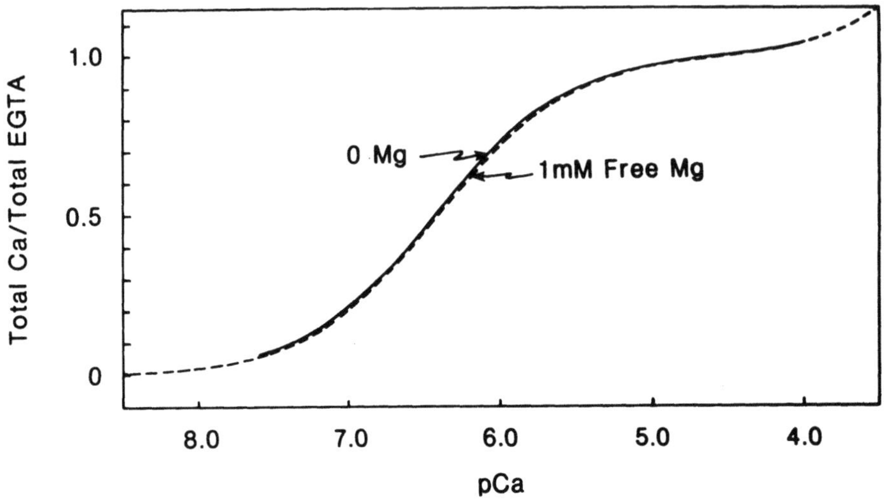

Figure 1. Calculated total Ca:total EGTA ratios as a function of pCa at two fixed levels of free Mg^{2+}. Other conditions are: 2 m*M* total EGTA, 20°C, pH 7.0, and 0.1 *M* ionic strength.

Ca^{2+} binding to EDTA is influenced by Mg^{2+}. An interesting consequence of the relative affinities of EDTA for Ca^{2+} and Mg^{2+} is shown in Figure 3, where total Mg was fixed at 1 m*M* (1/2 total EDTA). Note that now the pCa range where [total Ca]/[total EDTA] ratios fall between 0.1 and 0.9 is almost twice as wide as when free Mg^{2+} is fixed.

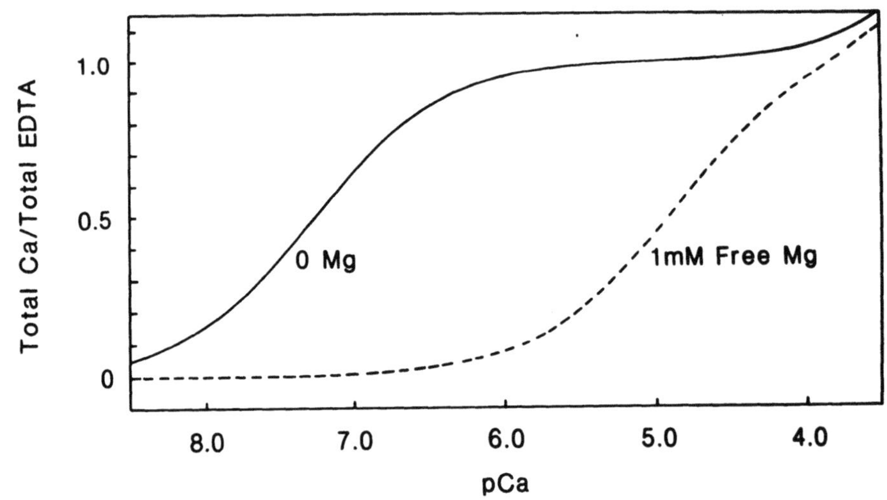

Figure 2. Calculated total Ca:total EDTA ratios as a function of pCa at two fixed levels of free Mg^{2+}. Other conditions are: 2 m*M* total EDTA, 20°C, pH 7.0, and 0.1 *M* ionic strength.

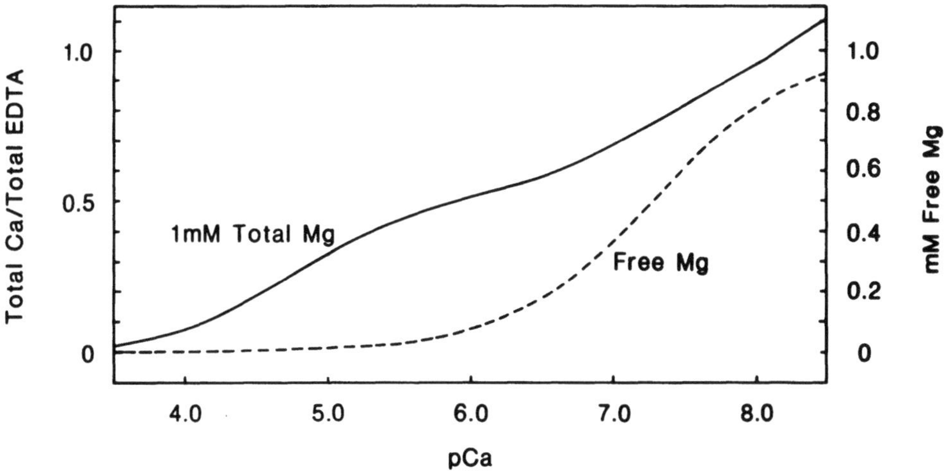

Figure 3. Calculated total Ca:total EDTA ratios as a function of pCa at constant total Mg. Conditions are as in Figure 2 except that total Mg = 1 m*M* (50% total EDTA). The free Mg^{2+} levels at each pCa are indicated on the right ordinate.

IV. INTERACTION WITH ATP

ATP is another common constituent in biological systems. Because this nucleotide binds all of the cations mentioned above, its presence will affect their free concentrations. Table III contains the stability constants reported by Martell and Smith (1974) for H^+, K^+, Na^+, Mg^{2+}, and Ca^{2+} binding to ATP at 0.1 *M* ionic strength. Note that these values were measured at 25°C, whereas those for EGTA and EDTA (Table I) were determined at 20°C. We have not included ΔH values for ATP, since the reported values were measured at zero ionic strength (Martell and Smith, 1974). Furthermore, many different sets of ATP stability constants have been reported [for example, Fabiato and Fabiato (1979) and Storer

Table III. Stability Constants for H^+, K^+, Ca^{2+}, and Mg^{2+} Binding to ATP at 25°C and 0.1*M* Ionic Strength

Ligand·metal complex	log *K* (25°C)
K_{HA} = HA/H·A	6.51
K_{H_2A} = H_2A/H·HA	4.06
K_{KA} = KA/K·A	1.0
K_{CaA} = CaA/Ca·A	3.77
K_{CaHA} = CaHA/Ca·HA	1.95
K_{MgA} = MgA/Mg·A	4.06
K_{MgHA} = MgHA/Mg·HA	2.10

[a] Data from Martell and Smith (1974), Volume 2.

and Cornish-Bowden (1976)]. It is therefore important that the conditions of the experiment dictate which ATP stability constants are to be used.

Equations 8–10 can be expanded to include ATP by following the conventions used above. First, an equation for total ATP (A_T) is written, and then the appropriate terms are added to eqs. 9 and 10. Finally, expressions for total Na (Na_T) and total K (K_T) are written. Since the constants for K and Na are similar, many times only one equation is written, say for K_T, and in the calculations K_T is set equal to total K + total Na. We adopt this simplification in writing the following set of equations:

$$A_T = A \cdot (a_H + K \cdot a_K + Ca \cdot a_{Ca} + Mg \cdot a_{Mg}) \tag{11}$$

$$E_T = E \cdot (e_H + K \cdot e_K + Ca \cdot e_{Ca} + Mg \cdot e_{Mg}) \tag{12}$$

$$K_T = K \cdot (1 + A \cdot a_K + E \cdot e_K) \tag{13}$$

$$Ca_T = Ca \cdot (1 + A \cdot a_{Ca} + E \cdot e_{Ca}) \tag{14}$$

$$Mg_T = Mg \cdot (1 + A \cdot a_{Mg} + E \cdot e_{Mg}) \tag{15}$$

where

$$a_H = 1 + H \cdot K_{HA} \cdot (1 + H \cdot K_{H_2A})$$

$$a_K = K_{KA} \cong K_{NaA}$$

$$a_{Ca} = K_{CaA} + H \cdot K_{HA} \cdot K_{CaHA}$$

$$a_{Mg} = K_{MgA} + H \cdot K_{HA} \cdot K_{MgHA}$$

$$K_T = \text{total K} + \text{total Na}$$

$$e_K = K_{KE}$$

and all other variables as defined previously.

The method used for solving eqs. 11–15 also depends on which of the ten variables are specified. The most straightforward solution is obtained by specifying the free cation concentrations K^+ (and Na^+), Ca^{2+}, Mg^{2+}, and the total ligand concentrations A_T and E_T. Equations 11 and 12 can then be solved for A and E, enabling a direct evaluation of K_T, Ca_T, and Mg_T from eqs. 13–15.

Sometimes it is desirable to specify the substrate (either $CaATP^{2-}$ or $MgATP^{2-}$) concentration instead of free ATP or total ATP. The first step in this problem is to calculate free ATP using the appropriate relationship in Table III before solving for A_T in eq. 11. For example, if constant [$MgATP^{2-}$] is desired, then A = $[MgATP^{2-}]/(K_{MgA} \cdot [Mg^{2+}])$. This enables the effects of varying metal or pH to be measured independent of substrate level.

V. CALCULATIONS

Although many elegant computer programs have been written to solve the complex equilibria involving multiple ligands and metals, we would like to present a very simple yet powerful program written in FORTRAN IV to solve eqs. 11–15. This program easily can be expanded to handle more ligands and metals independent of whether "free" or "total" concentration of metals and ligands are specified. A listing of the program "TABLE" is given in the Appendix at the end of the chapter.

This program calculates the total amount of Ca in each of a series of solutions at various pCa levels with fixed total EGTA, ATP, K, and Mg at pH 7.0 and 25.0°C (lines 70–130). The function "SADJ" (lines 1130–1200) is used to adjust the EGTA stability constants for the assay temperature. The ATP constants are not temperature adjusted because ΔH values are not known at this ionic strength, and the temperature is 25°C. Note that all proton constants are increased by 0.11 log units ("SINC," line 130), reflecting an ionic strength of 0.1 *M*.

This program illustrates how to handle calculations when either free or total cation values are held constant. Whenever a total cation value is specified, the program must solve eqs. 11–15 at each pCa level by an iterative method. Thus, there are two looping procedures in the program. The first varies pCa (lines 550–1020), whereas the other solves the complex equilibria at each pCa (lines 670–960).

The first step in solving eqs. 11–15 iteratively is to assign [free cation] values (lines 570–620). Thereafter, each iteration uses the current values for Ca, Mg, and K to calculate new values for E and A (lines 670–680), which are then used to update the estimates of Mg and K (lines 770–780). The previous Mg and K values, saved in lines 720–730, are compared with their current values to test the precision of each new estimate (lines 890–960). In spite of the fact that this program will give precise (± 0.001%) estimates of Mg and K in about 13 iterations, we have included an iteration counter to handle the potential problem of nonconvergence (lines 830–840). The line printer output of this program follows the listing. The last column indicates the number of iterations required at each pCa.

In summary, we have shown how to write a set of equations that describe the complex equilibria present in solutions containing multiple ligands and metals. Methods were given showing how temperature and ionic strength effects can be incorporated into the calculations. Finally, a simple computer program, written in FORTRAN IV, was presented, which easily can be adapted to the specific needs of each investigator. The usefulness of this program increases dramatically when it is used as a recipe generator to calculate the volumes of various stock solutions needed to mix each test solution.

APPENDIX

```
C     PROGRAM TABLE
C
      REAL K,KO,MG,MGO
C
C DEFAULT VALUES FOR ASSAY COMPOSITION AND CONDITIONS
C
      TEGTA = 0.002          !TOTAL EGTA   (MOLAR)
      TATP  = 0.002          !TOTAL ATP        "
      TK    = 0.090          !TOTAL K          "
      TMG   = 0.003          !TOTAL MG         "
      TEMP  = 25.0           !ASSAY TEMPERATURE (CELSIUS)
      PH    = 7.0            !  "   PH
      SINC  = 0.11           !CONCENTRATION TO MIXED CONSTANTS AT 0.1 M
C
C CALCULATE EGTA COEFFICIENTS EH, EC, EM
C
      SHE  = SADJ(TEMP, 9.47, -5.8, 20.0) + SINC
      SH2E = SADJ(TEMP, 8.85, -5.8, 20.0) + SINC
      SH3E = 2.66 + SINC
      SH4E = 2.00 + SINC
      EH = 1.0 + (((10.0**(SH4E-PH) + 1.0)*10.0**(SH3E-PH) + 1.0)
     1   *10.0**(SH2E-PH) + 1.0)*10.0**(SHE-PH)
      SCE  = SADJ(TEMP, 10.97, -8.1, 20.0)
      SCHE = 5.29 + SINC
      EC = 10.0**SCE + 10.0**(SCHE+SHE-PH)
      SME  = SADJ(TEMP, 5.21, 5.0, 20.0)
      SMHE = 3.36 + SINC
      EM = 10.0**SME + 10.0**(SMHE+SHE-PH)
C
C CALCULATE ATP COEFFICIENTS AH, AC, AM, AK
C
      SHA  = 6.51 + SINC
      SH2A = 4.06 + SINC
      AH = 1.0 + (10.0**(SH2A-PH) + 1.0)*10.0**(SHA-PH)
      SCA  = 3.77
      SCHA = 1.95 + SINC
      AC = 10.0**SCA + 10.0**(SCHA+SHA-PH)
      SMA  = 4.06
      SMHA = 2.1 + SINC
      AM = 10.0**SMA + 10.0**(SMHA+SHA-PH)
      AK = 10.0**1.0
C
C OUTPUT ASSAY CONDITIONS AND SETUP HEADING
C
   10 WRITE(6,11) TEGTA, TK, TATP, TMG, PH, TEMP
   11 FORMAT(1H0, 31X, 'FINAL ASSAY CONDITIONS' /
     1 19X, 'ANION TOTALS', 24X, 'CATION TOTALS' /
     2 17X, 'EGTA', 1PE12.2, 23X, 'K', E12.2 /
     3 17X, 'ATP ', E12.2, 22X, 'MG', E12.2 //
     4 17X, 'ASSAY PH', 0PF8.2, 17X, 'TEMPERATURE', F8.1 //
     5 17X, 'PCA', 9X, 'FREE MG', 9X, 'FREE CA', 8X, 'TOTAL CA')
C
C CALCULATE TOTAL CA FROM PCA 3.5 TO 8.0 BY 0.1 PCA INCREMENTS
C
      DO 200 I=35, 80, 1
      PCA = FLOAT(I)/10.0
      CA  = 10.0**(-PCA)
C
```

```
C START EACH CYCLE WITH [FREE CATION] = [TOTAL CATION]
C
          MG   = TMG
          K    = TK
          ITER = 0
C
C CALCULATE [FREE ANION] USING CURRENT [FREE CATION] VALUES
C
  110     E = TEGTA/(EH + CA*EC + MG*EM)
          A = TATP/(AH + K*AK + CA*AC + MG*AM)
C
C SAVE OLD VALUE OF EACH [FREE CATION] BEING CALCULATED
C
          MGO = MG
          KO  = K
C
C CALCULATE NEW [FREE CATION] VALUES
C
          MG  = TMG/(1.0 + E*EM + A*AM)
          K   = TK/(1.0 + A*AK)
          TCA = CA*(1.0 + E*EC + A*AC)
C
C INCREMENT COUNTER "ITER" & CHECK ITS VALUE
C
          ITER = ITER + 1
          IF(ITER .GT. 100) GO TO 190
C
C CHECK TO SEE IF EACH CALCULATED [FREE CATION] VALUE HAS CONVERGED
C
          Z = MG - MGO
          IF(MG .EQ. 0.0) GO TO 170
          Z = Z/MG
  170     IF(ABS(Z) .GT. 0.0001) GO TO 110
C
          Z = K - KO
          IF(K .EQ. 0.0) GO TO 180
          Z = Z/K
  180     IF(ABS(Z) .GT. 0.0001) GO TO 110
          GO TO 200
C
  190     WRITE(6,191)
  191     FORMAT('0ITERATION LIMIT EXCEEDED.  VALUES HAVE NOT CONVERGED')
C
  200     WRITE(6,201) PCA, MG, CA, TCA
  201     FORMAT(F21.2, 1P3E16.3)
          STOP
          END
C
C ADJUST STABILITY CONSTANT BASED UPON ASSAY TEMPERATURE
C       TEMP   ASSAY TEMPERATURE
C        PKA   LOG10 OF THE STABILITY CONSTANT
C         DH   ENTHALPY CHANGE PER DEGREE C
C          T   TEMPERATURE AT WHICH PKA AND DH WERE DETERMINED
C
          FUNCTION SADJ(TEMP, PKA, DH, T)
C
          DATA X/2.3025851/          !LOGE(10.0)
          DATA R/1.96985E-3/         !UNIVERSAL GAS CONSTANT
C
          SADJ = PKA + DH*(TEMP-T)/(X*R*(T+273.2)**2)
          RETURN
          END
```

FIXED ASSAY CONDITIONS

ANION TOTALS		CATION TOTALS	
EGTA	2.00E-03	K	9.00E-02
ATP	2.00E-03	MG	2.00E-03

ASSAY PH 7.00 TEMPERATURE 25.0

PCA	FREE MG	FREE CA	TOTAL CA	ITERATIONS
3.50	1.410E-03	3.162E-04	2.497E-03	11
3.60	1.385E-03	2.512E-04	2.359E-03	11
3.70	1.364E-03	1.995E-04	2.319E-03	12
3.80	1.346E-03	1.585E-04	2.254E-03	12
3.90	1.332E-03	1.259E-04	2.201E-03	12
4.00	1.320E-03	1.000E-04	2.158E-03	12
4.10	1.311E-03	7.943E-05	2.123E-03	12
4.20	1.303E-03	6.310E-05	2.094E-03	13
4.30	1.297E-03	5.012E-05	2.070E-03	13
4.40	1.291E-03	3.981E-05	2.049E-03	13
4.50	1.287E-03	3.162E-05	2.031E-03	13
4.60	1.284E-03	2.512E-05	2.014E-03	13
4.70	1.281E-03	1.995E-05	1.998E-03	13
4.80	1.278E-03	1.585E-05	1.983E-03	13
4.90	1.276E-03	1.259E-05	1.966E-03	13
5.00	1.274E-03	1.000E-05	1.948E-03	13
5.10	1.272E-03	7.943E-06	1.927E-03	13
5.20	1.271E-03	6.310E-06	1.903E-03	13
5.30	1.269E-03	5.012E-06	1.875E-03	13
5.40	1.267E-03	3.981E-06	1.841E-03	13
5.50	1.265E-03	3.162E-06	1.802E-03	13
5.60	1.262E-03	2.512E-06	1.754E-03	13
5.70	1.260E-03	1.995E-06	1.699E-03	13
5.80	1.256E-03	1.585E-06	1.634E-03	13
5.90	1.253E-03	1.259E-06	1.559E-03	13
6.00	1.249E-03	1.000E-06	1.474E-03	13
6.10	1.245E-03	7.943E-07	1.380E-03	13
6.20	1.240E-03	6.310E-07	1.277E-03	13
6.30	1.235E-03	5.012E-07	1.167E-03	13
6.40	1.231E-03	3.981E-07	1.054E-03	13
6.50	1.226E-03	3.162E-07	9.386E-04	13
6.60	1.221E-03	2.512E-07	8.252E-04	13
6.70	1.216E-03	1.995E-07	7.163E-04	13
6.80	1.212E-03	1.585E-07	6.143E-04	13
6.90	1.208E-03	1.259E-07	5.209E-04	13
7.00	1.205E-03	1.000E-07	4.372E-04	13
7.10	1.202E-03	7.943E-08	3.637E-04	13
7.20	1.199E-03	6.310E-08	3.001E-04	13
7.30	1.197E-03	5.012E-08	2.460E-04	13
7.40	1.195E-03	3.981E-08	2.005E-04	13
7.50	1.193E-03	3.162E-08	1.626E-04	13
7.60	1.192E-03	2.512E-08	1.314E-04	13
7.70	1.191E-03	1.995E-08	1.058E-04	13
7.80	1.190E-03	1.585E-08	8.495E-05	13
7.90	1.190E-03	1.259E-08	6.807E-05	13
8.00	1.189E-03	1.000E-08	5.445E-05	13

REFERENCES

Boyd, S., Bryson, A., Nancollas, G. H., and Torrance, K. 1965. Thermodynamics of ion association. Part XII. EGTA complexes with divalent metal ions. *J. Chem. Soc., 5*:7353–7358.

Fabiato, A., and Fabiato, F. 1979. Calculator programs for computing the composition of the solutions containing multiple metals and ligands used for experiments in skinned muscle cells. *J. Physiol. (Paris), 75*:463–505.

Martell, A. E., and Smith, R. M. 1974. *Critical Stability Constants*, Volumes 1–4. Plenum Press, New York.

Storer, A. C., and Cornish-Bowden, A. 1976. Concentration of $MgATP^{2-}$ and other ions in solution: Calculation of the true concentrations of species present in mixtures of associating ions. *Biochem. J., 159*:1–5.

Tsien, R. Y. 1980. New calcium indicators and buffers with high selectivity against magnesium and protons: Design, synthesis, and properties of prototype structures. *Biochemistry, 19*:2396–2404.

Chapter 7

Study of Cardiac Autonomic Receptors by Radiolabeled Ligand Binding Assays

Allan S. Manalan,* Larry R. Jones, Henry R. Besch, Jr., and August M. Watanabe*

Department of Medicine and Department of Pharmacology and Toxicology
Indiana University School of Medicine,
Krannert Institute of Cardiology, and
*The Veterans Administration Medical Cente
Indianapolis, Indiana

I. INTRODUCTION

The development of radioligand binding assays to study directly neurotransmitter and hormone receptors has heralded a new era of discovery of the properties and regulation of these receptors and the effectors with which they interact. In the area of cardiovascular pharmacology, application of radioligand binding techniques has facilitated significant advances in the study of receptors found in cardiac tissues, most notably the receptors of the sympathetic and parasympathetic divisions of the autonomic nervous system. β-Adrenergic receptors in cardiac muscle have been studied most extensively by these techniques, and substantial research has also been done on muscarinic cholinergic receptors. Reports of application of radioligand binding techniques to the study of cardiac α-adrenergic receptors have been less abundant, perhaps as a result of technical difficulties associated with the relatively less satisfactory available radiolabeled ligands.

Although the general principles of radioligand binding assays are applicable to the analysis of cardiac autonomic receptors, certain specific considerations

Present address for Allan S. Manalan: Cardiovascular Institute, Department of Medicine, Michael Reese Hospital and Medical Center, Chicago, Illinois.

complicate the design and interpretation of experiments involving myocardial membranes. This chapter discusses various aspects of the use of radioligand binding techniques specifically to study autonomic receptors in cardiac muscle. The emphasis is on practical considerations involved in the assay of membrane bound receptors. For more comprehensive discussions of radioligand binding assays, the reader is referred to several recent review articles (Boeynaems and Dumont, 1975; Cuatrecasas and Hollenberg, 1976; Maguire *et al.*, 1977; Ross *et al.*, 1977; Hoffman and Lefkowitz, 1980; Watanabe *et al.*, 1982).

II. RECEPTOR SOURCES

Judicious selection and careful characterization of a suitable receptor-containing preparation is crucial to the successful application of radioligand binding techniques to the study of cardiac autonomic receptors. Although radioligand binding techniques have been applied to the study of diverse experimental preparations, cardiac autonomic receptors have been studied most extensively utilizing homogenates of myocardium or membrane preparations derived from these homogenates. This section focuses on the uses of these broken-cell preparations prepared from myocardium.

The simplest receptor-containing preparation from heart is the crude homogenate of myocardial tissue. Advantages of the myocardial homogenate include its ease of preparation and its convenience for studying small amounts of myocardial tissue. In theory, its preparation in a single step minimizes the likelihood of alterations of the functional properties of receptors that might result from a more extensive purification scheme. In practice, the utility of crude homogenates of myocardium for the detailed study of autonomic receptors is limited by several factors.

First, although β-adrenergic and muscarinic receptors are measurable in crude myocardial homogenates, receptor content in these preparations is relatively low (Figure 1). As a result, for canine ventricular myocardium, quantities of crude homogenate in the range of 0.2 to 0.6 mg of homogenate protein per assay tube are usually required for reliable quantitation of specific receptor binding when tritiated ligands are used. Inclusion of these relatively large amounts of crude homogenate in the assay mixture results in relatively high levels of nonspecific binding of radioligand to the large amount of nonreceptor material as well as a tendency toward greater variability of the replicate determinations of both total and nonspecific binding.

Second, the possible presence of endogenous receptor agonists and regulatory factors complicates analysis of radioligand binding experiments performed in unwashed crude myocardial homogenates. Persistence of endogenous autonomic receptor agonists potentially complicates determinations of receptor number as well as radioligand affinity. Likewise, possible persistence of bound Mg^{2+} or GTP in these homogenates makes the analysis of receptor regulation by exogenous ions or nucleotides difficult. Although problems associated with these endogenous soluble agents can be reduced by resorting to a large-volume incubation, the

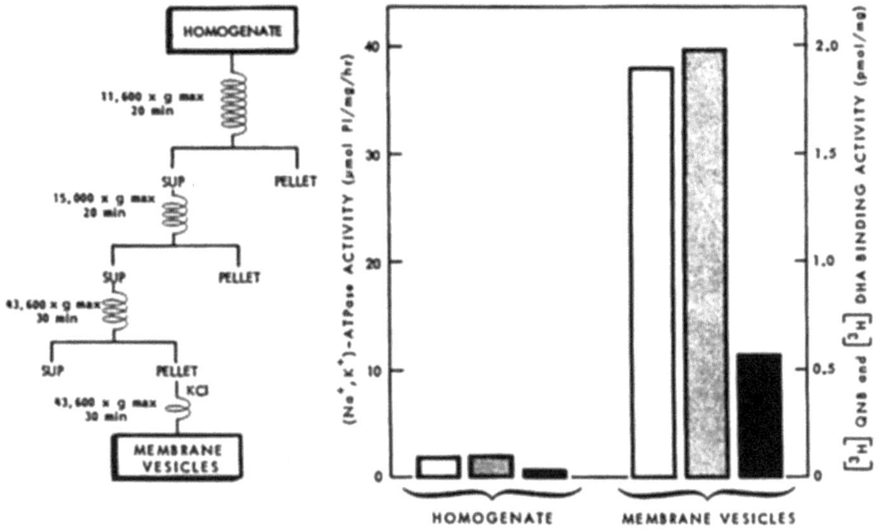

Figure 1. Preparation of membrane vesicles and quantitation of enrichment of receptor and nonreceptor markers. Preparation of tissue homogenates and subsequent isolation of membrane vesicle fractions were performed using a slight modification of the procedure previously described by Jones *et al.* (1979). All preparatory procedures were performed at 4°C. A 20% homogenate of canine ventricular myocardium was prepared by disrupting 25–35 g of tissue three times for 30 sec in 4 volumes of ice-cold 0.25 *M* sucrose, 30 m*M* histidine, with a Polytron® PT-20 at a setting of half-maximal speed. To obtain the membrane vesicle fraction from this crude homogenate, 20-min low-speed centrifugations at 11,600 × g_{max} and 15,000 × g_{max} were employed to remove larger tissue fragments, nuclei, and mitochondria. The membrane vesicle fraction was then sedimented at 43,600 × g_{max} for 30 min. Resuspension and recentrifugation of the membrane vesicles fraction in 0.6 *M* KCl were performed to remove adherent soluble proteins from myocardial membranes. Membrane vesicles were then resuspended in 0.25 *M* sucrose, 30 m*M* histidine and either used fresh on the day of preparation or stored frozen at −20°C until use. Quantitation of receptor and nonreceptor markers revealed parallel 20-fold enrichment of muscarinic receptor content {assessed with [^{3}H]quinuclidinyl benzilate ([^{3}H]QNB) ▨}, β-adrenergic receptor content {assessed with [^{3}H]dihydroalprenolol ([^{3}H]DHA) ■}, and activity of the sarcolemmal marker Na^+,K^+-ATPase (□) in the membrane vesicle fraction over that present in the homogenate.

problem of persistence as a result of high-affinity associations of these agonists or regulating factors with their respective binding sites is not so easily obviated. Nevertheless, if the limitations associated with this crude preparation are kept in mind, radioligand binding studies can be performed successfully in simple homogenates of myocardial tissue.

Various membrane-enriched fractions prepared from homogenates of cardiac tissue have been successfully utilized to study cardiac autonomic receptors. Preparation of a membrane vesicle fraction using a relatively simple differential centrifugation protocol (Jones *et al.*, 1979) results in substantial enrichment of both β-adrenergic and muscarinic receptors (Figure 1). Of course, accurate quantification of the level of enrichment of a given membrane fraction requires assessment not only of receptors but of nonreceptor markers as well, such as the Na^+,K^+-

ATPase of sarcolemma. The use of carefully characterized membrane-enriched fractions provides several advantages that facilitate study of autonomic receptors. First, repeated washing and the high-ionic-strength KCl extraction step would be expected to remove adherent soluble proteins and any loosely bound regulatory factors from the membrane fraction (Figure 1). Second, the substantial enrichment of receptor content attendant to even a simple centrifugation protocol allows accurate quantification of receptors utilizing only 50–150 μg protein per assay tube (Figure 1). The use of relatively small amounts of protein less contaminated by nonreceptor material results in reduction of nonspecific binding of radioligands as well as greater reproducibility of replicate determinations of total and nonspecific binding. In addition to their technical advantages in radioligand binding assays, appropriately prepared highly purified membrane-enriched fractions such as those described in the chapter by Jones and Besch (Chapter 1, this volume) demonstrate preservation of β-adrenergic receptor–adenylate cyclase coupling, making them useful for study of proximal mechanisms of cellular response to catecholamines (Jones *et al.*, 1980). (Coupling of muscarinic receptors to particulate guanylate cyclase has not been convincingly demonstrated in broken-cell preparations of heart.)

Despite the advantages afforded by the use of membrane vesicle fractions derived from myocardial tissue, several limitations must be taken into account in the interpretation of binding data obtained using these preparations. First, both structural and functional evidence supports the existence of membranes in vesicular form (Besch *et al.*, 1977; Jones *et al.*, 1980). As a result, free access of added regulatory factors (e.g., ions, guanine nucleotides) to their binding sites within sealed membrane vesicles cannot be assumed. Similarly, despite the washing attendant to membrane purification, the possible persistence of endogenous agents (receptor agonists, guanine nucleotides, ions) either tightly bound or sequestered within the vesicles must be considered in the interpretation of studies of receptor regulation. Secondly, the possible alteration in the functional properties of autonomic receptors as a result of the purification scheme must also be considered. In this regard, it is advantageous to compare the functional properties of the receptors in purified preparations to those in crude homogenates to exclude artificial alterations in receptor characteristics attendant to purification steps.

Once a membrane-containing preparation has been selected, the preparation should be carefully characterized with respect to receptor density as well as to content of nonreceptor markers. Several enzymic and binding activities appear to be present in canine cardiac membrane vesicles derived from sarcolemma and absent from membrane vesicles derived from sarcoplasmic reticulum. Activities apparently confined to cardiac sarcolemma include Na^+,K^+-ATPase, sialic acid, adenylate cyclase, particulate cAMP-dependent protein kinase, as well as β-adrenergic and muscarinic receptors (Jones *et al.*, 1979, 1981). Assessment of nonreceptor as well as receptor markers affords the opportunity to quantify the level of sarcolemmal content of a given preparation, thus allowing quantitation of the extent of membrane purification by comparison with activities present in a crude homogenate. Such quantitative information is useful in determination of relative recoveries, thus facilitating detection of any losses of receptors attendant to a particular "purification" scheme. Quantitation of nonreceptor as well as receptor markers is an absolute requirement when comparing relative receptor densities in multiple membrane-containing samples (e.g., studies of regional distribution of receptors or studies of receptor density before and after experimental intervention) in order to insure that alterations in receptor number indeed reflect alterations in membrane density of receptors rather than alteration of receptor number merely as a result of alteration of membrane content of the preparations being compared (e.g., related to edema, cellular infiltration).

Receptor-containing preparations derived directly from myocardial tissue should be expected to reflect the cellular inhomogeneity inherent in a tissue source that contains multiple cell types. Fibrocytes, blood cells, vascular and neural elements, as well as myocytes present in cardiac tissue variously contribute to the content of the crude homogenate and subsequent membrane-enriched fractions prepared from myocardium. As a result, autonomic receptors present in these fractions may be contributed by more than one cell type, and alterations in receptor density may reflect changes in receptor contribution by any of these cell types. To avoid limitations inherent in the study of inhomogeneous preparations of intact tissue, tissue culture techniques can be utilized to isolate cell populations from cardiac tissue that are homogeneous with respect to cell type. These preparations can then be applied to study autonomic receptors in specific cell types (Lau *et al.*, 1980).

III. RADIOLIGAND CHARACTERISTICS

Following the initial reports of successful uses of radioligands in identifying autonomic receptors, a large number of pharmacological agents have been radiolabeled, and their utility in performing radioligand binding assays has been explored. Several criteria have been used to establish the presence of radioligand interaction with autonomic receptors: (1) appropriate affinity and specificity of radioligand binding, (2) appropriate kinetics of binding, (3) saturability, and (4) displacement by known receptor agonists and antagonists in accordance with their pharmacological potencies (Cuatrecasas and Hollenberg, 1976).

Because a sizable number of radioligands have been developed, characterized, and shown to meet these criteria, it is now possible to select among several available radioligands to suit a particular experimental problem.

In choosing an appropriate radioligand for a given application, several characteristics of the available radioligand preparations should be considered (Table I). From a technical standpoint, using a radioligand that displays high receptor affinity is advantageous in radioligand binding assays. With a high-affinity radioligand, appreciable numbers of receptors may be identified with the use of a very low concentration of radioligand, at which nonspecific binding of radioligand to nonreceptor elements is minimized. In addition, the slow dissociation rate of the radioligand:receptor complex attendant to the high-affinity interaction facilitates separation of free radioligand from bound radioligand. Likewise, radioligands possessing high specific activity allow detection of small receptor popu-

Table I. Characteristics of Radiolabeled Antagonists Utilized in Studies of Cardiac Autonomic Receptors

Radioligand	K_D (cardiac tissue) (p*M*)	Specific activity (Ci/mmole)	Pharmacological specificity	Receptor subtype selectivity	Remarks
[^{125}I]Iodohydroxybenzylpindolol	50–150[a,b]	2200	β-Adrenergic	Nonselective	Racemic Complex kinetics reported[c] "Inactive" (+)stereoisomer displays appreciable receptor affinity[d]
[^{3}H](−)Dihydroalprenolol	360–2500[e,f,g]	30–50	β-Adrenergic	Nonselective	*l*-Stereoisomer
[^{3}H](±)Carazolol	135[h]	25	β-Adrenergic	Nonselective	Racemic Complex kinetics reported[h] "Inactive" (+)stereoisomer displays appreciable receptor affinity[d,h]
[^{3}H](±)Quinuclidinyl benzilate	30[i]	30	Muscarinic		Racemic Complex kinetics reported[j,k] [^{3}H]*l*QNB Commercially available
[^{3}H]Dihydroergocryptine	2300–2900[e,l]	20–50	α-Adrenergic	Nonselective	
[^{3}H]WB4101	950–2000[l,m,n]	15–30	α-Adrenergic	α_1-selective	
[^{3}H]Prazosin	580[g]	30	α-Adrenergic	α_1-selective	

[a] Lau *et al.* (1980).
[b] Hedberg *et al.* (1980).
[c] Ross *et al.* (1977).
[d] Burgisser *et al.* (1981).
[e] Williams and Lefkowitz (1978).
[f] U'Prichard *et al.* (1978).
[g] Karliner *et al.* (1979).
[h] Manalan *et al.* (1981).
[i] Fields *et al.* (1978).
[j] Galper *et al.* (1977).
[k] Jarv *et al.* (1979).
[l] Briley *et al.* (1979).
[m] U'Prichard and Snyder (1979).
[n] Raisman *et al.* (1979).

lations or fractional occupancy of more substantial receptor populations even in the presence of extremely low radioligand concentrations.

Of the radioligand preparations suitable for study of autonomic receptors, some are radiolabeled preparations of the pharmacologically active stereoisomer, whereas others consist of a racemic mixture containing the two stereoisomers, both of which are radiolabeled. Although autonomic receptor binding studies can be successfully performed with racemic radioligands, the presence of the biologically inactive radiolabeled stereoisomer represents a potential source of nonspecific binding. More significantly, for the extremely high-affinity radioligands such as $[^{125}I](\pm)$iodohydroxybenzylpindolol and $[^{3}H](\pm)$carazolol, the relatively less active stereoisomers nevertheless display high affinity for β-adrenergic receptors (Figure 2) (Burgisser *et al.*, 1981; Manalan *et al.*, 1981). Thus, especially under assay conditions in which receptor concentration is high, binding of the less active stereoisomers to β-adrenergic receptors may contribute appreciably to the total radioligand binding (Burgisser *et al.*, 1981). The contribution of extremely high-affinity binding of the "active" stereoisomer and high-affinity binding of the "less active" stereoisomer may result in anomalous saturation curves, which may be misinterpreted if the possible contribution of both stereoisomers is not appreciated. These practical as well as theoretical disadvantages can be avoided by using radiolabeled preparations containing only the active stereoisomers.

Results of radioligand binding studies have confirmed the existence of subtypes of both α- and β-adrenergic receptors. Examination of receptor-containing preparations derived from myocardium reveals the presence of a small population of β_2-adrenergic receptors as well as a large population of β_1-adrenergic receptors existing within the same tissue (Hancock *et al.*, 1979; Minneman *et al.*, 1979; Manalan *et al.*, 1981). Similarly, coexistence of α_1 and α_2 receptors in rat myocardium has been suggested (Briley *et al.*, 1979; Raisman *et al.*, 1979), although certain details remain controversial (U'Prichard and Snyder, 1979). In heart, it is possible that the various α- and β-adrenergic receptor subtypes reside on different cell types and thus subserve different physiological functions (Lau *et al.*, 1980). Accordingly, in certain experimental situations, it may be desirable to examine a single receptor subtype. Although no pharmacological agent appears to be completely specific for a given receptor subtype, several agents display significant subtype selectivity, making them useful in the study of autonomic receptor subpopulations. Cardiac autonomic receptor subpopulations can be studied indirectly by examination of competition of an unlabeled subtype-selective agent with a nonselective radioligand for binding to autonomic receptors (Figure 3). Alternatively, by use of an appropriate radiolabeled subtype-selective agent, the presence of a given receptor subtype can be examined directly.

Perhaps the most problematic issue in designing radioligand binding assays involves the choice between using radiolabeled agonist and radiolabeled antagonist for studying autonomic receptors. The use of radiolabeled agonists possesses obvious theoretical advantages, affording the opportunity for direct examination of the kinetics of agonist-specific receptor regulation by guanine nucleotides and ions. In addition, the use of radiolabeled agonist allows direct verification of its

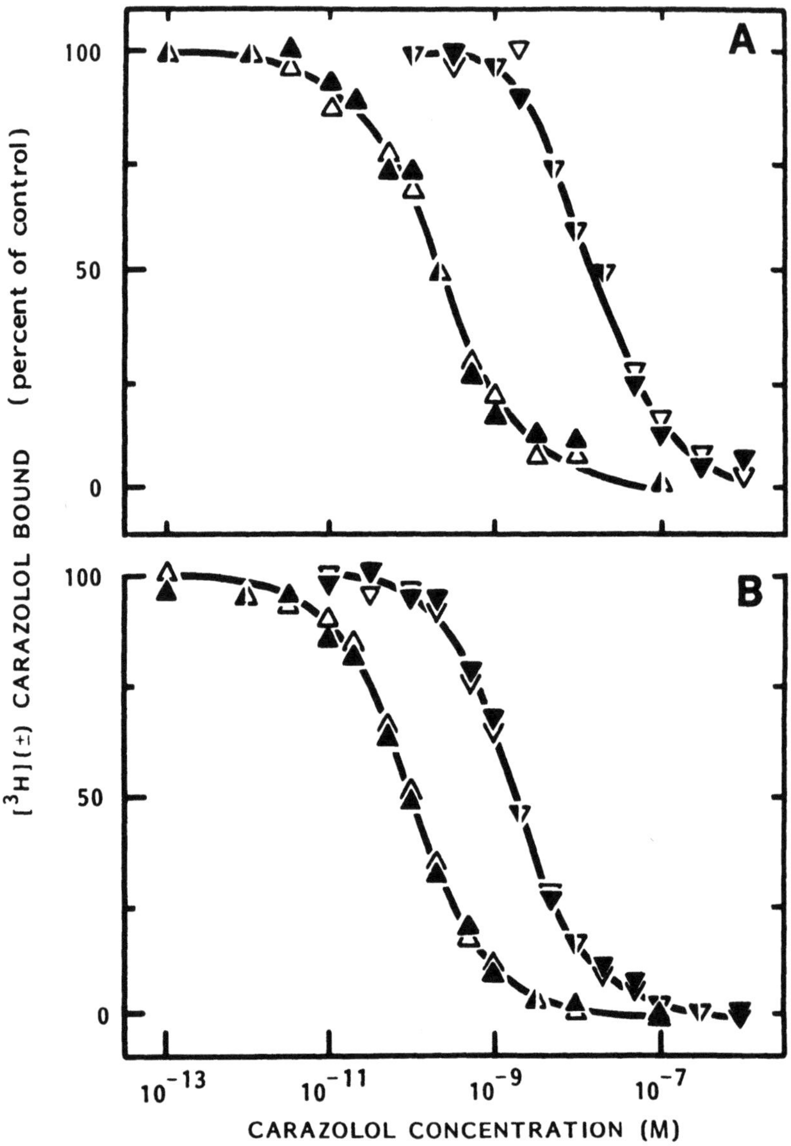

Figure 2. Stereospecificity of the interaction of carazolol with β-adrenergic receptors present in membrane vesicles derived from canine ventricular myocardium (panel A; predominantly β_1 subtype) and canine lung (panel B; predominantly β_2 subtype). Membrane vesicles (approximately 100 μg protein) were incubated in 5 ml of medium containing 50 m*M* tris buffer (pH 7.5 at 22°C), 9 m*M* $MgCl_2$, 1 m*M* ascorbic acid, $[^3H]$(±)carazolol, and the indicated concentrations of unlabeled stereoisomers. Incubations were conducted at 37°C for 60 min, a reaction time that allowed complete equilibration of $[^3H]$(±)carazolol binding. Reactions were terminated by rapid filtration through Whatman GF/C filters. Filters were rinsed with four 5-ml aliquots of ice-cold 50 m*M* tris buffer containing 9 m*M* $MgCl_2$. Filters were then dried and suspended in 10 ml Aquasol II, and retained radioactivity was determined by liquid scintillation counting. All determinations of total and nonspecific binding were performed in triplicate. Specific binding was taken as that binding that was displaceable by 20 μ*M* (±)propranolol. In this figure, $[^3H]$(±)carazolol specifically bound has been plotted as a function of competing concentrations of unlabeled stereoisomers of carazolol. $[^3H]$(±)Carazolol binding has been expressed as a percentage of binding

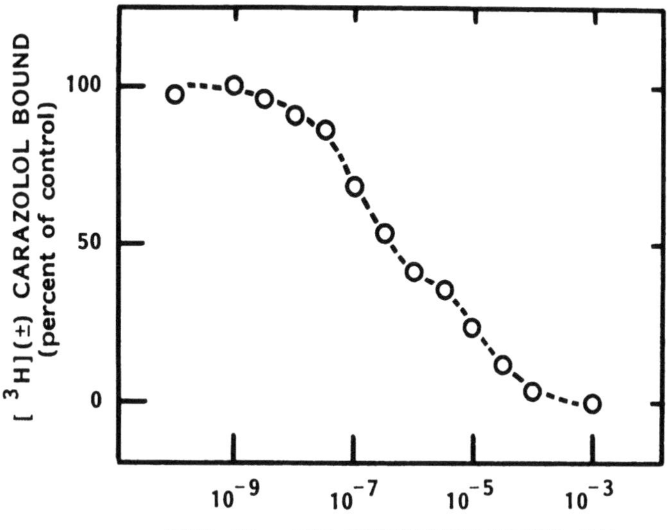

Figure 3. Demonstration of coexisting β_1- and β_2-adrenergic receptor subtypes by examination of competition of the highly β_1-selective antagonist EMD33-512 with [^{3}H](±)carazolol for binding to β-adrenergic receptors. Membrane vesicles were incubated in 5 ml of medium containing 50 m*M* tris buffer (pH 7.5 at 22°C), 9 m*M* $MgCl_2$, 1 m*M* ascorbic acid, [^{3}H](±)carazolol, and the indicated concentrations of EMD33-512. Assays were conducted as described in legend for Figure 2. Specific [^{3}H](±)carazolol binding, expressed as a percentage of binding in the absence of competing drug, has been plotted as a function of competing EMD33-512 concentration. [^{3}H](±)Carazolol concentration was 240 p*M*. For purposes of illustration, this competition curve has been generated using a mixture of membrane vesicles derived from canine ventricular myocardium and canine lung. The resultant β-adrenergic receptor population consists of a mixture of approximately 60% β_1-adrenergic receptors and 40% β_2-adrenergic receptors. The resultant biphasic competition curve is a consequence of EMD33-512 competition with [^{3}H](±)carazolol for binding to β_1-adrenergic receptors (apparent at EMD33-512 concentrations in the range 10^{-8} to 10^{-6} *M*) and β_2-adrenergic receptors (apparent at EMD33-512 concentrations in the range 10^{-6} to 10^{-3} *M*). Such binding data are amenable to analysis utilizing various computer-based techniques, as briefly described in the text.

biological properties and direct correlation between receptor occupancy and proximate biochemical responses. Unfortunately, the successful use of radiolabeled agonists to identify β_1-adrenergic receptors present in myocardial tissue has not yet been reported. Accordingly, studies of agonist interaction with β-adrenergic receptors in myocardium have been approached indirectly by examination of agonist competition with radiolabeled antagonist for binding to receptors.

in the absence of competing agent. *S*(−)Carazolol (△,▲); *R*(+)carazolol (▽,▼). As expected for these β-adrenergic antagonists, presence (closed symbols) or absence (open symbols) of 10^{-4} *M* 5′-guanylylimidodiphosphate had no effect on the position or configuration of competition curves for either stereoisomer. Slope factors (negative of Hill coefficient) derived from competition curves were approximately 1.0, consistent with simple antagonist competition (see text). For these competition curves, [^{3}H](±)carazolol was present at a concentration of approximately twice its K_D to facilitate graphic comparison of experimental results obtained in the two preparations. Inhibition constants derived according to the method of Cheng and Prusoff (1973) were: for myocardium, *S*(−)carazolol 7.0 × 10^{-11} *M*, *R*(+)carazolol 4.2 × 10^{-9} *M*; and for lung, *S*(−)carazolol 2.3 × 10^{-11} *M*, *R*(+)carazolol 5.1 × 10^{-10} *M*.

IV. PRACTICAL CONSIDERATIONS OF THE BINDING ASSAY

Once an appropriate receptor-containing preparation is prepared and a suitable radioligand selected, specific conditions of the radioligand binding assay must be chosen according to several obvious considerations. The specific radioligand binding to receptors should be linear with respect to receptor concentration over the range of protein concentrations utilized. When very-high-affinity radioligands (e.g., [^{3}H]quinuclidinyl benzilate, [^{3}H]carazolol) are used at low concentrations, appreciable binding of radioligand to receptors may lead to significant decreases in free radioligand concentration during the incubation. Under these conditions, changes in free radioligand concentration can be minimized most easily by use of increased incubation volumes (1–5 ml), thus allowing identification of a similar receptor number (specific binding) without significant alteration of free radioligand concentration. For equilibrium studies, the time of incubation should be selected on the basis of careful kinetic analysis to insure complete equilibration of binding. It should be noted that, assuming a simple model of radioligand (L) interaction with receptor (R),

$$R + L \underset{k_{-1}}{\overset{k_{+1}}{\rightleftharpoons}} RL \tag{1}$$

the approach of radioligand binding ($[RL]_t$ at time t) to equilibrium ($[RL]_{eq}$) derived from the integrated second order rate law,

$$[RL]_t/[RL]_{eq} = 1 - e^{-(k_{+1}[L] + k_{-1})t} \tag{2}$$

is a function of both the association rate constant k_{+1} and the dissociation rate constant k_{-1} as well as the radioligand concentration (Maguire *et al.*, 1977). For the very-high-affinity radiolabeled antagonists, k_{-1} is by necessity low, dictating the relatively lengthy equilibration time (e.g., 40–60 min) seen with low concentrations of these agents.

Following an appropriate incubation time, free radioligand must be separated from bound radioligand before receptor binding can be quantified. For membrane-bound cardiac autonomic receptors, although both equilibrium dialysis and centrifugation techniques can be utilized, simple filtration through glass fiber filters has proven to be the easiest and most practical method for accomplishing removal of free radioligand and quantitative recovery of bound radioligand. Unfortunately, no technique accomplishes a complete removal of all radioligand that is not bound to a specific receptor, and such persistence of unbound radioligand adherent to sample or filter support is termed nonspecific binding. This nonspecific radioligand binding, which is kinetically instantaneous, nonsaturable, and nondisplaceable by specific receptor agonists or antagonists, can be practically quantified by conducting parallel incubations in the presence of appropriate saturating concentrations of competing unlabeled pharmacological agents. In this regard, when the separation of free from bound radioligand is accomplished by filtration, filters are then washed with aliquots of buffer solution as appropriate to reduce maximally this nonspecific binding without altering recovery of specifically bound radioligand.

V. EXPERIMENTAL DESIGN AND DATA ANALYSIS

In order to obtain useful data, radioligand assays are designed within the framework of an experimental model of radioligand:receptor interaction. The simplest model of interaction, involving the reversible association of a single receptor molecule (R) with a single radioligand molecule (L) to form a radioligand:receptor complex (RL)

$$R + L \underset{k_{-1}}{\overset{k_{+1}}{\rightleftharpoons}} RL \tag{1}$$

serves as the usual basis for the design of initial experiments necessary to characterize a receptor binding assay. In this equation, k_1, the second-order association rate constant, and k_{-1}, the first-order dissociation rate constant, are defined by

$$d[RL]/dt = k_{+1}([R][L]) - k_{-1}([RL]) \tag{3}$$

At equilibrium, when $d[RL]/dt = 0$,

$$k_{+1}[R]_{eq}[L]_{eq} = k_{-1}[RL]_{eq} \tag{4}$$

the dissociation constant, K_D, is defined as

$$K_D \equiv k_{-1}/k_{+1} = [R]_{eq}[L]_{eq}/[RL]_{eq} \tag{5}$$

In order to reduce this equation to a form readily applicable to the analysis of binding data, the following substitutions are made:

$$[R]_T = [R]_{eq} + [RL]_{eq} \tag{6}$$

$$[L]_T = [L]_{eq} + [RL]_{eq} \approx [L]_{eq} \tag{7}$$

Note that the second assumption applies only when incubation conditions are such that radioligand is present in great excess, so that no appreciable change in free radioligand concentration occurs during the binding reaction. With these substitutions, mathematical rearrangement yields an equation analogous to the Michaelis–Menten equation of enzyme kinetics:

$$[RL]_{eq}/[R]_T = [L]_T/(K_D + [L]_T) \tag{8}$$

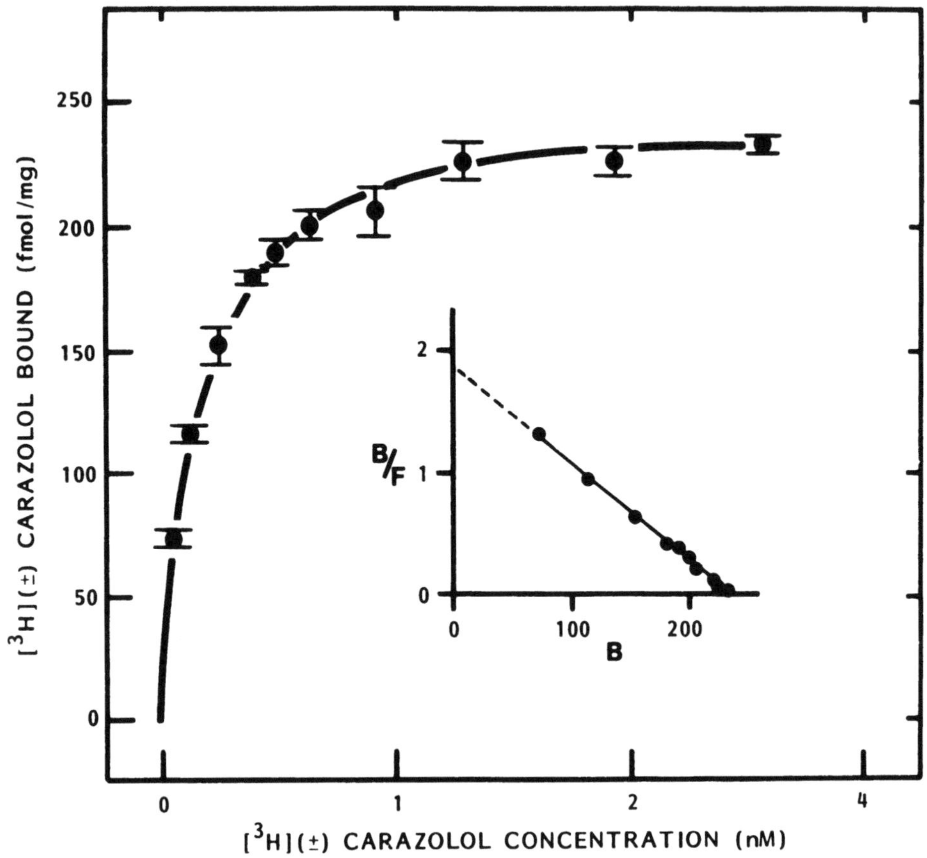

Figure 4. Saturation curve and Scatchard analysis of specific binding of $[^3H](\pm)$carazolol to β-adrenergic receptors present in membrane vesicles derived from canine ventricular myocardium. Membrane vesicles (approximately 100 μg protein) were incubated in 1 ml of medium containing 50 m*M* tris buffer (pH 7.5 at 22°C), 9 m*M* $MgCl_2$, 1 m*M* ascorbic acid, and indicated concentrations of $[^3H](\pm)$carazolol. Assays were conducted as described in legend for Figure 2. Specific binding was taken as that binding that was displaceable by 20 μ*M* (±)propranolol. Error bars are ±1 standard error of the difference. Parameters derived from Scatchard analysis of $[^3H](\pm)$carazolol binding to myocardial β-adrenergic receptors include a dissociation constant (K_D) of 1.35×10^{-10} *M* and a receptor total of 243 fmoles/mg protein.

Since total radioligand concentration $[L]_T$ is defined, and the equilibrium concentration of bound radioligand $[RL]_{eq}$ can be experimentally obtained, determination of radioligand binding as a function of free radioligand concentration enables calculation of the two parameters of this model: total receptor concentration, $[R]_T$, and the dissociation constant, K_D, an index of receptor affinity. Although these parameters can be approximated from graphic analysis of the rectangular hyperbolic plot of radioligand bound as a function of free radioligand concentration (Figure 4), analysis of these saturation curves has been facilitated by a simple mathematical transformation of binding data according to a rearrangement of the above equation:

$$[RL]_{eq}/[L]_T = -(1/K_D)[RL]_{eq} + [R]_T/K_D \tag{9}$$

analogous to the approach of Scatchard to the analysis of interactions between ions and proteins (Scatchard, 1949). Thus, if the proposed model of a reversible association of radioligand with receptor applies, and incubation conditions have been adjusted such that free radioligand concentration remains constant throughout the incubation, then Scatchard plots of $[RL]_{eq}/[L]_T$ as a function of $[RL]_{eq}$ should be linear with slope $-1/K_D$ and x-intercept $[R]_T$. Nonlinear Scatchard plots suggest either that the working model of radioligand:receptor interaction does not apply or that assumptions inherent in the mathematical derivation are not satisfied experimentally because of methodological problems.

Several causes of convex-upward Scatchard plots include positive cooperativity, incomplete recovery of bound radioligand, zero-order inactivation of radioligand, radiolabeled contaminant, and separation of free from bound radioligand prior to equilibrium (Boeynaems and Dumont, 1975). Causes of concave-upward Scatchard plots include negative cooperativity as well as the existence of two receptor populations with differing radioligand affinity (Boeynaems and Dumont, 1975). Obviously, the possibility of methodological problems must be carefully explored to avoid false interpretations of nonlinear Scatchard plots.

Once the K_D for a radioligand has been determined, receptor affinity for unlabeled agents can then be derived indirectly by analysis of the ability of these unlabeled agents to compete with the radioligand for binding to receptors. Assuming a model of simple competition between radioligand and unlabeled agent for a single population of receptor sites, the inhibition constant, K_i, of the unlabeled agent (analogous to the dissociation constant) is given by

$$K_i = IC_{50}/(1 + [L]_T/K_D) \tag{10}$$

where IC_{50} is the concentration of unlabeled agent that results in half-maximal attenuation of radioligand binding, $[L]_T$ is the concentration of radioligand, and K_D is the dissociation constant of the radioligand:receptor complex (Cheng and Prusoff, 1973). Thus, plots of radioligand binding as a function of competing agent allow identification of the IC_{50} for that agent, from which calculation of the K_i can be readily accomplished. This technique is useful for correlating the affinity of the radiolabeled ligand (by Scatchard analysis) with that of its unlabeled counterpart and for establishing the stereospecificity of the ligand:receptor interaction (Figure 2). Moreover, examination of a series of known pharmacological agonists and antagonists by this technique establishes the pharmacological specificity of the receptor population being studied. In addition, the use of unlabeled pharmacological agents displaying substantial selectivity for autonomic receptor subtypes has allowed indirect quantitative assessment of the relative contribution of the two receptor subpopulations present in a given assay (see below, Figure 3).

In analysis of equilibrium radioligand binding studies, the Hill plot has been empirically employed to mathematize the observed complex interaction of agonists with their receptor:effector complexes. The Hill model (Hill, 1910), originally proposed to account for the shape of oxyhemoglobin binding curves, assumes the overall reaction of *n* molecules of ligand (L) with each receptor (R)

$$R + nL \overset{K'}{\rightleftharpoons} RL_n \tag{1a}$$

Based on this model, mathematical derivation pursued by analogy to that described above yields

$$[RL_n]_{eq}/[R]_T = [L]_T^n/K' + [L]_T^n \tag{8a}$$

The logit transformation of this equation

$$\log\{[RL_n]_{eq}/([R]_T - [RL_n]_{eq})\} = n \log[L]_T - \log K' \tag{11}$$

provides the basis for the quasilinearized Hill plot of $\log\{[RL_n]_{eq}/([R]_T - [RL_n]_{eq})\}$ as a function of $\log[L]_T$.

Although the Hill plot has theoretical shortcomings, its application to the analysis of radioligand binding studies provides a simple, empirical, mathematical description of agonist–receptor interactions that do not exhibit Michaelis–Menten kinetics (see Cornish-Bowden and Koshland, 1975). Based on Hill analysis of radioligand competition curves, slope factors (negative of Hill coefficient) for antagonist competition are approximately 1, consistent with simple Michaelis–Menten kinetics. Slope factors substantially less than 1 observed for agonist competition with radiolabeled antagonist for binding to receptors in guanine-nucleotide-depleted membranes are mathematical manifestations of the complex nature of agonist : receptor interaction.

In the characterization of any radioligand binding assay, information derived by equilibrium binding studies is complemented by analysis of the kinetics of the interaction of radioligand with receptors. As is the case for equilibrium studies, the approach to kinetic analysis involves construction of a theoretical model of ligand : receptor interaction, which is then tested experimentally. Initial experiments are generally directed toward testing a simple model of radioligand (L) interaction with receptors (R):

$$R + L \underset{k_{-1}}{\overset{k_{+1}}{\rightleftharpoons}} RL \tag{1}$$

whose rate law is defined as the sum of a second-order association reaction (eq 3) and a first-order dissociation reaction (eq 4):

$$d[RL]/dt = k_{+1}[R][L] - k_{-1}[RL] \tag{12}$$

The assumption that radioligand is present in great excess (eq. 7) simplifies the mathematical derivation of the integrated rate law, a linearized form of which is amenable to experimental testing:

$$\ln([RL]_{eq}/\{[RL]_{eq} - [RL]_t\}) = (k_{+1}[L]_T + k_{-1})t \qquad (13)$$

To test the proposed kinetic model of ligand:receptor interaction, experimental data quantifying the formation of radioligand:receptor complex as a function of time are plotted in derived fashion. If the proposed kinetic model of a reversible bimolecular binding reaction is valid, plots of $\ln([RL]_{eq}/\{[RL]_{eq} - [RL]_t\})$ versus time would be expected to be linear, with slope equal to $k_{+1}[L]_T + k_{-1}$. Analysis of a series of such plots obtained utilizing several different radioligand concentrations ($[L]_T$) allows construction of a linear plot of the form $k_{observed} = k_{+1}[L]_T + k_{-1}$, from which the kinetic parameters k_{+1} and k_{-1} can be derived. It should be noted that determination of k_{-1} by this method is possible only when the quantity $k_{+1}[L]_T$ is not extremely large in comparison to k_{-1}. In practice, accurate estimates of these kinetic parameters are complemented by specific experimental analysis of the dissociation reaction as well. Experimentally, following preincubation of radioligand with receptors, the association reaction is blocked, either by dilution or by addition of excess unlabeled antagonist, such that further association of radioligand with receptors becomes negligible (see Boeynaems, 1976). Subsequent quantitation of radioligand:receptor complex as a function of time ($[RL]_0$ at time = 0; $[RL]_t$ at time t) allows independent determination of the first-order dissociation rate constant k_{-1}, defined by the first-order dissociation rate law. Once again, experimental data are plotted in transformed fashion, according to the integrated form:

$$\ln([RL]_t/[RL]_0) = -k_{-1}t$$

If experimental data conform to the proposed first-order dissociation model, then plots of $\ln([RL]_t/[RL]_0)$ versus time would be expected to be linear, with slope providing an independent estimate of $-k_{-1}$. Notably, assuming that methodological difficulties have been excluded, nonlinearity of these derived kinetic plots implies that the proposed model of simple reversible interaction of ligand with receptor does not account for the experimental data. In these instances, alternative models to account for the observed binding kinetics are then developed and experimentally tested. In this regard, observed binding kinetics for very-high-affinity ligands, including $[^{125}I]$iodohydroxybenzylpindolol, $[^3H]$quinuclidinyl benzilate, and $[^3H]$carazolol, appear to be inconsistent with a simple reversible bimolecular interaction, and alternative kinetic models have been required to account for available data (Ross *et al.*, 1977; Galper *et al.*, 1977; Jarv *et al.*, 1979; Manalan *et al.*, 1981). Denaturation of receptors occurring over the extended incubation times remains a possible alternative explanation that must be considered in evaluation of these data. Nevertheless, if the kinetic properties of these high-affinity radioligands are appreciated, radioligand binding assays can be successfully designed and interpreted.

The quantitative analysis of complex radioligand binding data has been facilitated by the use of computer modeling techniques (see, for example, DeLean *et al.*, 1978). Although details concerning computer applications are beyond the scope of this chapter, the most general computer-based approach involves the application of statistical methods to the evaluation of a series of hypothetical models of radioligand:receptor interaction (Hancock *et al.*, 1979). Based on statistical analysis, the mathematical model that best accounts for the experimental data is identified and its parameters calculated.

Various computer-modeling or computer-assisted techniques have been applied to the study of cardiac autonomic receptors. As a notable example, computer-based analysis of radioligand binding data suggests the existence of both β_1- and β_2-adrenergic receptor subtypes in preparations derived from cardiac tissue. The results of these computer assisted analyses in various species suggest cardiac β_1/β_2 receptor ratios of (rat) 85%/15%, (dog) 85%/15%, and (frog) 20%/80% (Hancock *et al.*, 1979; Minneman *et al.*, 1979; Manalan *et al.*, 1981). As noted above, the coexistence of β_1- and β_2-adrenergic receptors may reflect the cellular inhomogeneity of cardiac tissue. Indeed, in primary cultures of neonatal rat cardiac cells, β_1 receptors appear to be localized to myoblasts, whereas β_2-adrenergic receptors reside on fibroblasts (Lau *et al.*, 1980).

VI. CONCLUSION

The application of radioligand binding techniques has facilitated significant improvements in the understanding of cardiac autonomic receptor function. In the future, it is anticipated that radioligand binding techniques will enjoy even more widespread application to the study of cardiovascular pharmacology. It has been the purpose of this chapter to summarize briefly certain practical issues that must be confronted in the rational design and appropriate interpretation of radioligand binding studies. For more comprehensive discussions of radioligand binding assays, the reader is referred to several recent review articles (Boeynaems and Dumont, 1975; Cuatrecasas and Hollenberg, 1976; Maguire *et al.*, 1977; Ross *et al.*, 1977; Hoffman and Lefkowitz 1980; Watanabe *et al.*, 1982).

ACKNOWLEDGMENTS

Original research sited in this chapter was supported by the Herman C. Krannert Fund, by grants HL18795, HL06308, and HL07182 from the National Heart, Lung and Blood Institute of the National Institutes of Health, and by the American Heart Association, Indiana Affiliate. Dr. Manalan was the recipient of a National Research Service Award HL06159 from the National Heart, Lung and Blood Institute.

REFERENCES

Besch, H. R., Jr., Jones, L. R., Fleming, J. W., and Watanabe, A. M. 1977. Parallel unmasking of latent adenylate cyclase and (Na^+,K^+)-ATPase activities in cardiac sarcolemmal vesicles. *J. Biol. Chem., 252*:7905–7908.

Boeynaems, J. M. 1976. Comparison of the effects of chemical and isotopic dilution on the dissociation of bound labelled ligands. *Anal. Biochem.*, *70*:366–376.

Boeynaems, J. M., and Dumont, J. E. 1975. Quantitative analysis of the binding of ligands to their receptors. *J. Cyclic Nucleotide Res.*, *1*:123–142.

Briley, M. S., Langer, S. Z., and Story, D. F. 1979. Binding studies on alpha-adrenoceptors and muscarinic cholinoceptors in rat ventricle: Effect of chemical sympathectomy. *Br. J. Pharmacol.*, *66*:90P.

Burgisser, E., Hancock, A. A., Lefkowitz, R. J., and DeLean, A. 1981. Anomalous equilibrium binding properties of high-affinity racemic radioligands. *Mol. Pharmacol.*, *19*:205–216.

Cheng, Y.-C., and Prusoff, W. H. 1973. Relationship between the inhibition constant (K_I) and the concentration of inhibitor which causes 50 percent inhibition (I_{50}) of an enzymatic reaction. *Biochem. Pharmacol.*, *22*:3099–3108.

Cornish-Bowden, A., and Koshland, D. E., Jr. 1975. Diagnostic uses of the Hill (logit and Nernst) plots. *J. Mol. Biol.*, *95*:201–212.

Cuatrecasas, P., and Hollenberg, M. D. 1976. Membrane receptors and hormone action. *Adv. Protein Chem.*, *30*:251–451.

DeLean, A., Munson, P. J., and Rodbard, D. 1978. Simultaneous analysis of families of sigmoidal curves: Application to bioassay, radioligand assay, and physiological dose–response curves, *Am. J. Physiol.*, *235*:E97.

Fields, J. Z., Roeske, W. R., Morkin, E., and Yamamura, H. I. 1978. Cardiac muscarinic cholinergic receptors: Biochemical identification and characterization. *J. Biol. Chem.*, *253*:3251–3258.

Galper, J. B., Klein, W., and Catterall, W. A. 1977. Muscarinic acetylcholine receptors in developing chick heart. *J. Biol. Chem.*, *252*:8692–8699.

Hancock, A. A., DeLean, A. L., and Lefkowitz, R. J. 1979. Quantitative resolution of beta-adrenergic receptor subtypes by selective ligand binding: Application of a computerized model fitting technique. *Mol. Pharmacol.*, *16*:1–9.

Hill, A. V. 1910. The possible effects of the aggregation of the molecules of hemoglobin on its dissociation curves, *J. Physiol.* (*Lond.*), *40*:iv–vii.

Hedberg, A., Minneman, K. P., and Molinoff, P. B. 1980. Differential distribution of beta-1 and beta-2 adrenergic receptors in cat and guinea pig heart. *J. Pharmacol. Exp. Ther.*, *213*:503–508.

Hoffman, B. B., and Lefkowitz, R. J. 1980. Radioligand binding studies of adrenergic receptors: New insights into molecular and physiological regulation. *Ann. Rev. Pharmacol. Toxicol.*, *20*:581–608.

Jarv, J., Hedlung, B., and Bartfai, T. 1979. Isomerization of the muscarinic receptor-antagonist complex. *J. Biol. Chem.*, *254*:5595–5598.

Jones, L. R., Besch, H. R., Jr., Fleming, J. W., McConnaughey, M. M., and Watanabe, A. M. 1979. Separation of vesicles of cardiac sarcolemma from vesicles of cardiac sarcoplasmic reticulum. *J. Biol. Chem.*, *254*:530–539.

Jones, L. R., Maddock, S. W., and Besch, H. R., Jr. 1980. Unmasking effect of alamethicin on the (Na^+,K^+)-ATPase, beta-adrenergic receptor-coupled adenylate cyclase, and cAMP-dependent protein kinase activities of cardiac sarcolemmal vesicles. *J. Biol. Chem.*, *255*:9971–9980.

Jones, L. R., Maddock, S. W., and Hathaway, D. R. 1981. Membrane localization of myocardial type II cAMP dependent protein kinase activity. *Biochim. Biophys. Acta*, *641*:242–253.

Karliner, J. S., Barnes, P., Hamilton, C. A., and Dollery, C. T. 1979. Alpha$_1$-adrenergic receptors in guinea pig myocardium: Identification by binding of a new radioligand, [^{3}H]prazosin. *Biochem. Biophys. Res. Commun.*, *90*:142–149.

Lau, Y. H., Robinson, R. B., Rosen, M. R., and Bilezikian, J. P. 1980. Subclassification of beta-adrenergic receptors in cultured rat cardiac myoblasts and fibroblasts. *Circ. Res.*, *47*:41–48.

Maguire, M. E., Ross, E. M., and Gilman, A. G. 1977. Beta-adrenergic receptor: Ligand binding properties and the interaction with adenylyl cyclase. *Adv. Cyclic Nucleotide Res.*, *8*:1–83.

Manalan, A. S., Besch, H. R., Jr., and Watanabe, A. M. 1981. Characterization of [^{3}H]($\pm$)carazolol binding to beta-adrenergic receptors: Application to study of beta-adrenergic receptor subtypes in canine ventricular myocardium and lung. *Circ. Res.*, *49*:326–336.

Minneman, K. P., Hegstrand, L. R., and Molinoff, P. B. 1979. Simultaneous determination of beta-1 and beta-2-adrenergic receptors in tissues containing both receptor subtypes. *Mol. Pharmacol.*, *16*:34–46.

Raisman, R., Briley, M., and Langer, S. Z. 1979. Specific labelling of postsynaptic $alpha_1$ adrenoceptors in rat heart ventricle by ^{3}H-WB4101. *Naunyn Schmiedebergs Arch. Pharmacol., 307*:223–226.

Ross, E. M., Maguire, M. E., Sturgill, T. W., Biltonen, R. L., and Gilman, A. G. 1977. Relationship between the beta-adrenergic receptor and adenylate cyclase. *J. Biol. Chem., 252*:5761–5775.

Scatchard, G. 1949. The attractions of proteins for small molecules and ions. *Ann. N.Y. Acad. Sci., 51*:660–672.

U'Prichard, D. C., and Snyder, S. H. 1979. Distinct alpha-noradrenergic receptors differentiated by binding and physiological relationships. *Life Sci., 24*:79–88.

U'Prichard, D. C., Bylund, D. B., and Snyder, S. H. 1978. (±)[^{3}H]epinephrine and (−)[^{3}H]dihydroalprenolol binding to beta-1 and beta-2 noradrenergic receptors in brain, heart, and lung membranes. *J. Biol. Chem., 253*:5090–5102.

Watanabe, A. M., Jones, L. R., Manalan, A. S., and Besch, H. R., Jr. 1982. Cardiac autonomic receptors: Recent concepts from radiolabelled ligand binding studies. *Circ. Res., 50*:161–174.

Williams, R. S., and Lefkowitz, R. J. 1978. Alpha-adrenergic receptors in rat myocardium: Identification by binding of [^{3}H]dihydroergocryptine. *Circ. Res., 43*:721–727.

Chapter **8**

Indicators of Calcium and Calcium Fluxes in Muscle, Its Subcellular Systems, and in Model Membranes

J. David Johnson, Denise E. Robinson, Laura A. Wittenauer, and Douglas A. Fugman

Department of Pharmacology and Cell Biophysics
University of Cincinnati College of Medicine
Cincinnati, Ohio

I. INTRODUCTION

The fundamental role of calcium and calcium fluxes in the mediation and regulation of a wide variety of both intra- and intercellular events is now widely recognized. It participates and indeed regulates cellular events as seemingly diverse as cell shape, cell–cell communication, glandular secretion, neurotransmitter release, flagellar motions, and muscle contraction. Coincident with our increasing awareness of the role of Ca^{2+} in cellular function and dysfunction, there has been an increase in the number and sophistication of Ca^{2+} indicators to measure and accurately report Ca^{2+} and rapid Ca^{2+} fluxes as they occur in their many diverse biological systems.

An ideal Ca^{2+} indicator would give a large, easily observable signal that was specific for Ca^{2+} over other metals in the concentration range of interest. Its response should be relatively insensitive to possible chemical changes within the

Present address for J. David Johnson and Laura A. Wittenauer: Department of Physiological Chemistry, Ohio State University Medical Center, Columbus, Ohio. Present address for Denise E. Robinson: Department of Pharmacology, Georgetown University, Washington, D.C. Present address for Douglas A. Fugman: Department of Anatomy and Cell Biology, University of Cincinnati College of Medicine, Cincinnati, Ohio.

cell, including ionic strength and pH. The response of the ideal indicator to Ca^{2+} would be sufficiently rapid and reversible to allow it to report rapid Ca^{2+} fluxes accurately. The indicator should be nonperturbing to the cell and cellular function, and it should not, in itself, alter [Ca^{2+}] or the Ca^{2+} flux. Finally, the ideal indicator should be readily available, stable, and easily deliverable to regions of the cell where we wish to probe for calcium.

This chapter discusses a variety of Ca^{2+} indicators and considers how well each fulfills the above criteria for an ideal Ca^{2+} indicator. We also discuss a new class of biological indicators of Ca^{2+} consisting of Ca^{2+}-binding proteins that have been labeled with fluorescent probe molecules, which undergo large, rapid Ca^{2+}-specific fluorescence changes. Finally, we describe methods that allow us to incorporate Ca^{2+} indicators into liposomes, providing a model membrane system for studying Ca^{2+} fluxes in membranes and providing possibilities for liposome-mediated delivery of indicators to intact muscle.

II. METALLOCHROMIC AND METALLOFLUORIC Ca^{2+} INDICATORS

A. Arsenazo III

Arsenazo III [0-(1,8dihydroxy-3,6-disulfonaphthylene-2,7-bisazo)-bis-benzenearsonic acid] (Arz III) is a metallochromic indicator that exhibits a large and fairly selective shift in its absorption spectrum when it complexes with Ca^{2+} (Michaylova and Ilkova, 1971). In the absence of metal, its visible absorption spectrum has an absorption maximum near 550 nm. The addition of millimolar amounts of Mg^{2+} shifts this absorption maximum to ~580 nm. The addition of Ca^{2+} produces rather dramatic changes in Arz III absorption, with two new peaks at ~600 and 658 nm (Michaylova and Ilkova, 1971; see Figure 3). With dual-wavelength absorption spectroscopy and the correct wavelength pair (675–685 nm), the response of Arz III is quite selective for Ca^{2+} (Scarpa *et al.*, 1978). The absorption changes with Ca^{2+}·Arz III complex formation are very large ($\Delta\epsilon \cong$ 25 $mM^{-1} \cdot cm^{-1}$ at 650, 685 nm and $\cong$13 $mM^{-1} \cdot cm^{-1}$ at 675, 685 nm), and its response has been reported to be linear with [Ca^{2+}] in the range 0.05 μM to 200 μM under the appropriate conditions (Ohnishi, 1978).

Although it had been generally assumed that Ca^{2+}·Arz III formed a 1:1 complex with an association constant near 2–7 $\times$ 10^4 M^{-1} (Scarpa *et al.*, 1978a; Michaylova and Ilkova, 1971; Dipolo *et al.*, 1976), it now appears that at higher [Arz III], a Ca^{2+}·Arz III complex of 1:2 molar ratio forms (Thomas, 1979). The apparent affinity of Ca^{2+} is ~3.3 $\times$ 10^3 M^{-1} for the first Arz III and ~1.7 $\times$ 10^5 M^{-1} for Ca^{2+} binding the second molecule of Arz III (Thomas, 1979). On the other hand, Mg^{2+} forms only a 1:1 complex with a $K_a \cong 1.4 \times 10^2$ M^{-1}. Thus, the $Ca^{2+}:Mg^{2+}$ selectivity of Arz III will increase with increasing concentrations of Arz III.

Although Arz III is one of the most sensitive of Ca^{2+} indicators, its rather high Ca^{2+} binding constant make it an exceptionally strong Ca^{2+} sink. At high Arz III concentrations and low [Ca^{2+}], it will bind significant amounts of Ca^{2+}

and seriously affect the free [Ca^{2+}] in the medium. For example, Ohnishi (1978) has shown that with 40 μM Arz III and 5 μM Ca^{2+}, ~76% of the total Ca^{2+} is bound to Arz III. Thus, arsenazo (particularly at high dye concentrations) would not give an accurate picture of free Ca^{2+} (at low concentrations).

The high association constant of Ca^{2+}·Arz III would also indicate that Ca^{2+} removal from Arz III may be relatively slow. The association rate constant of Ca^{2+}·Arz III has been estimated to be ~4.4×10^6 M^{-1}·sec^{-1}, whereas its dissociation rate constant is much slower, near 85 sec^{-1} (Ogawa *et al.*, 1980). Thus, although Ca^{2+} binding to Arz III produces changes in its absorption that are quite rapid, Ca^{2+} removal from Arz III and the associated absorption changes are really quite slow (85 sec^{-1}). Arsenazo III may not, therefore, be adequate for monitoring even moderately rapid Ca^{2+} fluxes.

Arsenazo III has another serious drawback in that the groups comprising its Ca^{2+}-coordination sites can be protonated, resulting in large absorption changes as a function of pH. The absorption changes in Arz III appear to be more sensitive to changes in pH in some cases than to changes in Ca^{2+}. Arsenazo III has been shown to have a deteriorating effect on the sarcoplasmic reticulum (Ogawa *et al.*, 1980). It has enjoyed extensive use in monitoring Ca^{2+} and Ca^{2+} fluxes in a variety of biological systems including squid axons, neurons, photoreceptors, mitochondria, sarcoplasmic reticulum, and muscle fibers (see Thomas, 1979; Scarpa *et al.*, 1978a; Baylor *et al.*, 1979).

B. Murexide

Murexide (ammonium purpurate) was first introduced by Ohnishi and Ebashi (1963,1964) as a metallochromic indicator for Ca^{2+}. In the absence of Ca^{2+}, it has an absorption band centered near 520 nm. Although millimolar amounts of Mg^{2+} have little influence on murexide absorbance, calcium produces a blue shift in its absorption maximum to 490 nm. With dual-wavelength spectroscopy and an appropriate wavelength pair for murexide (i.e., 500, 544 nm or 507, 540 nm), Ca^{2+} concentrations may be measured accurately (without interference from Mg^{2+}) and with a range of linearity from ~1 to 200 μM Ca^{2+} using 100 μM murexide (Ohnishi, 1978). Murexide has a relatively small change in extinction of $\Delta\epsilon$ = ~6.1 mM^{-1}·cm^{-1} (Ogawa *et al.*, 1980; Scarpa *et al.*, 1978a) and a rather low affinity for Ca^{2+} [K_{Ca} ~280 M^{-1} (Ohnishi, 1978) or K_{Ca} ~400 M^{-1} (Geier, 1968)]. For this reason, murexide has a low sensitivity to Ca^{2+}, and relatively high concentrations of murexide must be used to achieve an adequate Ca^{2+} signal (0.1 m*M* to 3 m*M*).

The low affinity of murexide for Ca^{2+} does, however, prove to be advantageous in some regards. Murexide does not act as a high-capacity Ca^{2+} sink (as does arsenazo), and, therefore, it does not significantly perturb the free [Ca^{2+}] it monitors. Furthermore, Ca^{2+} binds to murexide at a rate of $\geq 6 \times 10^7$ M^{-1} sec^{-1} (Geier, 1968), and assuming a K_{Ca} of 280 M^{-1}, the dissociation rate of Ca^{2+} from murexide would be in the range of 2×10^5 sec^{-1}. Thus, murexide (unlike Arz III) would be able to monitor extremely rapid Ca^{2+} fluxes because of these rapid Ca^{2+} exchange rates.

Murexide shows a sharp increase in its Ca^{2+} affinity above neutral pH, it is sensitive to ionic strength (Ohnishi *et al.*, 1978), and the dye itself is quite labile in aqueous solution (unlike arsenazo).

It has been suggested that murexide interacts with the membrane of sarcoplasmic reticulum (Blayney *et al.*, 1977), but we (Johnson and Schwartz, 1978) and others (Ogawa *et al.*, 1980) find that it provides an accurate measure of Ca^{2+} uptake and release in fragmented SR without serious perturbation of the system.

Recently (Ohnishi, 1978), tetramethylmurexide (TMX) was introduced as a Ca^{2+} indicator. Its spectral responses and specificity for Ca^{2+} are similar to those of murexide, but TMX is more sensitive to Ca^{2+}, with a $\Delta\epsilon$ of $\sim$12.8 $mM^{-1}\cdot cm^{-1}$ at the 507, 544 nm wavelength pair (Ogawa *et al.*, 1980), and its affinity for Ca^{2+} is similar [K_{Ca} $\sim$360 M^{-1} (Ohnishi, 1978)] to that of murexide. The major advantage of TMX is its increased sensitivity to Ca^{2+} and its relative insensitivity to pH. Although TMX is also somewhat more stable in aqueous solution than MX, it also appears to be more permeable to the sarcoplasmic reticulum during Ca^{2+} uptake (Ogawa, 1980). Murexide has been used to monitor Ca^{2+} fluxes in sarcoplasmic reticulum (Ohnishi and Ebashi, 1964), mitochondria (Mela and Chance, 1968), muscle (Jöbsis and O'Connor, 1966), and cell suspensions (Cittadini *et al.*, 1971).

C. Antipyrylazo III

Scarpa *et al.* (1978a,b) introduced antipyrylazo III (APIII) as a metallochromic Ca^{2+} indicator for use in biological systems. Magnesium does not produce any change in absorbance above 670 nm, whereas Ca^{2+} produces an increase in antipyrylazo III absorption at 650 and 700 nm. Calcium transients may be measured using the wavelength pair 675, 690 nm or 720, 790 nm without interference from Mg^{2+} (Scarpa *et al.*, 1978a,b). Its affinity for Ca^{2+} is intermediate between the K_{Ca} of murexide and that of arsenazo, being $\sim 6.5 \times 10^3$ M^{-1} (assuming a 1:1 complex), and its difference molar absorption coefficient is $\Delta\epsilon = 6.5$ $mM^{-1}\cdot cm^{-1}$ using the 720, 790 nm wavelength pair (Ogawa *et al.*, 1980). Thus, the changes in absorption or sensitivity of antipyrylazo III to Ca^{2+} are smaller than those of Arz III and greater than those of MX or TMX. It is sensitive to $\sim$0.5 μM Ca^{2+}, and its absorption changes are linear with Ca^{2+} up to $\sim$100–200 μM (Scarpa *et al.*, 1978a).

Antipyrylazo III, like arsenazo III, is sensitive to pH and ionic strength. It does not, however, appear to have a significant affinity for many biological membranes, nor does it produce any serious perturbation of SR or mitochondrial function (Scarpa *et al.*, 1978b). The rate of Ca^{2+} exchange with antipyrylazo III (like its Ca^{2+} affinity) is intermediate between those of MX and Arz III. It appears to be sufficiently fast for measurements of Ca^{2+} transients that occur in the millisecond range (Scarpa *et al.*, 1978b).

Recently, it has been suggested that antipyrylazo, like Arz III, forms 1:1 and 1:2 molar complexes of $Ca^{2+}\cdot$AP III. Thus, AP III may have species that have higher binding constants and slower dissociation rate constants than those reported. This could represent a serious problem for its use at high dye concentrations.

Antipyrylazo III has been used to monitor Ca^{2+} fluxes across SR, mitochondria, chromaffin vesicles (Scarpa *et al.*, 1978b), and in skeletal muscle fibers (Kovács *et al.*, 1979).

D. Chlorotetracycline

The peptide antibiotic chlorotetraclycline (CTC) was introduced by Caswell and Hutchison (1971a) as a fluorescent chelate probe for divalent cations. Fluorescence of CTC (ex. 380, emiss. 530 nm) is enhanced when it chelates divalent cations such as Mg^{2+} or Ca^{2+} as well as when it is placed in a more nonpolar medium. It is maximally fluorescent, therefore, when it chelates Ca^{2+} or Mg^{2+} while it is membrane bound. Although CTC has a higher affinity for Mg^{2+} than for Ca^{2+} in aqueous solution, in a nonpolar medium, the situation is reversed. Caswell and Hutchison (1971b) have reported a K_{Mg} of $3.7 \times 10^3\ M^{-1}$ and K_{Ca} of $2.3 \times 10^3\ M^{-1}$ for CTC in aqueous solution and a K_{Mg} of $4 \times 10^4\ M^{-2}$, K_{Ca} of $1.1 \times 10^5\ M^{-1}$ for CTC in a more nonpolar solution (i.e., 70% methanol). Thus, CTC fluorescence has some specificity for "membrance-bound" Ca^{2+} (Caswell and Warren, 1972).

Its calcium affinity is low enough that CTC should have a rapid exchange rate with Ca^{2+}. Chlorotetracycline has been used to monitor Ca^{2+} fluxes produced by sarcoplasmic reticulum (Caswell and Warren, 1972; Carvalho and Carvalho, 1977), mitochoncria (Caswell and Hutchison, 1971; Schuster and Olson, 1974), red cell ghost, and nerve cells (Hallet *et al.*, 1972). Use of CTC is limited by the fact that its fluorescence is enhanced by binding of Ca^{2+} or Mg^{2+} and by the interaction of CTC with the biological membrane itself. It has been shown that the amount of CTC bound to the SR membrane increases with increasing Ca^{2+} uptake (Carvalho and Carvalho, 1977). The fluorescence increases that occur with Ca^{2+} uptake in these systems are not, therefore, unambiguous indicators of Ca^{2+} fluxes. Further, the degree of perturbation produced by CTC binding to biological membranes is uncertain. It is likely that at high enough concentrations of CTC, chlorotetracycline in itself may influence Ca^{2+} uptake or release.

Despite these limitations, CTC does provide a convenient means of monitoring Ca^{2+} fluxes across biological membranes even in the presence of Mg^{2+}. Figure 1 compares the fluorescence changes in CTC and S-TnC_{DANZ} (to be discussed later) during Ca^{2+} uptake and release in rabbit skeletal sarcoplasmic reticulum (RSSR). ATP-stimulated Ca^{2+} uptake produces an increase in CTC fluorescence since with Ca^{2+} accumulation, more Ca^{2+} is bound to the membrane-bound CTC probe molecule. With Ca^{2+} release from the SR vesicle, the Ca^{2+} concentration near the membrane-bound probe is decreased, and the fluorescence intensity decays accordingly. Thus, CTC is useful in reporting Ca^{2+} ions near the inner surface of the SR membrane. Although CTC is membrane permeable, it has not been used to monitor calcium transients in intact fibers, a use for which it seems particularly well suited.

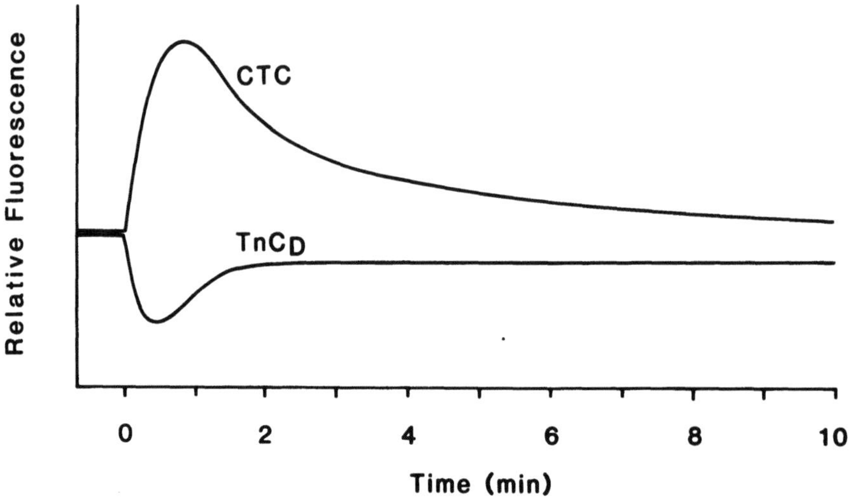

Figure 1. Calcium uptake and release in rabbit skeletal SR as monitored by chlorotetracycline fluorescence and TnC_{DANZ} fluorescence. Conditions: 0.8 mg/ml RSSR, 20 μM added Ca^{2+}, 3 mM $MgCl_2$ in 10 mM tris-maleate, pH 6.8, 100 mM KCl with 2 μM S-TnC_{DANZ} or 10 μM chlorotetracycline. At time zero, Ca^{2+} uptake was stimulated by the addition of 0.5 mM ATP, resulting in the rise in CTC fluorescence at 510 nm and the decrease in S-TnC_{DANZ} fluorescence at 520 nm. Spontaneous Ca^{2+} release then results in the subsequent decrease in CTC fluorescence and increase in TnC_{DANZ} fluorescence. Excitation was at 340 and 380 nm for TnC_{DANZ} and CTC, respectively.

III. BIOLOGICAL INDICATORS OF CALCIUM

A. Aequorin

Aequorin is the best-known member of a class of bioluminescent proteins (molecular weight ~20,000) that emit blue light as a function of bound Ca^{2+}. Since the initial suggestion of Shimomura *et al.* (1963), aequorin has enjoyed extensive use as a biological Ca^{2+} indicator.

Aequorin is particularly useful because of its high sensitivity to Ca^{2+}. Under the appropriate conditions, its luminescence increases linearly with pCa from 7.0 to 4.0 (Allen *et al.*, 1977). It is most successfully used, however, in determining intracellular calcium in the range 10^{-7} to 10^{-5} M and has a limited utility for measuring changes in large extracellular Ca^{2+} pools. Since Ca^{2+} may be detected with only femtomole quantities of aequorin, and aequorin has ~3 Ca^{2+}-binding sites with K_{Ca} ~6×10^4 M^{-1} (Blinks, 1978), under normal conditions, aequorin should not produce a large perturbation of the Ca^{2+} fluxes it reports.

Aequorin emits light only in the presence of Ca^{2+}, so there is essentially zero background, a particularly attractive feature for a Ca^{2+} indicator. Because aequorin generates light in the presence of Ca^{2+}, its "Ca^{2+} signal" is very easy to detect, making it particularly useful for Ca^{2+} measurements in the small volumes of biological cells and fibers.

Although the aequorin light reaction is specific for Ca^{2+} among biologically relevant divalent cations, Mg^{2+} can compete with Ca^{2+} and influence the Ca^{2+}

dependence of aequorin emission. Like most indicators, a variety of environmental conditions such as salt concentration, temperature, and pH influence the Ca^{2+}–aequorin reaction (see Blinks, 1978).

Aequorin is somewhat limited in measuring the true time course of very rapid increases in Ca^{2+}. This is because of the ~7 to 11-msec delay between Ca^{2+} binding and aequorin light emission (Hastings *et al.*, 1969). This delay time would introduce serious distortions in aequorin's report of very rapid Ca^{2+} transients.

Aequorin is also handicapped by the irreversibility of its Ca^{2+}-induced luminescence reaction. Once aequorin has seen Ca^{2+} and emitted light, it is not responsive to further Ca^{2+} (in the absence of a regenerating system). This not only requires caution to keep aequorin Ca^{2+}-free during its preparation, handling, and storage, but it means that aequorin's luminescence reports Ca^{2+} binding but not Ca^{2+} removal from the protein. The aequorin signal will continue to diminish after repeated challenges of Ca^{2+}.

In spite of these limitations, aequorin has been extremely useful in monitoring Ca^{2+} and Ca^{2+} transients in many living cells, including skeletal (Ridgway and Ashley, 1967), cardiac (Allen and Blinks, 1978), and smooth (Neering and Morgan, 1980; Fay *et al.*, 1979) muscle.

B. Fluorescent Calcium Binding Proteins: Dansylaziridine-Labeled Troponin C

Troponin C is a 17,000-dalton protein that may easily be isolated in large quantities from rabbit back skeletal muscle (Potter and Gergely, 1974). It is the Ca^{2+} receptor for the regulation of skeletal muscle contraction. Troponin C contains four Ca^{2+}-binding sites. Two sites, the Ca^{2+}–Mg^{2+} sites, bind Ca^{2+} and Mg^{2+} competitively [K_{Ca} ~$2 \times 10^7 M^{-1}$; K_{Mg} ~$4 \times 10^3 M^{-1}$ (Potter and Gergely, 1975)]. The two remaining sites, the Ca^{2+}-specific regulatory sites, are specific for Ca^{2+} (K_{Ca} ~$5 \times 10^5 M^{-1}$), and Ca^{2+} exchange with these sites serves to regulate the interaction of actin with myosin and muscle contraction (Potter and Gergely, 1975).

Troponin C may be easily labeled at methionine-25 with the fluorescent probe molecule dansylaziridine to produce TnC_{DANZ} (Johnson *et al.*, 1978). This TnC_{DANZ} undergoes a twofold increase in its fluorescence when Ca^{2+} binds to the Ca^{2+}-specific sites of TnC (see Figure 2). This fluorescence increase is Ca^{2+} specific and occurs over the free Ca^{2+} range from pCa 7.0 to pCa 4.0 (see inset of Figure 2). Magnesium binding to the Ca^{2+}–Mg^{2+} sites of TnC produces a ~20% decrease in TnC_{DANZ} fluorescence but does not affect the fluorescence increase occurring with Ca^{2+} binding to the Ca^{2+}-specific sites. Thus, a large Ca^{2+}-specific fluorescence increase occurs with Ca^{2+} and Ca^{2+} fluxes in a very biologically relevant range of Ca^{2+}.

Fluorescence stopped-flow studies (Johnson *et al.*, 1979) of the rate of these Ca^{2+}-induced fluorescence changes in TnC_{DANZ} indicate that Ca^{2+} binds to the Ca^{2+}-specific sites of TnC and produces this fluorescence increase extremely rapidly (within the 2.4-msec mixing time of the instrument; ≥500 sec^{-1}). EGTA or EDTA can remove Ca^{2+} from the Ca^{2+}-specific sites and reverse these flu-

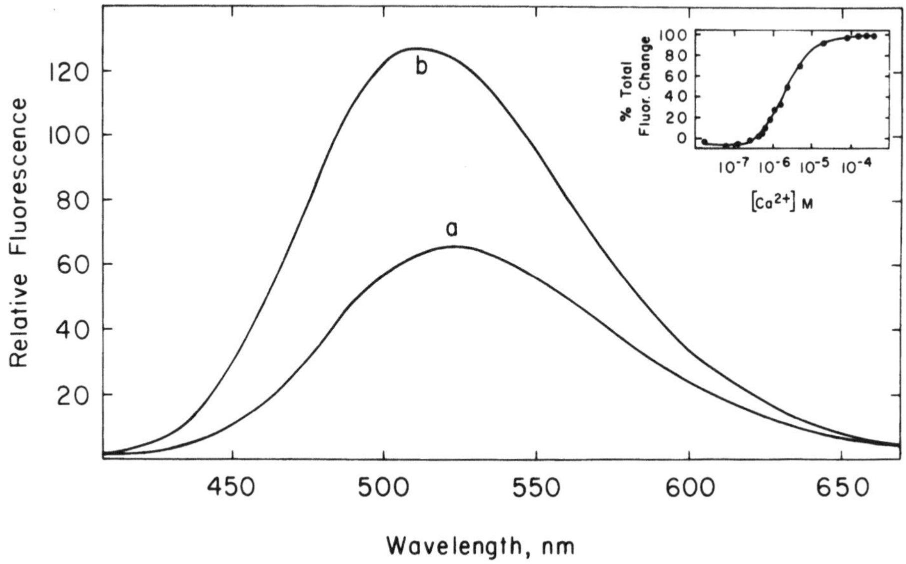

Figure 2. The fluorescence of TnC_{DANZ} in the absence (a) and presence (b) of 3×10^{-4} *M* Ca^{2+}. The inset shows the Ca^{2+} dependence of this 2.1-fold fluorescence increase. Conditions: 3 μ*M* TnC_{DANZ} in 10 m*M* potassium phosphate, 90 m*M* KCl, and 2 m*M* EGTA, pH 7.0. The Ca^{2+} titration was conducted as described by Johnson *et al.* (1978).

orescence increases with a half-time of 2–3 msec or a rate of ~300 sec^{-1}. Thus, Ca^{2+} exchange with the Ca^{2+}-specific sites of TnC and the associated fluorescence changes in TnC_{DANZ} occur very rapidly; TnC_{DANZ} is, therefore, sufficiently rapid to monitor even very rapid Ca^{2+} fluxes in muscle or other biological systems.

The fluorescence changes in TnC_{DANZ} may be used to monitor Ca^{2+} uptake and release in subcellular systems of muscle including the sarcoplasmic reticulum and mitochondria (Johnson and Schwartz, 1978). In the presence of Ca^{2+} and SR, TnC_{DANZ} fluorescence at 520 nm is high (Figure 1). When ATP is added to stimulate Ca^{2+} uptake by the SR, Ca^{2+} is removed from TnC_{DANZ}, and its fluorescence decreases with Ca^{2+} uptake. As spontaneous Ca^{2+} release occurs from the SR, Ca^{2+} once again binds to TnC_{DANZ} to produce the observed time-dependent fluorescence increase. Thus, TnC_{DANZ} provides an excellent means of monitoring Ca^{2+} regulation by these subcellular systems of muscle.

Perhaps because it is a natural component of muscle, TnC_{DANZ} is nonperturbing to these systems. It is a water-soluble protein and does not bind to natural membranes (SR or mitochondria) either in the presence or absence of Ca^{2+}, as determined by ultracentrifugation (J. D. Johnson, unpublished observations). Further, Ca^{2+} uptake in SR as measured by the murexide method, ^{45}Ca binding, and TnC_{DANZ} fluorescence are all both qualitatively and quantitatively similar. Finally, with this technique and Ca^{2+} regulation by SR, we are mimicking a fundamental process in the regulation of muscle contraction, i.e., the flow of Ca^{2+} between the sarcoplasmic reticulum and the regulatory sites of troponin C. This Ca^{2+} flow may easily be monitored by TnC_{DANZ} fluorescence.

IV. ENCAPSULATION OF TnC_{DANZ} AND Arz III INTO LIPOSOMES

Our efforts to incorporate Ca^{2+} indicators into liposomes have been prompted from two fronts. First, the studies of Leung (1980) and Leung *et al.* (1977) have suggested that nonpermeable dye molecules including 6-carboxyfluorescein and IAANS [2-(4′-iodoacetamidoanilino)-napthalene-6-sulfonic acid] encapsulated in liposomes could be delivered to intact muscle fibers via a liposome–muscle fiber fusion process. Liposomes could, therefore, provide a convenient means of introducing Ca^{2+} indicators or any nonpermeable molecule into intact muscle fibers. Secondly, having a Ca^{2+} indicator inside of a liposome would provide us with a convenient means of monitoring perturbations of lipid structure (by lipases, ionophores, detergents, etc.) or action of biological Ca^{2+} pumps or channels that allow Ca^{2+} entry into these model membranes. For these studies, we chose S-TnC_{DANZ} and Arz III as Ca^{2+} indicators for many of the reasons listed previously. The liposomes of choice should be well characterized in terms of their preparation techniques, homogeneity, and stability and should be single lamellar. For this reason, we chose to prepare small, unilamellar vesicles by the tip sonication technique with egg phosphatidylcholine as the main lipid constituent.

A. Preparation of S-TnC_{DANZ} Liposomes and Arz III Liposomes

Small unilamellar vesicles containing TnC_{DANZ} or Arz III were prepared by microtip sonication of lipid plus indicator. Typically, 20 mg of egg phosphatidylcholine was dissolved with 10% molar ratio of cholesterol and stearylamine in chloroform. This solution was N_2 dried, lyophilized to remove organic solvent, and layered with 1.5 ml of 10 mg/ml TnC_{DANZ} in 10 m*M* MOPS, 90 m*M* KCl, and 2 m*M* EGTA or 10 mg of purified Arz III (Sigma grade I) in 10 m*M* tris-Cl, 100 m*M* KCl, pH 7.4. These solutions were sonicated under N_2 for 10 min at force 3.5 on a Heat Systems Sonicator (Model W-225R) at 42°C. The cleared sonicated solution was centrifuged at 45,000 rpm for 30 min to remove any large multilamellar vesicles or particles, and the generally small pellet was discarded. The supernatants from the TnC_{DANZ} and Arz III preparations were applied to an A-5 M column (75 × 2 cm) or a G-25 column (30 × 1.5 cm), respectively, to separate free indicator from lipid vesicles. In each case, the lipid vesicles with incorporated indicators came in the void volume, well separated from free indicator. These lipid peaks (usually about 5–7 ml) were then used as TnC_{DANZ} liposomes or Arz III liposomes and generally contained ~0.25 mg TnC_{DANZ}/mg lipid or 0.01 mg Arz III/mg lipid, representing a trapping efficiency of ~18% or 1%, respectively.

B. Effect of Ca^{2+} and Lipid Perturbation on Indicator Liposomes

Figure 3 shows the effects of the sequential additions of Ca^{2+}, detergent, and EGTA to each encapsulated indicator. The initial spectrum of each (curve 1) is indicative of Ca^{2+} free indicator. Addition of Ca^{2+} (curve 2) produces essentially no change in TnC_{DANZ} fluorescence or Arz III absorption. Addition of de-

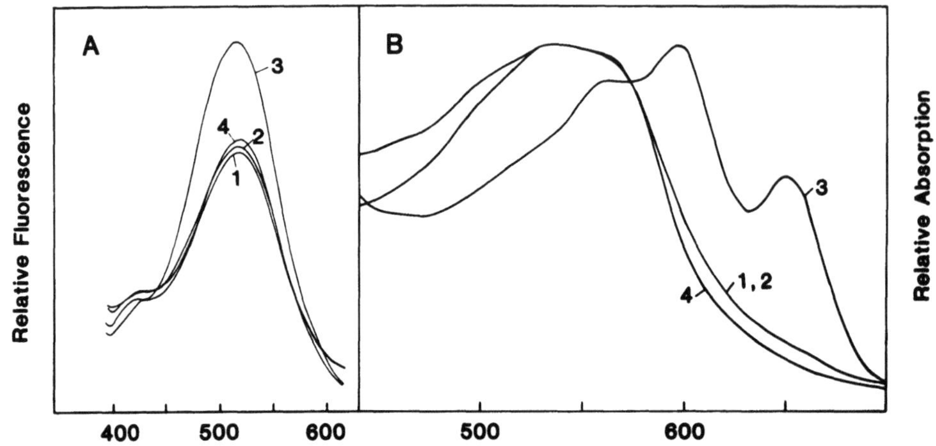

Figure 3. The effect of sequential additions of Ca^{2+}, detergent, and EDTA on TnC_{DANZ} liposome fluorescence and Arz III liposome absorption. Inset A: Initial fluorescence spectrum of TnC_{DANZ} liposomes (1); spectrum after the subsequent additions of 2 m*M* Ca^{2+} (2); 5 μl of 20% $C_{12}E_9$ detergent (3); and 20 m*M* EDTA (4). Solution was 0.2 ml of TnC_{DANZ} liposomes prepared with egg phosphatidylcholine, 10% cholesterol, and 10% stearylamine (~1.7 mg/ml in phospholipid in 1 ml total volume of 10 m*M* tris-Cl, pH 7.4, 0.9% NaCl, 1 m*M* EDTA, and 0.01% Na-azide. Excitation was at 340 nm on a Perkin–Elmer 650-10S ratio-recording spectrofluorometer. Inset B: Initial absorption spectrum of Arz III liposomes (1); spectrum after the subsequent addition of 100 μ*M* Ca^{2+} (2); 5 μl of 20% $C_{12}E_9$ detergent (3); and 10 m*M* EDTA (4). Solution was 0.1 ml of Arz III liposomes (2 mg/ml in phospholipid) in 1 ml total volume of 10 m*M* tris-Cl, pH 7.4, 100 m*M* KCl.

tergent to these liposomes (curve 3) allows Ca^{2+} to bind to TnC_{DANZ} or Arz III, producing the observed changes in TnC_{DANZ} fluorescence and Arz III absorption that are characteristic of indicator–Ca^{2+} complex formation. These changes are readily reversed by the addition of EDTA (curve 4). Thus, when TnC_{DANZ} or Arz III is encapsulated in these liposomes, it is protected from external Ca^{2+}. When the lipid barrier is broken by detergents, Ca^{2+} readily complexes with the indicator, producing the observed spectral changes.

Any perturbation of lipid structure that allows Ca^{2+} entry across the membrane may be easily monitored. Calcium ionophores such as X537A, A23187, and ionomyocin facilitate Ca^{2+} entry and produce fluorescence and absorption changes similar to those produced by detergents. Thus, as a model membrane system, liposome-encapsulated Ca^{2+} indicators provide a very convenient means of monitoring the action, stoichiometry, and specificity of various ionophores for Ca^{2+} (i.e., TnC_{DANZ} liposomes report Ca^{2+} entry, whereas Arz III liposomes report either Ca^{2+} or Mg^{2+} entry, depending on the wavelengths being monitored).

Lipases and phospholipases are known to disrupt lipid membranes by hydrolyzing their lipids and phospholipids. Their action on these liposomes may be easily followed by the fluorescence or absorption changes they produce with TnC_{DANZ} liposomes or Arz III liposomes, respectively, when Ca^{2+} crosses the disrupted membrane to complex with indicator. Figure 4 shows the action of phospholipase A_2 on Arz III liposomes. Phospholipase A_2 action results in a time-

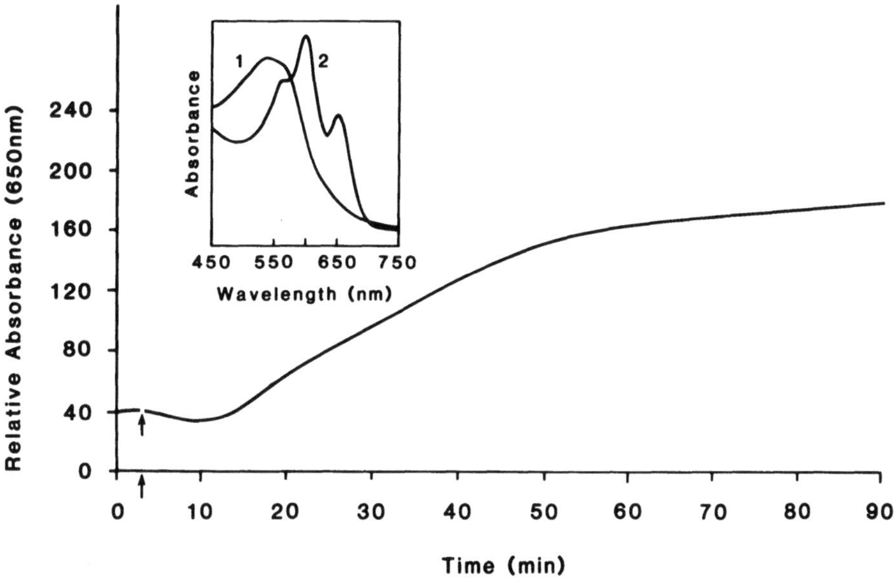

Figure 4. Effect of phospholipase A_2 on Arz III liposome absorption. At the time indicated by the arrow, phospholipase A_2 (20 μg/ml) was added to Arz III liposomes (0.28 mg/ml in phospholipid) in 10 m*M* tris-Cl, 100 m*M* KCl, pH 7.4, pCa 3.0, and the increase in absorption at 650 nm was followed as a function of time. The inset shows the initial absorption spectrum of Arz III liposomes after the addition of Ca^{2+} (1) and their absorption spectrum after PLA_2 treatment (2).

dependent increase in Arz III 650-nm absorption that is characteristic of Ca^{2+} binding to indicator (see inset, Figure 4); TnC_{DANZ} liposomes behave essentially the same way, and the time-dependent action of PLA_2 may be easily monitored by its fluorescence increase.

These liposomes are useful, therefore, as a model system for studying the action of lipases and phospholipases on artificial membranes with variable lipid composition.

The activities of detergents or drugs suspected of being lipophilic and or lytolytic may be easily tested for their ability to disrupt a liposome (of any lipid composition) and allow Ca^{2+} to complex with indicator. Liposomes with encapsulated indicators and external Ca^{2+} may be titrated with detergents, and the concentration dependence of their disruption of the vesicle may be followed by the associated fluorescence or absorption changes. With detergents such as Na-deoxycholate, we find that once a certain critical concentration is reached (i.e., ~0.04% for 0.08 mg/ml TnC_{DANZ} liposomes in 10 m*M* tris-HCl, 100 m*M* KCl, and 200 μ*M* Ca^{2+}), the disruption (fluorescence increase) occurs spontaneously in a time-dependent fashion to completion. Thus, both the concentration dependence and time dependence of vesicle disruption may be followed by fluorescence.

Other exciting possibilities that we are currently exploring include reconstitution of the Ca^{2+}-ATPase of sarcoplasmic reticulum membrane (i.e., the Ca^{2+} pump) with liposomes containing Ca^{2+} indicators. In this way, we could easily

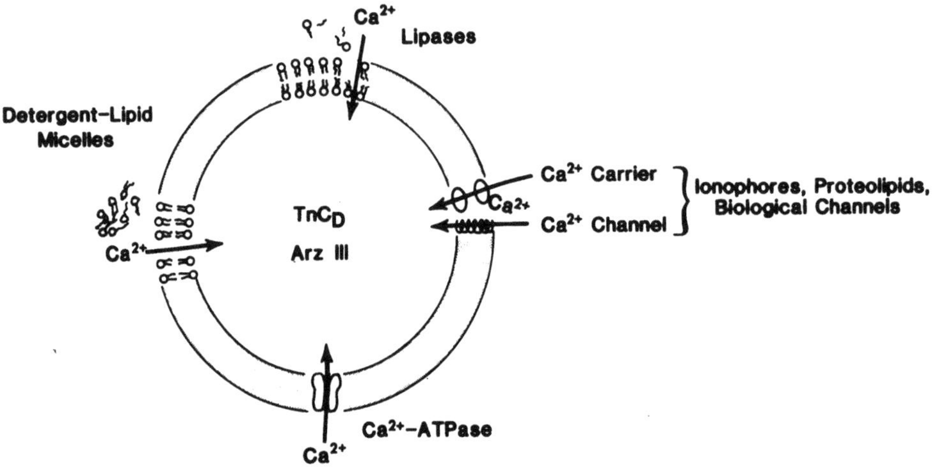

Figure 5. A schematic diagram of possible mechanisms of Ca^{2+} influx into "indicator liposomes." A bilayer lipid membrane with encapsulated TnC_{DANZ} or Arz III is shown. Calcium may enter through "holes" in the membrane or complete membrane disruption produced by phospholipases, lipases, or detergents; by passive transport utilizing Ca^{2+} carriers, Ca^{2+} channels, or Ca^{2+} pores; or by active transport across the bilayer by Ca^{2+} pumps.

monitor Ca^{2+}-pumping activity as Ca^{2+} is actively accumulated inside the SR vesicle.

In general, any perturbation of lipid structure such as formation of Ca^{2+} channels, pores, carriers, or active transport systems in the lipid bilayer could be monitored. The action of these various agents on the production of Ca^{2+} influx in these indicator liposomes is represented schematically in Figure 5. All of these processes may be easily followed using Arz III liposomes or TnC_{DANZ} liposomes in the presence of external Ca^{2+} to monitor the inward Ca^{2+} fluxes produced by any of these processes.

V. LIPOSOMAL DELIVERY TO INTACT MUSCLE FIBERS

Studies by Leung (1980) and Leung *et al.* (1977) have suggested that fluorescent dyes including 6-carboxyfluorescein and IAANS may be incorporated into liposomes and delivered to intact muscle fiber bundles via a liposome–muscle fiber fusion process. These studies point out the possibility of introducing any chemical or macromolecule into an intact muscle fiber or bundle after its encapsulation into the appropriate liposome. In this manner, chemicals that alter specific biochemical and mechanical functions of muscle could be introduced, and their action on the various functions of muscle could be examined in the intact fiber. Further, if Ca^{2+} indicators could be delivered to intact fibers via this process, then Ca^{2+} transients could be studied and related directly to tension production in intact excitable fibers.

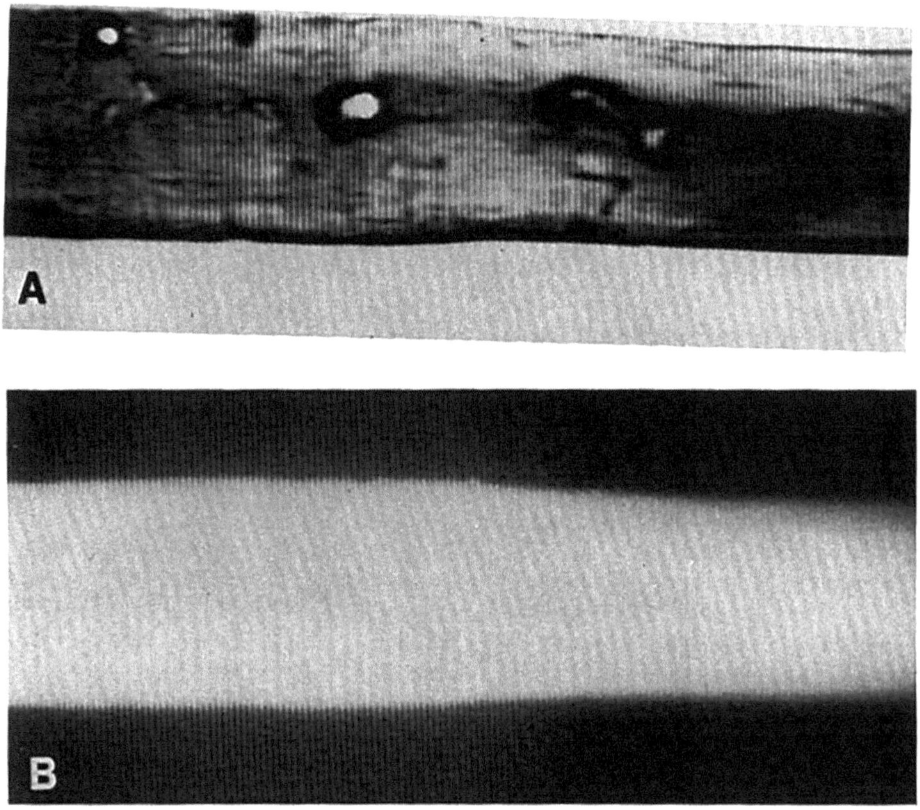

Figure 6. Liposomal delivery of 6-CF dye into an intact single muscle fiber. A: A photomicrograph (×250) of a single muscle fiber. B: A fluorescence photomicrograph of the same fiber now illuminated with ultraviolet light through the A filter cube of a Leitz Diavert fluorescence microscope. The fiber shows an intense green fluorescence characteristic of 6-CF. The fiber initially showed no fluorescence, and this photograph was taken after 1 hr of incubation with 6-CF liposomes before rinsing.

When it is possible to fuse Ca^{2+} indicator liposomes with intact skeletal muscle or myocytes and deliver Ca^{2+} indicators into the intact cell, then the Ca^{2+} fluxes that regulate muscle contraction and relaxation may be easily monitored by fluorescence or transmitted light microscopy. The effect of various pharmacological agents on these fundamental processes in muscle may then be examined in the context of the intact living cell. We are currently pursuing these possibilities with our TnC_{DANZ} and Arz III liposomes.

The feasibility of a liposome-mediated delivery process is documented by our preliminary studies with 6-carboxyfluorescein (6-CF) encapsulated in dipalmitoyl phosphatidylcholine lipid vesicles. The 6-CF fluorescence is self-quenched by the high concentration (~0.075 *M*) of dye in the liposome. When the liposome fuses with a muscle fiber, dye enters the muscle fiber and is tremendously diluted into the large volume of the fiber. This results in the fiber becoming much more fluorescent than the background 6-CF liposomes. Figure 6A shows a photomicrograph of a single muscle fiber from frog semitendinosis. Figure 6B shows the fluorescence of the same fiber after 1-hr incubation with 0.5 mg/ml of 6-CF liposomes. The fiber shows an intense green fluorescence over the background 6-CF liposome fluorescence. The fluorescence of the fiber is even more dramatic when the liposome incubating solution is washed off. The fluorescence does not wash out of the fiber, nor does the free dye stain the fiber. Further studies of these fluorescent muscle fibers indicate that its cell membrane remains intact and is nonpermeable to Ca^{2+} and that the 6-CF dye has actually entered the intact fiber and stained the contractile proteins.

Since Ca^{2+} indicators S-TnC_{DANZ} and Arz III may also be incorporated into these liposomes, we should be able to deliver them to intact muscle fibers by similar liposome fusion techniques. This will open the possibility of monitoring Ca^{2+} transients in intact living single fibers.

ACKNOWLEDGMENT

We wish to acknowledge the support of the Muscular Dystrophy Association of America.

Note added in proof: While this manuscript was in press, R. Y. Tsien (*Nature 290*:527, 1981) developed a very useful class of calcium indicators. These quin-2-tetraacetoxymethylesters bind calcium with high affinity (K_d = 115 n*M*) in 1:1 stoichiometry with 5-fold selectivity over Mg^{2+} to produce a large fluorescence increase. Their esters can permeate the cell where they are hydrolyzed, resulting in the intracellular trapping of a calcium-selective fluorescent indicator. These compounds will undoubtedly have great potential for monitoring calcium and calcium fluxes in a variety of living cells.

REFERENCES

Allen, D. G., and Blinks, J. R. 1978. Calcium transients in aequorininjected frog cardiac muscle. *Nature, 273*:509–513.

Allen, D. G., Blinks, J. R., and Prendergast, F. G. 1977. Aequorin luminescence: Relation of light emission to calcium concentration—A calcium-independent component. *Science, 196*:996–998.

Baylor, S. M., Chandler, W. K., and Marshall, M. W. 1979. Arsenazo III signals in singly dissected frog twitch fibres. *J. Physiol.* (*Lond.*), *287*:23P–24P.

Blayney, L. O., Thomas, J., Muir, J., and Henderson, A. 1977. Critical reevaluation of murexide technique in the measurement of calcium transport by cardiac sarcoplasmic reticulum. *Biochim. Biophys. Acta, 470*:128–133.

Blinks, J. R. 1978. Measurement of calcium ion concentrations with photoproteins. *Ann. N.Y. Acad. Sci. 307*:71–85.

Carvalho, C. A. M., and Carvalho, A. P. 1977. Fluorimetric monitoring of calcium binding to sarcoplasmic reticulum membranes. *Biochim. Biophys. Acta, 468*:21–30.

Caswell, A. H., and Hutchison, J. D. 1971a. Visualization of membrane bound cations by a fluorescent technique. *Biochem. Biophys. Res. Commun., 42*:43–49.

Caswell, A. H., and Hutchison, J. D. 1971b. Selectivity of cation chelation to tetracyclines: Evidence for special conformation of calcium chelate. *Biochem. Biophys. Res. Commun., 43*:625–630.

Caswell, A. H., and Warren, S. 1972. Observation of calcium uptake by isolated sarcoplasmic reticulum employing a fluroescent chelate probe. *Biochem. Biophys. Res. Commun., 46*:1757–1763.

Cittadini, A., Scarpa, A., and Chance, B. 1971. Kinetic evidence for Ca^{2+} uptake by intact Ehrlich ascites tumor cells. *FEBS Lett., 18*:98–102.

Dipolo, R. O., Requena, J., Brinley, F. J., Mullins, L. J., Scarpa, A., and Tiffert, T. 1976. Ionized calcium concentrations in squid axons. *J. Gen. Physiol., 67*:433–467.

Fay, F. S., Shlexin, H. H., Granger, W. C., and Taylor, S. R. 1979. Aequorin luminescence during activation of single isolated smooth muscle cells. *Nature, 280*:506–508.

Geier, G. 1968. Die Kineti der Murexid-Komplex Bildung mit Kationen verschiedenen Koordination scharakters. Eine untersuchung mittels der Temperatur sprung-Relaxations Methode. *Helv. Chim. Acta, 51*:94–105.

Hallet, M., Schneider, A. S., and Carbone, E. 1972. Tetracycline fluorescence as calcium-probe for nerve membranes with some model studies using Erythrocyte ghosts. *J. Membr. Biol., 10*:31–44.

Hastings, J. W., Mitchell, G., Mattingly, P. H., Blinks, J. R., and van Leeuwen, M. 1969. Response of aequorin bioluminescence to rapid changes in calcium concentration. *Nature, 222*:1047–1050.

Jöbsis, F. F., and O'Connor, M. J. 1966. Calcium release and reabsorption in the sartorius muscle of the toad. *Biochem. Biophys. Res. commun., 25*:246–252.

Johnson, J. D., and Schwartz, A. 1978. Dansylaziridine-labeled troponin C: A new fluorescent "physiological" probe for Ca^{2+} regulation by sarcoplasmic reticulum. *J. Biol. Chem., 253*:5243–5246.

Johnson, J. D., Collins, J. H., and Potter, J. D. 1978. Dansylaziridine-labeled troponin C. A fluorescent probe of Ca^{2+} binding to the Ca^{2+}-specific regulatory sites. *J. Biol. Chem., 253*:6451–6458.

Johnson, J. D., Charlton, S. C., and Potter, J. D. 1979. A fluorescence stopped-flow analysis of Ca^{2+} exchange with troponin C. *J. Biol. Chem., 254*:3497–3502.

Kovács, L., Rios, E., and Schneider, M. F. 1979. Calcium transients and intramembrane charge movement in skeletal muscle fibres. *Nature, 279*:391–396.

Leung, J. 1980. Liposomes: Effect of temperature on their mode of action on single frog skeletal muscle fibers. *Biochim. Biophys. Acta, 597*:427–432.

Leung, J., and Putnam, S., 1977. Transporting an impermeable fluorence dye into frog skeletal muscle fibers using artificial liposomes, *Proc. Int. Union Physiol. Sci., XIII*:441.

Mela, L., and Chance, B. 1968. Spectrophotometric measurements of the kinetics of Ca^{2+} and Mn^{2+} accumulation in mitochondria. *Biochemistry, 7*:4059–4063.

Michaylova, V., and Ilkova, P. 1971. Photometric determination of micro amounts of calcium with arsenazo III. *Anal. Chim. Acta, 53*:194–198.

Neering, I. R., and Morgan, K. G. 1980. Use of aequorin to study Neering excitation–contraction coupling in mammalian smooth muscle. *Nature, 288*:585–587.

Ogawa, Y., Harafuji, H., and Kurebayashi, N. 1980. Comparison of the characteristics of four metallochromic dyes as potential calcium indicators for biological experiments. *J. Biochem.* (*Tokyo*), *87*:1293–1303.

Ohnishi, S. T. 1978. Characterization of the murexide method: Dual wavelength spectrophotometry of cations under physiological conditions. *Anal. Biochem., 85*:165–179.

Ohnishi, T., and Ebashi, S. 1963. Spectrophotometrical measurement of instantaneous calcium binding of the relaxing factor of muscle. *J. Biochem.* (*Tokyo*), *54*:506–511.

Ohnishi, T., and Ebashi, S. 1964. The velocity of calcium binding of isolated sarcoplasmic reticulum. *J. Biochem.* (*Tokyo*), *55*:599–603.

Potter, J. D., and Gergely, J. 1974. Troponin, tropomyosin, and actin interactions in the Ca^{2+} regulation of muscle contraction. *Biochemistry, 13*:2697–2703.

Potter, J. D., and Gergely, J. 1975. The calcium and magnesium binding sites on troponin and their role in the regulation of myofibrillar adenosine triphosphatase. *J. Biol. Chem., 250*:4628–4633.

Ridgway, E. G., and Ashley, C. C. 1967. Calcium transients in single muscle fibers. *Biochem. Biophys. Res. Commun., 29*:229–234.

Scarpa, A., Brinley, F. J., Tiffert, T., and Dubyak, G. R. 1978a. Metallochromic indicators of ionized calcium. *Ann. N.Y. Acad. Sci., 307*:86–111.

Scarpa, A., Brinley, F. J., and Dubyak, G. 1978b. Antipyrylazo III, a "middle range" Ca^{2+} metallochromic indicator. *Biochemistry, 17*:1378–1386.

Schuster, S. M., and Olson, M. S. 1974. Studies of the energy dependent uptake of divalent metal ions by beef heart mitochondria. *J. Biol. Chem., 249:*7151–7158.

Shimomura, O., Johnson, F. H., and Saiga, Y. 1963. Microdetermination of calcium by aequorin luminescence. *Science, 140:*1339–1340.

Thomas, M. V. 1979. Arsenazo III forms 2:1 complexes with Ca and 1:1 complexes with Mg under physiological conditions. *Biophys. J., 25:*541–548.

Venkatakrishnan, R., Leung, J., Mason, D. T., and Wikman-Coffelt, J. 1979. Liposome for the transport of an impermeable fluorescent dye into muscle fibers. *Biochem. Med. 21:*209–214.

Chapter 9

Isolated Heart Preparations Perfused or Superfused with Balanced Salt Solutions

Ingrid L. Grupp and Gunter Grupp

Departments of Pharmacology and Cell Biophysics, Physiology, and Internal Medicine (Division of Cardiology)
University of Cincinnati College of Medicine
Cincinnati, Ohio

I. INTRODUCTION

Hearts of small laboratory animals (rats, guinea pigs, small rabbits, and cats) are frequently used for either isolated work-performing (antegrade or anagrade perfused) or Langendorff (retrograde perfused) heart preparations. Muscle strips from the atria and strips and/or papillary muscles from the ventricles of these hearts provide excellent specimens for heart muscle preparations immersed in or superfused with balanced salt solutions (BSS). Muscle strip preparations, especially atrial and ventricular trabeculae preparations and Purkinje fibers, are also used from dog, sheep, and pig hearts and, occasionally, from small portions of human hearts excised during open-heart surgery. The long-term viability of the preparations is greatly enhanced by the prevention of intravascular coagulation of blood and by removal of blood from the heart tissues at the time of sacrifice. For this reason, we always pretreat the experimental animals, including dogs, with intraperitoneal (i.p.) or intravenous (i.v.) injections of 5000 IU heparin/kg body weight and wash out, immediately after sacrifice, the coronary arterial and venous system with warm or cold BSS, dependent on the type of preparation we use (see below).

II. MUSCLE STRIP PREPARATIONS

Isolated strip or papillary muscle preparations (depending on the size of the heart) are procured from left atria and right ventricles of rats, guinea pigs, cats, and rabbits. Right atrial tissues are excluded except for experiments in which drug effects on spontaneous pacemaker activity are needed and where the presence of ganglion cells is of importance. The animals are anesthetized i.v. with 20 mg/kg sodium pentobarbital and heparanized (5000 U USP/kg) to prevent postmortem intravascular coagulation of blood, especially in the coronary arteries. To preserve maximal myocardial function and exclude transient hypoxemia during sacrifice, the animals are artifically respirated with room air mixed with O_2 throughout the procedure. After opening of the chest, the hearts are removed and immediately suspended in a Langendorff apparatus for retrograde perfusion of the coronary system with warm Krebs–Henseleit solution. The atrial and ventricular strips and/or papillary muscles are then dissected from the suspended and perfused hearts. The dissected preparations are mounted in a bath chamber with a volume of 70 ml. We try to avoid the severe trauma of the guillotine or head or neck blows and prefer a quick superficial but sufficient use of anesthetics, since we wash out the myocardium via the coronary system during the entire duration of the strip dissection, removing the remnants of the anesthetic in the most efficient way possible.

A. Selection of Preparation

1. Atrial Tissue

Most atria of small laboratory animals make excellent preparations since they are usually thin enough to permit easy O_2 diffusion in the oxygenated bath. Left and right atria can be easily distinguished, and most atria are big enough to allow for two or more uniformly sized strips. Sometimes whole left atria are preferred, especially when the tissues are also to be used for biochemical analysis. When whole left atria are used with strong-current field stimulation, neural tissue or ganglionic cells in the atria may affect the outcome of studies of inotropy (Grupp et al., 1982). For point stimulation, the tissue holder used will determine the size and shape of the preparation, since one end of the strip must cover both punctate electrodes, which deliver the current for stimulation of the preparations. Atrial strips can be cut long enough to allow easy recording of contractile force without the noise and interference of high amplification of the electronic signal. In experiments in which two bath chambers are used simultaneously, each half of an atrium can be placed in a different bath, allowing for the observation of different effects in the same atrium. On the other hand, one strip each of a left and of a right atrium of the same animal can be observed in the same chamber.

2. Ventricular Tissue

Some species, especially cat and guinea pig, have thin, elongated papillary muscles less than 1 mm in diameter. These are ideal specimens for observations on ventricular tissue. Other species have very small papillary muscles (rat) or short and thick ones (rabbit). In these cases, strip preparations from ventricles instead of papillary muscles may have to be used. The ventricular strips must be thin enough for sufficient oxygenation and long enough for satisfactory recording

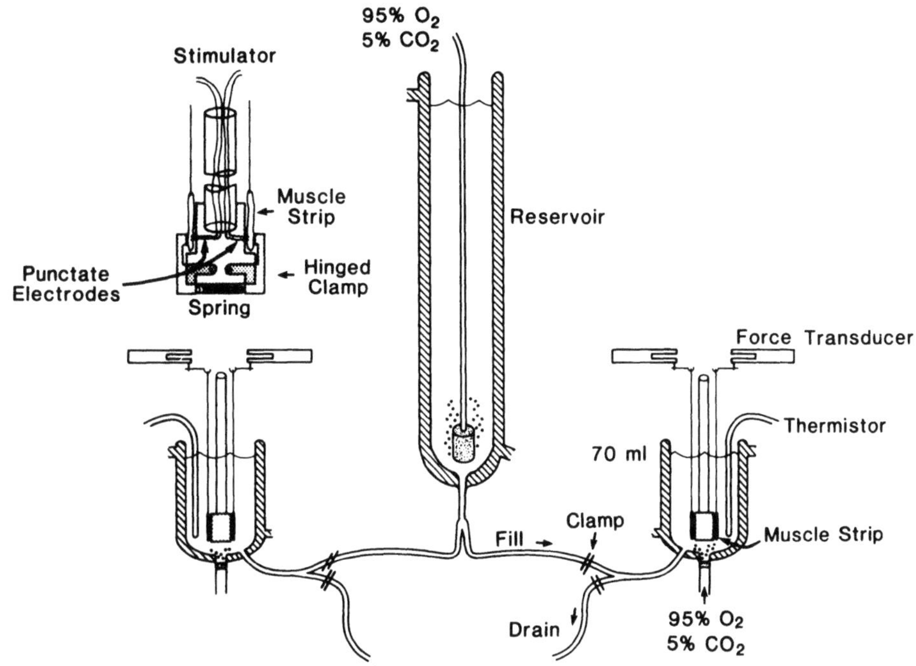

Figure 1. Schematic drawing of a setup for two muscle chambers accomodating two strips each. Left upper corner: magnification of the muscle holder.

of contractile force. Most often, when papillary muscles can not be cut in half lengthwise, good ventricular preparations can be cut from the right ventricular outflow tract near the pulmonary artery, cutting the long axis of the strip in parallel with the flow direction. Strips exceeding 1 mm thickness can not be sufficiently oxygenated in a continuously contracting heart preparation. The higher the bath temperature and frequency of contraction, the smaller the necessary thickness. Sufficient oxygenation can be crudely estimated by increasing stimulation frequency. Alternating heights of contractions (''pulsus alternans'') will occur at relatively low frequencies (relative to species and temperature) when oxygenation is insufficient. The absence of alternation of contractile force, especially at frequencies well above the frequency of the intended experiment, will give some but not absolute assurance of sufficient oxygenation.

B. Mounting of Strips

It is most convenient to use electrode–clamp holders that accommodate two strip preparations (Figure 1, upper left side; see also Blinks, 1965; Levy, 1971). One clamp each can be used to fix one end of the strip firmly on top of the two punctate electrodes, which are used to stimulate the strip. The other end of the strip is connected to the mechanical arm of a force transducer via a silk thread. The force transducer should be mounted on a plate whose distance from the clamp can be crudely adjusted by a rack and pinion and finely adjusted by a micrometer. This adjustment shortens or lengthens the strips mechanically and is used to determine the length–tension relationship of each strip. The micrometer is also used to set the resting tension of each strip to be maintained throughout the experiment. In most preparations, the resting tension at maximal active tension (L_{max}) will be between 0.7 and 1.2 g. It is best, therefore, to set the initial resting tension below but close to 1.0 g. In most preparations, the resting tension originally set will remain relatively constant. Preparations in which resting tension changes more than 30% during an experiment should be discarded, unless such changes occur as a consequence of drug action, i.e., the Ca^{2+} blockers.

C. Stimulation

Because of the spread of excitation in a functional syncytium over all fibers, the initiating impulse should be delivered through punctate electrodes. This arrangement allows for the least current to be used to stimulate the strips. Although in heart muscle, in contrast to skeletal muscle, the strength of the stimulus does not determine the number of fibers stimulated, the strength of the stimulus may influence contractile force of the heart muscle strip via current-dependent release of transmitter stored in the heart muscle (e.g., catecholamines; Levy, 1975, Figure 21). Therefore, a change in the strength of the stimulus during an experiment should be avoided. Sometimes field stimulation using large-surface electrode plates and high-current stimulation is required. In these cases, the possibility of current-dependent changes in contractile force cannot be excluded (see above).

D. Constancy of Temperature, Frequency, and Ion Composition

Since Sidney Ringer's classic paper 100 years ago on ion composition and Blinks's and Koch-weser's classic review (1963) of the significance of frequency, temperature, and species for cardiac contraction 20 years ago, it is clear that predictions about the function of isolated heart preparations are hazardous. Therefore, it is of the essence to be constant and consistent during an experimental run. Much effort should be devoted to keeping temperature and frequency constant. Their constancy should be monitored continuously. Effects of alterations of temperature and/or frequency on the species and experimental conditions under study have to be determined anew for each instant. There should be no assumption or prediction. Since ion compositions of BSS vary from study to study and lab to lab, one should remain consistent within one's own laboratory. Most BSS, for instance, contain 1.8–2.5 m*M* Ca^{2+}. Some also have 0.5 m*M* Na-EDTA, thus reducing their effective Ca^{2+} concentration by that amount, yet Luellmann considers 0.9 m*M* Ca^{2+} as the "physiological concentration." The Mg^{2+} content varies from 0.1 to 1.2 m*M*, and K^+ from 2.5 to 5.9 m*M*. Each of these ions is considered of crucial importance for the consequences of contractile force regulation produced by inotropic agents. All of this speaks for the need to be consistent. Most frequently used is Krebs–Heseleit BSS (Table I, left column). Other Tyrode solutions are indicated in the middle and right columns of Table I.

Table I. Contents of Some Balanced Salt Solutions (mM)[a]

	Krebs–Henseleit	Godfraind	Erdmann
NaCl	118	137	137
KCl	4.7	2.3	4.98
$CaCl_2$	2.5	0.9	1.8
$MgSO_4$	1.2	0.105	1.05
KH_2PO_4	1.2	—	0.42
NaH_2PO_4	—	0.417	—
$NaHCO_3$	25.0	11.9	11.9
Glucose	5.5	5.5	10.0
NaEDTA	0.5		
Total K^+	5.9	2.3	5.4
Total Mg^{2+}	1.2	0.105	1.05
Total Ca^{2+}	2.0	0.9	1.8
pH	7.4	7.0	7.0

[a] We have used these three solutions in recent studies at 30, 35, and 37°C (Grupp *et al.*, 1981, 1982).

E. Desirability to Mount Atrial and Ventricular or Right and Left Atrial Strips in the Same Bath Chamber

Recently, reports have surfaced that atrial and ventricular myocardium of the same species respond differently to the same agent: examples are vanadate in the guinea pig (Grupp *et al.*, 1979), ouabain in the rat (Grupp *et al.*, 1981), and histamine in the rabbit heart (Johnson *et al.*, 1980). The same is true for histamine effects on left and right atria of guinea pigs and rabbits (McNeill and Verma, 1979).

F. Measurement and Recording of Contractile Force in Isolated Muscle Strip Preparations

In the beginning of each muscle strip experiment, zero tension, L_{max}, and resting tension of the mounted strip are established by stretching the strip with the micrometer adjustment. As the strip is stimulated, stretch is slowly increased until the first contractions become visible in the output records of the force transducer and the force differentiator, indicating gram force and gram/sec change in force during contraction and relaxation, respectively. As tension is increased, active tension, i.e., total tension minus resting tension, is monitored. L_{max} is recorded as maximum active tension. It is useful to do the experiments at a constant point of the length–tension curve either at L_{max} or a fixed percentage of L_{max} or a fixed resting tension below L_{max}. It should be routine to record both developed force and df/dt. Both records support each other yet may give different information.

III. ISOLATED PERFUSED HEART PREPARATIONS

For isolated perfused work-performing heart preparations or for Langendorff retrograde-perfused heart preparations, hearts from rats, guinea pigs, small rabbits, and small cats can be used. In principle, the hearts are prepared as described in the previous paragraph using the same precautions and preparations.

The basic perfusion system for both preparations was originally described by Neely *et al.* (1967) for rat hearts and modified by us for use in guinea pig, small rabbit, and cat hearts for simultaneous monitoring of both mechanical and electrical events (Wiester *et al.*, 1973). The diagram of the apparatus is seen in Figure 2. It consists of a working heart (antegrade or anagrade system) that is perfused via the left atrium (left panel), and the retrograde system, which perfuses the coronary vascular system retrogradely via the aorta (Langendorff preparation, right panel). The two systems can be used in the same heart by simply clamping off one system while the other is in use. This is accomplished by opening the venous return and aortic resistance lines and closing the retrograde flow line (broken line) and *vice versa*. Hence, transition from one system to the other can be done easily and quickly during the course of any experiment. Buffer solutions can be changed, heated, and oxygenated in one system while the other is in use; or buffer can be changed in either system during use if done carefully and gradually. Buffer solutions can potentially be recycled in either system.

Figure 3 shows an enlargement of the heart chamber, Figure 4 the heart after removal of the Plexiglas chamber, and Figure 5 the heart with its immediate attachments including cannulas, electrical connection, and the locations of pressure transducers. The photograph in Figure 6 shows the size and arrangement of the equipment.

The heart chamber is made of Lucite with openings cut into the sides so that cannulas and stimulating wires can exit (Figure 3). The chamber helps to keep the humidity and temperature up and to collect all the effluents from the pulmonary artery (= coronary outflow). The bottom of the chamber is closed except for the coronary flow exit. The plastic chamber is held in place by a size 8 stopper by friction and can be removed and replaced at any time. The stopper has two holes, which hold the two stainless steel cannulas for mounting the heart. Both cannulas are grooved to accommodate the ligatures to fit the aorta or the left atrium to the cannulas. The aortic and left atrial cannulas can be exchanged for larger sized cannulas for larger hearts. The atrial cannula (Figure 7) is modified so that left atrial pressure can be monitored inside the left atrium.

The pressure chamber to provide "elastic recoil" (see Figure 2 and top part of Figure 5) is constructed from the female portion of 14/35 standard taper joint. A plastic stopper allows the injection of 2.5 ml of air to produce the necessary elasticity for the otherwise rigid system (*Windkessel*).

A reservoir called "bubble trap" is specially made for the atrial inflow (venous return) in order to minimize any fluctuations in hydrostatic pressure. It holds 20 ml of buffer and has a wide overflow drain. The reservoir to the left of the trap in Figure 2 should hold 2 liters. There is also a reservoir for the retrograde

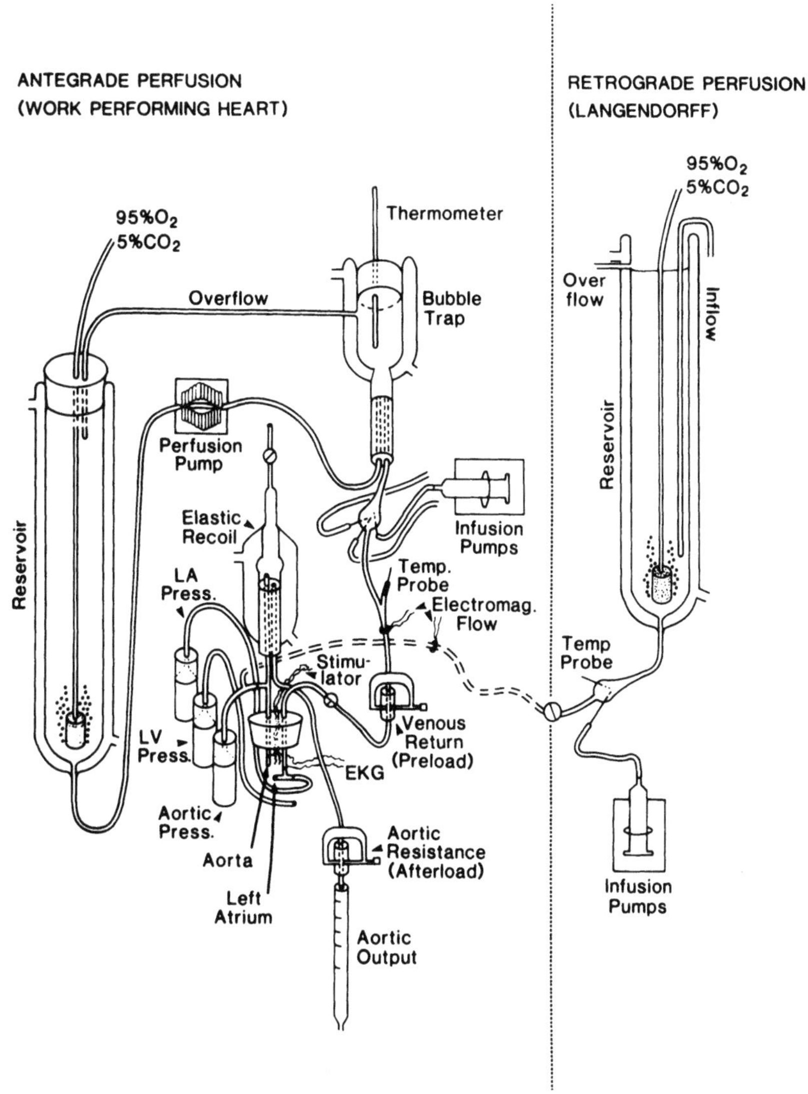

Figure 2. Schematic drawing of the working heart preparation (left of stippled line) and non-working (Langendorff) preparation (right of stippled line).

system (right panel of Figure 2). Coarse-porosity sintered glass filters are used to oxygenate the buffers in the reservoirs with 95% O_2 and 5% CO_2.

A. Sequence of Preparation

After the quick heparinization, introduction of anesthesia, and initiation of artificial respiration, the chest of the heart donor is opened through the left fourth intercostal space. The heart is quickly isolated after identification of the major

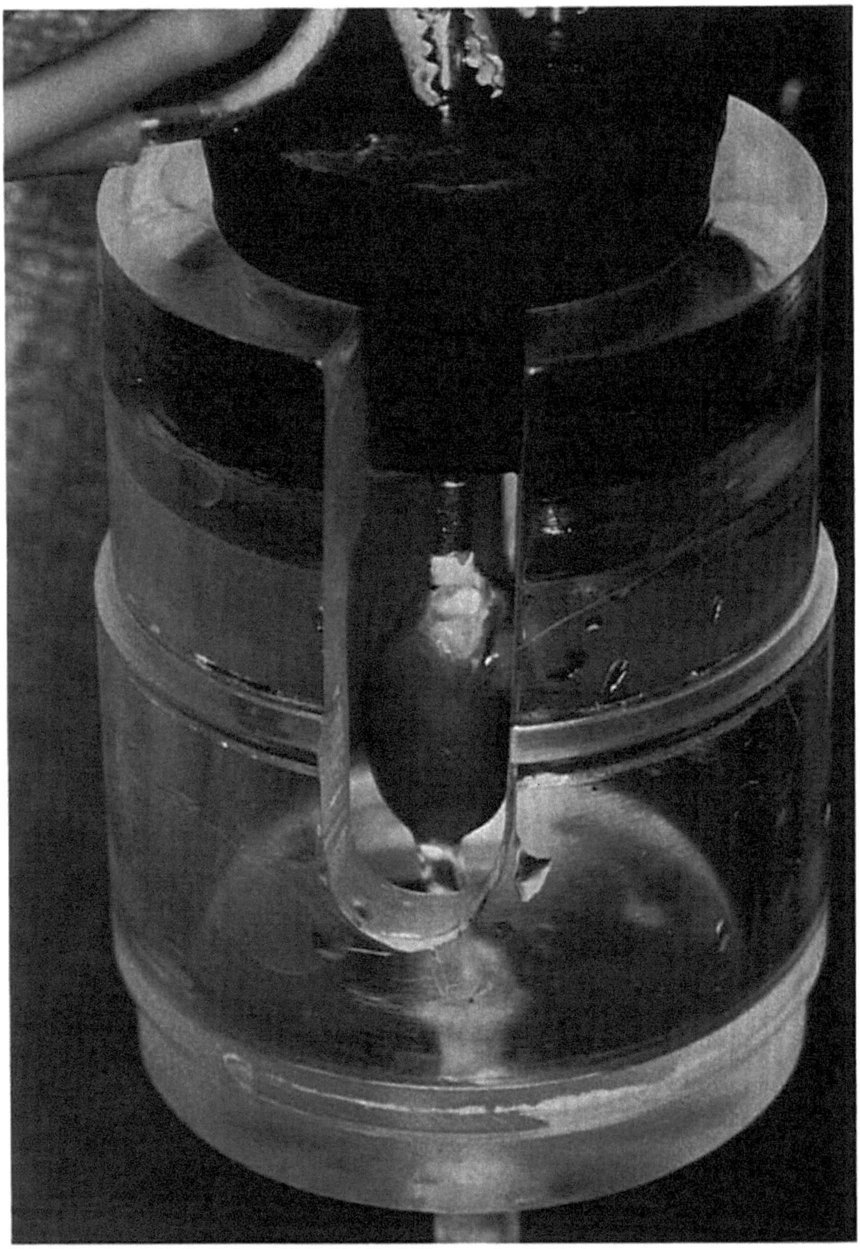

Figure 3. Plexiglas chamber surrounding the heart to collect coronary outflow and to keep heart warm and moist.

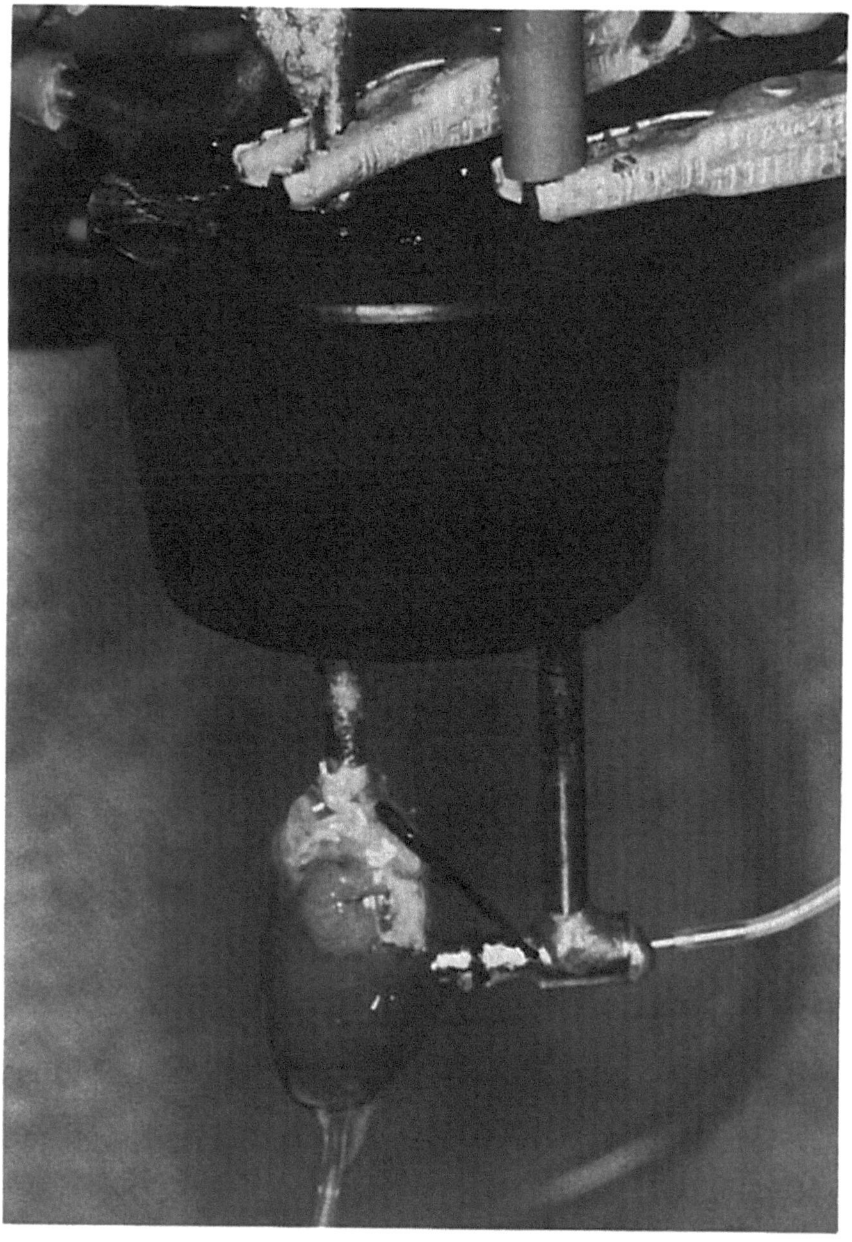

Figure 4. Isolated heart (Plexiglas chamber removed) suspended on aortic cannula. Note: two alligator clips above the rubber stopper for recording EKG and stimulation of the heart.

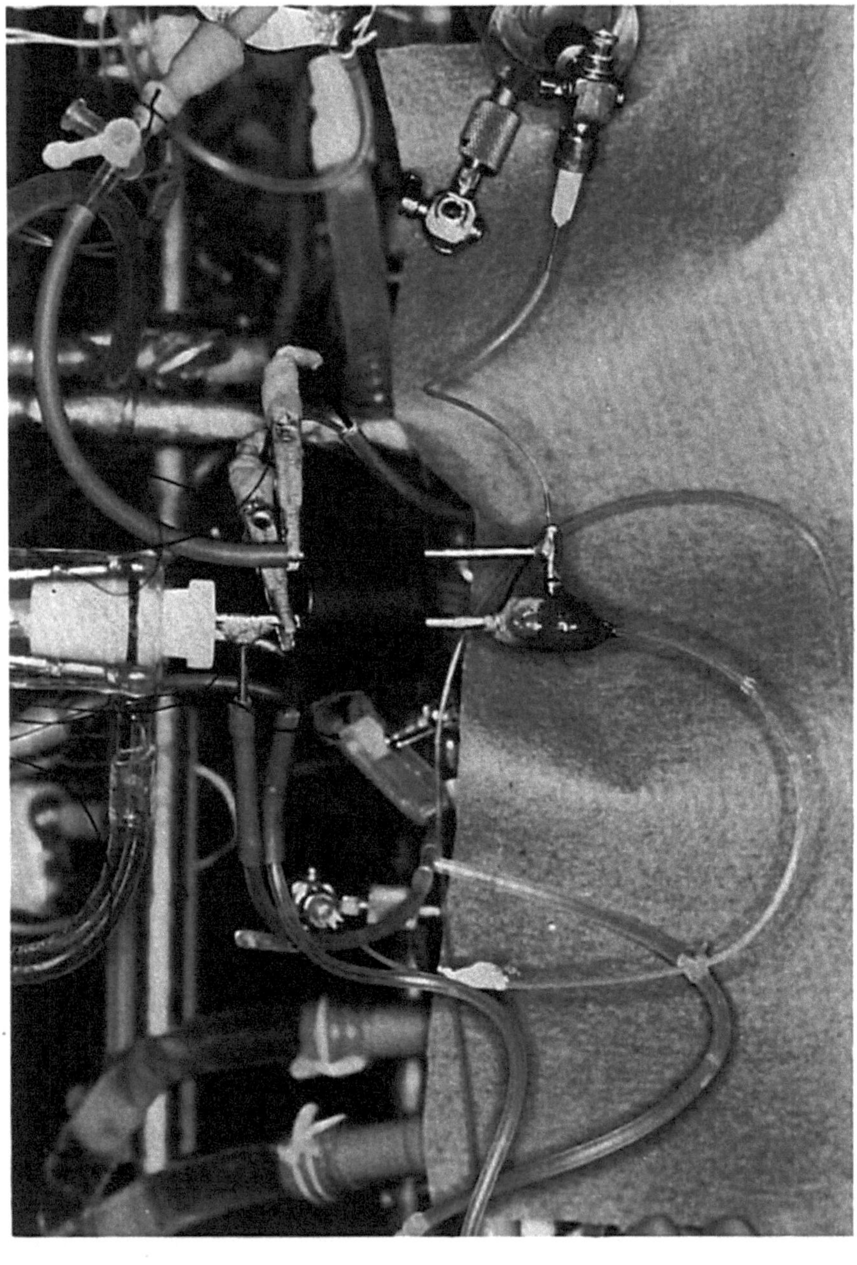

Figure 5. Close-up of isolated heart, aortic and left atrial cannulas, and alligator clips. Directly above the clips: elastic recoil chamber. Note also to the right of the heart the position of the left atrial pressure transducer, to be lined up exactly at the height of the heart.

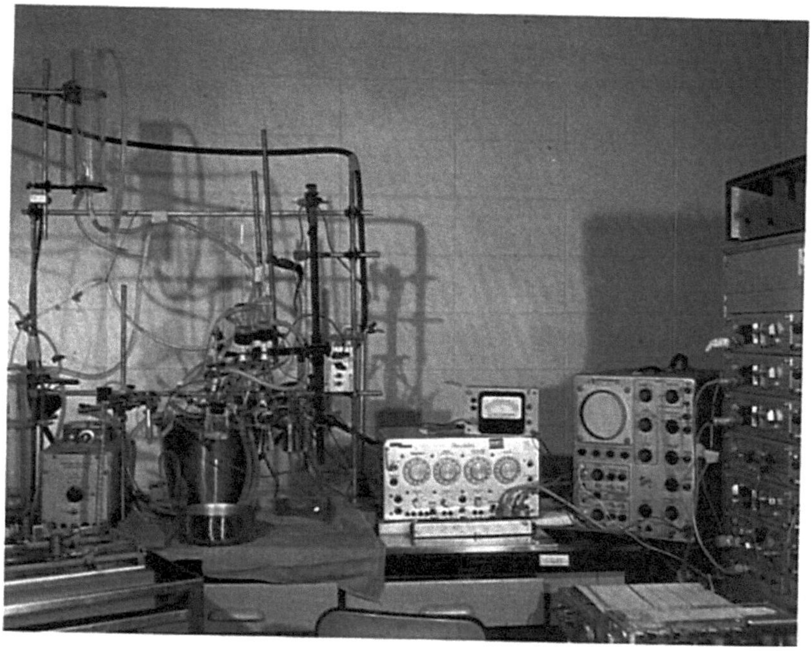

Figure 6. Overview of the setup of the isolated work-performing heart preparation.

vessels. The aorta is then opened, and the aortic cannula inserted. Retrograde perfusion is begun at this time and continued from then on. The retrograde perfusion line, which should have been recirculating at a slow rate, is, after connection to the aortic cannula, perfusing the coronary circulation with warm oxygenated buffer. The heart should contract vigorously. The time from the opening of the chest until full retrograde perfusion should not be more than 1 min.

At this time, the heart is rotated on the cannula in order to position the atrial cannula close to the opening into the left atrium. There are usually two pulmonary vein roots; the intervening tissue between them is cut to make the opening larger. Before the atrial cannula is connected, one end of the intraventricular catheter is put through the enlarged opening, gently pushed past the mitral valve, forced through the myocardium at the apex of the left ventricle, and connected to a pressure transducer. This leaves the other (flanched) end of the catheter lying within the cavity of the left ventricle. Intraventricular pressure and d*p*/d*t* readings originate from this location. The left atrial cannula can now be readied to be tied into the pulmonary vein opening. Flow in the left atrial cannula is set with a screw clamp at 35–40 ml/min. The left atrium is now slipped onto the cannula and fixed with a ligature. The integrity of the ligation is tested by filling the left atrium for about 1 sec. If the cannulation is done correctly, the left auricle will fill, intraventricular pressure will rise, and a small amount of buffer will exit the atrial pressure line. The three pressure cannulas are now connected to their pressure

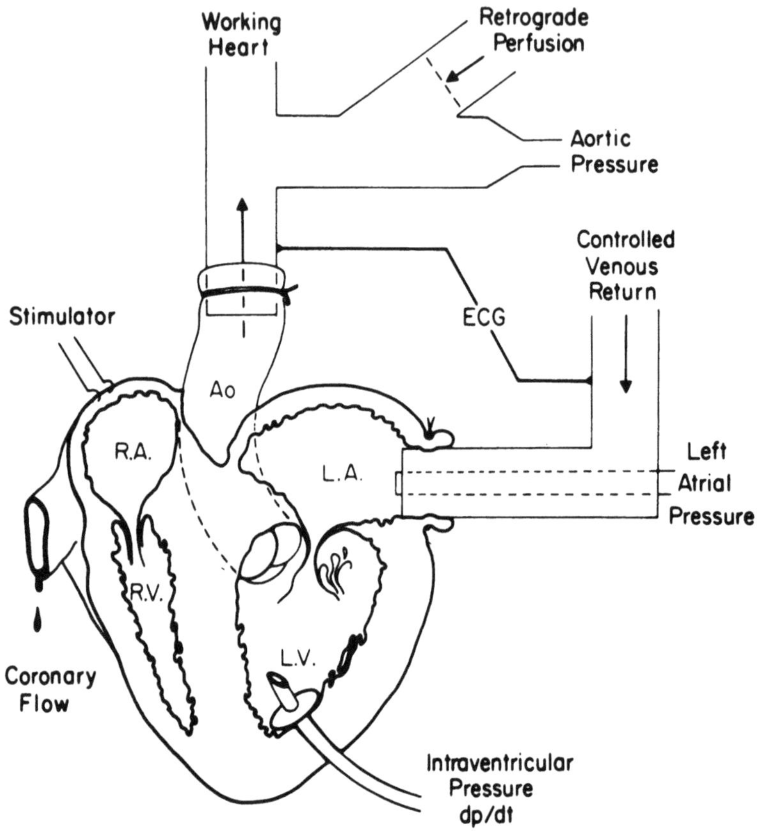

Figure 7. Flow scheme of the isolated work-performing and of the retrograde-perfused (Langendorff) heart preparations. In the work-performing heart, fluid flows from controlled venous return to left atrium (LA) to left ventricle (LV) through aorta (Ao) to Starling resistance ("working heart") and "coronary flow"; in the Langendorff preparation from "retrograde perfusion" to Ao to "coronary flow."

transducers, and the plastic heart chamber is put in place. A schematic flow diagram is presented in Figure 7.

Criteria for a good preparation to this point include regular beating, zero left atrial pressure, and a positive inotropic response when the left atrial bubble trap is turned on, i.e., venous return is started. The preparation up to this point should not have taken more than 10 min.

B. The Isolated Work-Performing Heart Preparation

The isolated work-performing heart preparation is initiated by clamping off the retrograde reservoir and opening the tubing to the aortic elastic recoil, the aortic resistance, and the left atrial bubble trap. Buffer entering the left atrium passes into the left ventricle, where ventricular contractions force the fluid through the aorta into the pressure chamber that is attached to the aortic cannula towards the aortic resistance (Starling resistance), where a "peripheral resistance" can

Table II. Recorded and Calculated Data from an Isolated, Work-Performing Heart Preparation[a]

Mechanical
* Arterial pressure; arterial pressure pulse; Starling resistance
* Intraventricular pressure; left ventricular end-diastolic pressure
* Intraventricular d*p*/d*t* (d*P*/d*t*), $dpdt_{max}$
Positive (contraction)
Negative (relaxation)
* Arterial d*p*/d*t*; mean arterial pressure
* Left atrial pressure; atrial pressure pulse
Heart rate (derived from EKG R–R interval or from pressure pulse)
* Aortic flow
* Coronary flow; coronary outflow, coronary resistance
* Constant, monitored venous return
Cardiac output: aortic flow + coronary flow
Total peripheral resistance (TPR): arterial *P*/cardiac output
Stroke volume: cardiac output/heart rate
Left ventricular work (kg): cardiac output × mean systemic pressure × 1.36 × 10^{-5}/dry weight of heart
Left ventricular stroke work: cardiac work/heart rate
* Contractile force with strain gauge arch; d*F*/d*t* of force
Electrical
* Electrogram; electrocardiogram
P–R interval: AV conduction time
QRS duration: spread of ventricular excitation
R–R interval: heart rate, heart rhythm
External pacing of atria and/or ventricles
Determination of excitability of heart: 1/stimulus strength
AV refractory period
Atrial and ventricular refractory period (interpolated beats)
Treppe; staircase; force–frequency relationship
Chemical
* ASTRUP: P_{O_2}; P_{CO_2}; pH
* Arteriovenous differences: O_2 consumption; substrate consumption; heat production

[a] Asterisks denote data recorded directly; other data are derived or calculated.

be adjusted with a micrometer screw clamp. Systolic aortic pressure should always exceed 50 mm Hg to guarantee sufficient coronary flow and perfusion pressure.

Aortic output can now be measured by closing the aortic output line at the bottom of the diagram in Figure 2 and observing the number of milliliters collected in 1 min. Coronary flow can either be collected for 1-min intervals in a graduated cylinder below the heart chamber or measured by weight with an electronic balance. All buffer collected can be returned to the oxygenation chamber for recycling. In most experiments, the buffer will be discarded.

The left atrial inflow (venous return) can be adjusted with another micrometer screw clamp so that there is an aortic output at the lowest possible atrial pressure.

Several tests of cardiac performance can be conducted with the isolated work performing heart (Table II).

In the *preload experiment*, venous return can be increased stepwise in small increments by opening the screw clamp on the venous return line. At each step, aortic pressure, intraventricular pressure, left atrial pressure, and d*p*/d*t* can be recorded, and aortic output and coronary flow can be measured. Increases in preload should be continued until cardiac output, d*p*/d*t*, and intraventricular pressure become constant or start to decline with each increase in mean left atrial pressure.

For the *afterload experiment*, the screw clamp on the left atrial inflow is set at a constant venous return. The afterload is produced by the screw clamp labeled "aortic resistance." This clamp is closed stepwise to produce small increases in intraventricular pressure. At each step, aortic output, coronary flow, and all pressure parameters (see above) are measured. The afterload is increased until the aortic output is reduced to only 1–2 ml/min. Thereafter, the afterload on the heart is released by gradually unscrewing the clamp until the control state is reestablished.

For an *aortic clamp experiment*, base-line aortic output and coronary flow measurements are made. Then, in the area just before the afterload clamp, the Tygon® tubing is occluded with a hemostat, which is left in place for 30–40 sec.

For *pacing experiments*, the atria are paced through the electrode clips connected to the metal cannulas with pulses of 0.5 msec duration and voltages 15% greater than threshold, usually 0.4–0.6 V, and varying frequencies. Since left atrial pressure, intraventricular pressure, d*p*/d*t*, aortic pressure, and sometimes contractile force are being recorded, the effectiveness of the heart's ability to follow a given pulse and the force/frequency relationship (staircase, *Treppe*) can be determined. Pacing is initiated at the natural frequency and slowly increased until impulses are being blocked at the AV node, at which point irregular beating occurs. The frequency is increased further until a 2 : 1 block is established and regular beating returned. Pacing frequency is increased further until irregularities again occur. At this time, the atria are no longer following the pace.

1. Measurements of Pressure and dp/dt

Pressures can be monitored by the use of the three Statham pressure transducers connected to low-level DC preamplifiers of polygraph recorders. The left atrial transducer (P-23 BC, range 0–50 mm Hg) should be calibrated with a water manometer on a full scale of 1–20 cm H_2O. The recording system, including the fluid-filled cannulas and catheters, should have a frequency response of at least 30 cps. Aortic and intraventricular pressures should be monitored with less sensitive pressure transducers (P-23 AC, range 0–750 mm Hg), which should be calibrated with a mercury manometer to full scales of 0–200 mm Hg. The recording system for the aortic pressure, including the fluid-filled cannulas and catheters, should have frequency responses of at least 40 cps with 2.5 ml of air in the pressure chamber. The intraventricular pressure system, including the fluid-filled cannula, should also have frequency response of the same magnitude. The degree of damping in each instance has to be determined empirically in order to obtain high-fidelity recordings.

If the frequency response is not satisfactory, different lengths and diameters of cannulas, catheters, or tubing should be tried until the appearance of the recorded pressure pulses is meaningful with respect to shape and responsiveness when abrupt changes are imposed on the heart. The volume of air in the pressure chamber plays an important role in the elasticity of the system. In our system, it was found that 2.5 ml of air was needed for the "best" pressure curves, but the elasticity provided by 2.5 ml of air was also an important factor in the overall ability of the heart to function, particularly for the maintenance of an effective coronary flow. With 1.0 ml of air in the pressure chamber, the heart showed marked deterioration before the experiment was completed. The illustrated system is overdamped with 1.0 ml of air and underdamped with 3.0 ml of air.

The first derivative of left ventricular pressure with respect to time (dp/dt) can be recorded by means of a linear differentiating circuit with a 1-msec time constant. A mercury manometer and a 502A dual-beam oscilloscope can be used for calibration of the signal.

Since mean left atrial pressure is used as the independent variable for most of the ventricular function curves, the reliability of this parameter is of primary concern. The transducer has to be carefully calibrated and rechecked frequently. It should be placed very near the heart and adjusted to the right height with a level. The zero reading must be checked again immediately following the establishment of the working heart experiment. If the zero has shifted more than 1.5 cm of H_2O, the working heart experiment should be discarded.

If the mitral valve is incompetent, the shape of the left atrial pressure waves changes, and intraventricular pressure becomes irregular.

2. *Measurement of Contractile Force and Contractility in Working Heart Preparations*

The working heart preparation offers the following parameters for the recording of contractile force and contractility: dp/dt derived from left ventricular pressure; Starling curves from left atrial pressure *vs.* cardiac output (coronary + aortic flow) or cardiac work (CO × aortic P); left ventricular and/or right ventricular contractile force and df/dt from strain gauge arches sewn to the free wall of the left and right ventricles; left and/or right ventricular volume from ultrasonic dimension crystals.

C. Retrograde Perfused Heart Preparations (Langendorff)

In some instances, most often when only information about responses of coronary flow is needed, the simpler Langendorff preparation is used. This preparation is also often used to prepare hearts for biochemical analysis. It should be recognized, however, that functional information is difficult to interpret in a nonworking heart preparation. Langendorff preparations may be marginally failing, yet the failure may not be recognized since neither atrial nor end-diastolic pressures are available for reference.

The Langendorff preparation can be established (see Figures 2 and 7) by closing the venous return and aortic resistance lines and opening the line to the retrograde reservoir. If a simple apparatus for retrograde perfusion of mammalian hearts is used, care has to be taken that the perfusion pressure, established by the height of the reservoir, remains constant all the time. This can only be achieved via a constant overflow in the reservoir and constant filling of the reservoir to keep the overflow going (see Figure 2, right panel). Constancy is also required for temperature, ion composition, P_{O_2}, P_{CO_2}, and pH. To avoid changing the perfusion fluids, drugs should be infused, using calibrated quantitative infusion pumps, just before the perfusion fluid enters the coronary system. Since coronary flow can be collected and measured and retrograde flow monitored with an electromagnetic flow meter, the exact molar concentration of infused drugs or infused ions (e.g., Ca^{2+} or K^{+}) can be calculated. Use of different concentrations of perfusate, different sizes of syringes, and different settings of the rate of volume delivery with the Harvard infusion pump allows a quantitative drug delivery over any desired range. The advantage of this approach is that drug delivery can be begun and ended cleanly without changing solutions and that all experimental parameters can be maintained on a constant level.

1. Measurement of Contractile Force and Contractility in Retrograde-Perfused Langendorff Heart Preparations

To record quantitative changes of contractile force in Langendorff preparations is more involved than in working heart preparations except when strain gauge arches sewn to the right and/or left ventricular wall are used to record isometric force and its derivative df/dt. In this case, a part of the right and/or left ventricular wall is stretched by the sutures fixing the strain gauge to the wall. This creates nearly isometric conditions to record contractile force and df/dt under close to quantitative conditions. No quantitative information can be derived from force measurements by connecting the apex of the heart to a force transducer, since it is not possible to create an isometric condition using the whole heart. Consequently, contractions recorded from the apex contain spatial movements of all ventricular walls in several directions, obviating any quantitative or even qualitative basis of measurements of contractile force.

Information on dp/dt from left ventricular pressure recordings can be used, but not without reservations. Catheter-tip balloons may or may not be an advantage. If the balloons fill the entire left ventricle, endocardiac compression of coronary supply is possible, and a false compliance (balloon) is added to one of the ventricles. If the balloon does not fill the ventricle volume, changes outside the balloon can occur with consequent changes in transmural balloon pressure. In addition, introduction of the balloon either can interfere with a valve or requires a major opening of the ventricular wall.

On the other hand, volume changes may occur with dp/dt is continuously recorded from a left ventricular pressure catheter without the use of a balloon. However, if these changes occur, they will be visible on the record as seen in the

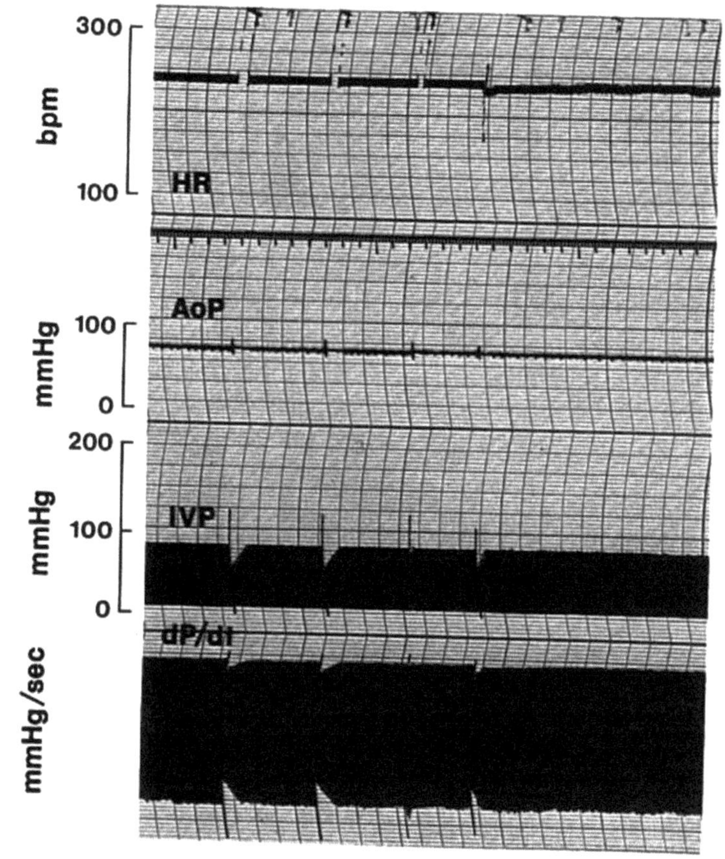

Figure 8. Accidental ventricular volume changes produced by extra systoles in the isolated guinea pig heart. HR, heart rate; AoP, aortic pressure; IVP, left ventricular pressure; d*P*/d*t*, differentiated IVP. Time in sec. Note four extra systoles in HR, IVP, and d*P*/d*t* record. The change produced by the extra systoles was corrected within less than 8 sec.

example in Figure 8. The record also will give an indication of whether the consequences of the volume change are or are not corrected within a few heart beats. We have found that in more than 95% of our preparations d*p*/d*t* could be recorded without a balloon with great reliability, and good information could be derived. In a few exceptions, the aortic valve did leak, and, therefore, the preparation had to be discarded. The leak was in all cases easily identified. The leak would also have interfered in the presence of a balloon. On the other hand, we frequently had difficulties with balloon-tipped catheters, even in preparations with easy installation and insertion of the balloons. It was our impression that small changes in contractile force could not be picked up quantitatively through the balloon recording, and we lost signals of positive inotropic effects that could be observed well with an unencumbered ventricle.

ACKNOWLEDGMENTS

Original work of the authors cited in this survey was supported in part by grants from the American Heart Association, Southwestern Ohio Chapter, and by NIH Program Project Grant PO1 HL 22619.

REFERENCES

Blinks, J. R. 1965. Convenient apparatus for recording contractions of isolated heart muscle. *J. Appl. Physiol.*, *20*:755–757.

Carrier, G. O., Luellmann, H., Neubauer, L., and Peters, T. 1974. The significance of a fast exchanging superficial calcium fraction for the regulation of contractile force in heart muscle. *J. Mol. Cell. Cardiol.*, *6*:333–347.

Grupp, G., Grupp, I., Johnson, C. L., Wallick, E. T., and Schwartz, A. 1979. Effects of vanadate on cardiac contraction and adenylate cyclase. *Biochem. Biophys. Res. Commun.*, *88*:440–447.

Grupp, G., Grupp, I. L., Ghysel-Burton, J., Godfraind, T., and Schwartz, A. 1982. Effects of very low concentrations of ouabain on contractile force of isolated guinea-pig, rabbit, and cat atria and right ventricular papillary muscles: An interinstitutional study. *J. Pharmacol. Exp. Ther.*, *220*:145–151.

Grupp, I. L., Grupp, G., and Schwartz, A. 1981. Digitalis-receptor desensitization in rat ventricle: Ouabain produces two inotropic effects. *Life Sci.*, *29*:2789–2794.

Johnson, J., and Grupp, G. 1980. Relationship between the positive inotropic effect of histamine and stimulation of cardiac adenylate cyclase in different species. *Fed. Proc.*, *39*:314.

Koch-Weser, J., and Blinks, J. R. 1963. The influence of the interval between beats on myocardial contractility. *Pharmacol. Rev.*, *15*:601–652.

Levy, J. V. 1971. Isolated atrial preparations. In: *Methods in Pharmacology*, pp. 77–104. Ed. by Schwartz, A. Appleton-Century-Crofts, New York.

McNeill, J. H., and Verma, S. C. 1979. Cardiac histamine receptors and cyclic AMP. Differences between guinea pig and rabbit heart. In: *Histamine Receptors*, pp. 271–284. Ed. by Yellin, T. O. Spectrum Publications, Jamaica, New York.

Neely, J. R., Liebermeister, H., Battersby, E. J., and Morgan, H. E. 1967. Effect of pressure development on oxygen consumption by isolated rat heart. *Am. J. Physiol.*, *212*:804–814.

Ringer, S. 1883. A further contribution regarding the influence of the different constituents of the blood on the contraction of the heart. *J. Physiol.* (*Lond.*) *4*:29–42.

Wiester, M. J., Bonventre, P. F., and Grupp, G. 1973. Estimate of myocardial damage induced by diphtheria toxin. *J. Lab. Clin. Med.*, *81*:354–364.

Chapter **10**

Derived Indices of Myocardial Function in Isolated Work-Performing Hearts

Gunter Grupp

Departments of Pharmacology and Cell Biophysics,
Physiology, and Internal Medicine (Division of Cardiology)
University of Cincinnati College of Medicine
Cincinnati, Ohio

I. INTRODUCTION

Quantitative measurements of the status of myocardial function and of changes in function produced by experimental conditions or agents are difficult to obtain. The difficulties increase when heart-to-heart comparisons are required. Clinically, the introduction and improvement of cardiac catheterization, electro- and echocardiography, and real-time radioopaque and radionuclide imaging have lessened the difficulty of this task somewhat. In animal experiments, greater quantitation has been attempted by direct measurements of pressures and their rates of change in most vessels and cavities of the heart and the circulatory system. Strain gauge arches and ultrasonic dimension crystals have been used to quantitate isometric force development (F), including rate change (dF/dt), and to accurately and directly determine wall thickness changes and diameter changes of heart chambers. In addition, information about isotonic contraction, velocity of contractile element shortening, velocity of circumferential fiber shortening, and maximum velocity of shortening can be obtained. Accurate and convenient flow and combined flow (cardiac output) measurements are possible. This information allows reliable calculation of preload and afterload, ventricular volumes and their changes, atrial and ventricular end-diastolic pressures, cardiac output, and stroke volume for a meaningful construction of Starling function curves. Calculations can be done of compliance of the heart (dP/dV), the modulus of elasticity during contraction (d*P*/d*l*), the velocity of shortening of the contractile element (V_{CE}), ejection fraction of the heart (*SV*/*EDV*), power (velocity × aortic *P*), acceleration of ejection of blood, and cardiac work (*SV* × aortic *P*).

Most indices of cardiac function are obtained at rest. In order to gain insight into the total range of cardiac function of an individual heart, particularly the limits to which it can be loaded and the maximal work it can perform, separate experiments with alterations of preload and of afterload should be conducted to assess the limits of the myocardial functional reserve available in an individual heart. Preload and afterload experiments are required, since it is well known that the volume work done during preload changes and the pressure work done during afterload changes put very different strains on the heart. In energetic terms, pressure load is about two to three times more expensive than volume load (see Figure 5 below).

II. ISOLATED HEART PREPARATIONS

The methods used and the apparatus required for a working heart preparation are described in detail elsewhere in this book (Chapter 9). In brief, it is necessary to protect the heart before and during the original preparations by light anesthesia with an anesthetic (e.g., pentobarbital) that can be easily washed out from the isolated heart, by preoperative heparinization with 5000 U or 5000 U/kg heparin i.p., and by artificial respiration with room air ± O_2 throughout the procedure. At the time of separation of the heart and transfer to the isolated perfusion apparatus, the aorta should be cannulated with a cannula connected to a perfusion reservoir filled with warm oxygenated Krebs–Henseleit Solution (KHS). A slow flow of KHS should be started before insertion of the cannula into the aorta, the opening of the cannula pointing towards the heart. At the moment of insertion, the venae cavae should be tied and then cut in order to begin retrograde perfusion of the coronary system of the heart to wash out blood, anesthetics, and other residues.

The heart can then be transferred to the working heart apparatus. One strain gauge arch each can be sewn to the free walls of the left and right ventricles. Since quantitative heart-to-heart comparisons of the status of cardiac function are intended, the stretch of ventricular myocardium and the placement of the strain gauge should be similar from experiment to experiment. Preliminary experiments with different measured ligature distances will be required to obtain an approximate length–tension curve. The ligature distance close to but just below the stretch producing maximum active tension (L_{max}) should be used for all experiments. It is best to first affix the threads used for the ligatures in an accurately measured distance to the preselected location of the ventricular wall. The strain gauge can then be attached and tested. To test the responsiveness of the strain gauge, extrasystoles can be initiated by irritating the ventricles with a probe. Special attention is required for calibrating and maintaining calibration of ultrasonic dimension crystals. Care has to be taken to avoid cross interference between electromagnetic flow probe and ultrasonic dimension crystal signals.

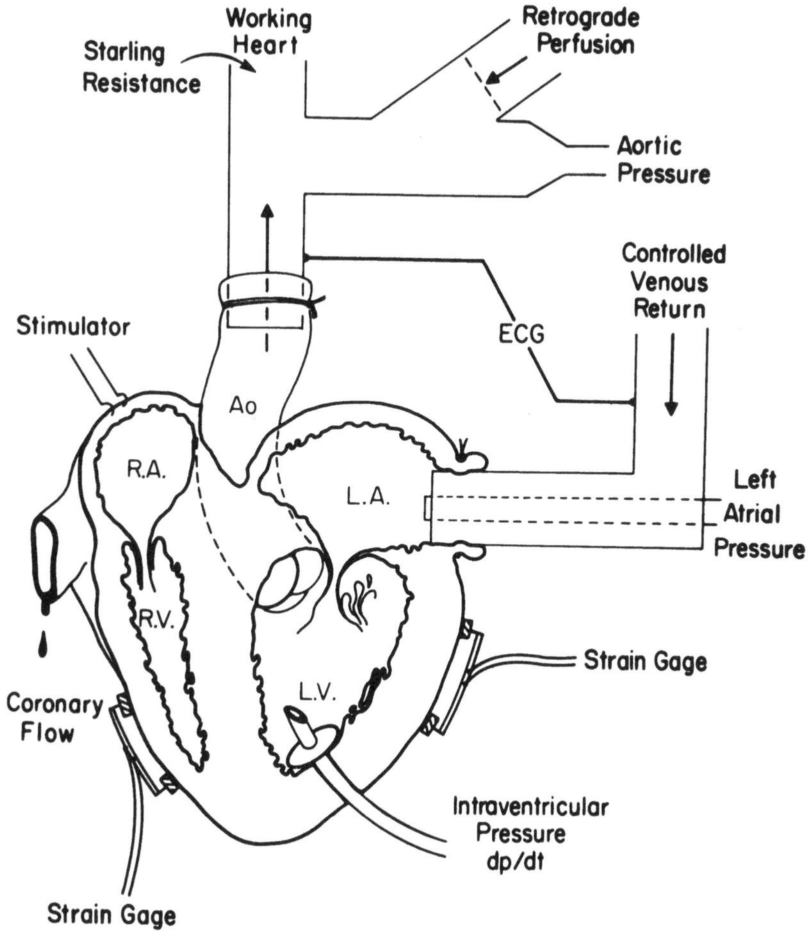

Figure 1. Schematic diagram of an isolated work-performing heart preparation. LA, RA, left or right atrium; LV, RV, left or right ventricle; Ao, aorta.

It is of great importance to pay attention to the quantitative aspects of calibration of pressure and force transducers and their differentiating circuits. The same is true for the electromagnetic flow meters and the devices used to measure collected flows (electronic balance, graduated collector).

III. EXPERIMENTAL APPROACH

The flow scheme of the isolated work-performing heart preparation is depicted in Figure 1. Well-oxygenated (Po_2 about 500; Pco_2 about 35; pH 7.5) Krebs–Henseleit solution at constant temperature (usually 30, 35, or 37°C) enters the left atrium via the cannula labeled "controlled venous return." The "venous return" is maintained constant by a finger pump regulated via a micrometer adjuster (preload adjusted) and an overflow and is continuously monitored by an electromagnetic flowmeter. Left atrial pressure is monitored through the venous return cannula with a low-range Statham pressure transducer (P-23 BC, 0–50 mm Hg range) and recorded with a low-level DC preamp on a full scale of 0–20 cm H_2O. Left ventricular pressure and aortic pressure are recorded through high-range Statham pressure transducers (P-23 AC, 0–750 mm Hg range) on a full scale of 0–200 mm Hg.

Flow continues to the left ventricle and is expelled as cardiac output through the aortic valve into the aorta. One part of cardiac output perfuses the coronary system and exits the heart through the open pulmonary artery to be collected and measured as "coronary flow." If O_2 consumption or substrate consumption of the beat should be measured, the "flow" can be collected through tubing tied into the pulmonary artery in a beaker under mineral oil. "Flow" can then be measured by the increase in weight of the beaker recorded from an electronic balance with digital readout. The other part of the cardiac output enters the elastic recoil (*Windkessel*) chamber where 2.5 ml of air provides the necessary "arterial" elasticity and recoil to maintain coronary flow throughout diastole. Flow then continues through an adjustable micrometer (aortic resistance, Starling resistance), which produces the afterload or peripheral resistance. The variable coronary and the constant Starling resistance form the total peripheral resistance. Coronary flow plus aortic flow equals cardiac output. Cardiac output and venous return should be identical; if not, the system has a leak. Furthermore, aortic and mitral valves must be fully functioning. Patency and tight closure can be tested by clamping the aortic catheter.

Left intraventricular pressure and its first derivative d*p*/d*t* are measured through flanged thin polyethylene tubing (PE90) that is inserted through the left pulmonary vein entering the left atrium and forwarded into the left ventricle at the time the mitral valve is open. The PE90 catheter is then forced through the apical wall of the left ventricle. The flanged end of the catheter then rests against the inner wall of the ventricle and holds the catheter in place. The advantages and disadvantages of recording d*p*/d*t* from this arrangement instead of from a balloon-tipped catheter are discussed elsewhere in this book (Chapter 9).

The left atrial and aortic cannulas are constructed from stainless steel and can, therefore, be used to record a lead I type EKG from the heart. The R-waves of the EKG can be used to instantaneously compute heart rate for a write-out on the polygraph recording all other parameters. The same electrodes, if a stimulus isolation unit is in the circuit, can serve as an external pacemaker.

A. Poststimulation and Postextrasystolic Potentiation: Staircase, Treppe, Paired Stimulation

Information about the status of cardiac function can be derived from the observation of the response of the force–frequency relationship by observing force and altering frequency. Maximum achievable contractile force can be observed with paired stimulation (Figure 2). With use of two interrelated stimulators, the frequency of stimulator 1 (S_1; 1 per sec, 1.0-sec stimulus interval, 60 beats per

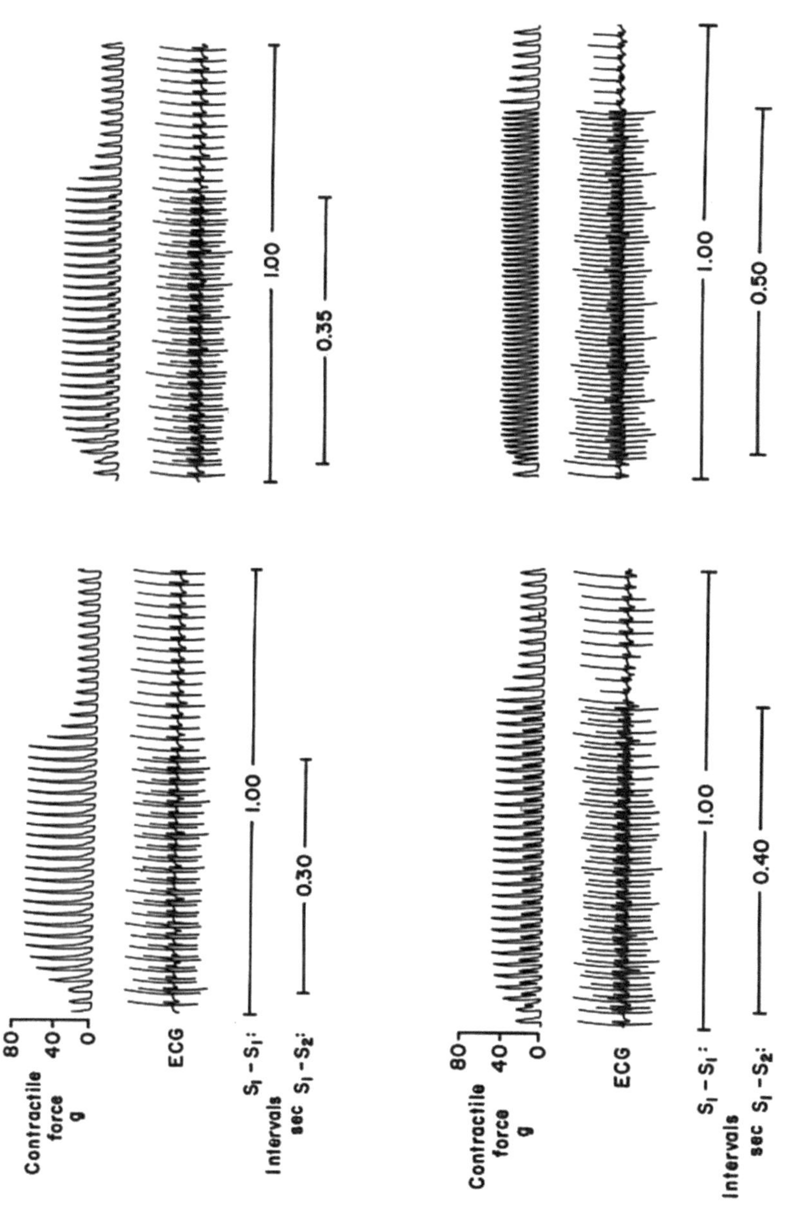

Figure 2. Effects of changes in intervals of stimuli on contractile force of the isolated heart. Strain gauge record of contractile force and placement of stimuli visible on ECG record. Constant S_1S_1 basal rate produced by stimulator 1. Intervals in sec S_1–S_2: use of stimulator 2 to shorten interval between S_1 and S_2 from 0.5 sec to 0.3 sec.

min) can be doubled by interposing another stimulus (S_2) from another stimulator exactly between two stimuli of S_1 (Figure 2, lower right corner), resulting in a rate of 120 bpm (0.5-sec stimulus interval). The higher frequency of 120 bpm leads to a higher contractile force, which is reached stepwise (staircase). When S_2 is terminated, poststimulation potentiation occurs (1 beat), and the staircase occurs in descending order. When S_2 is moved closer to S_1, from 0.5 sec to 0.4 sec (Figure 2, left lower corner), a stronger potentiation occurs, exceeding the staircase. By closing to 0.35 and 0.30 sec (Figure 2, right and left upper corners), maximum potentiation is achieved. In another experiment (Figure 3, upper record), maximum potentiation is achieved with 0.25- and 0.24-sec S_1–S_2 intervals. However, at 0.23 sec, the functional refractory period is approached, and at 0.22 it is completely reached, because the S_2 stimulus could no longer excite the ventricle. In still another experiment (Figure 3, lower record), S_1 interval of 1.0 sec is changed to 0.5 sec; staircase and an increased contractile force follow. S_2 interpolation to 0.22 sec produces maximum potentiation, which remains maximal to 0.19 sec. Functional refractory period under this condition is 0.18 sec.

To test the force–frequency (staircase) response in isolated hearts with higher frequencies, it is useful to stimulate the heart even during the control period at a slightly higher frequency than the basal heart rate. Stimulating at a lower frequency might produce irregularities. From the stimulated baseline, frequency should be increased by 0.5 cps for each step for 1 min until no or a negative response occurs. This should be followed by reduction in frequency by the same steps in reverse order.

B. Pressure and Volume Work as an Index for Myocardial Performance

In an isolated heart preparation equilibrated for 30 to 60 min, the test of the upper and lower limits of pressure and volume load should begin at the low end of the range. In all species, the lowest pressure should be just above 50 mm Hg aortic systolic pressure. The venous return (volume) must be different for different species: guinea pig heart (15–30 ml/min); rat heart (10–25); rabbit heart (30–60 ml/min); small cat heart (30–60 ml/min). These values are approximations; they may be different in some hearts. The example in this section is the isolated work-performing rabbit heart equilibrated for 30 min.

Venous return (volume) was first adjusted to about 30–35 ml/min. Following this, aortic resistance was adjusted to a systolic pressure of 52 mm Hg. At this point, the venous return measured with the electromagnetic flow meter has to equal the sum of coronary flow and aortic flow (cardiac output), indicating that there is no leak in the preparation. Figure 4 indicates some of the parameters recorded. From top to bottom (initial values in parentheses): heart rate or EKG (here, heart rate, 145 bpm); aortic pressure (here, 52/16, mean 40 mm Hg); left intraventricular pressure (here 54/0 mm Hg); + and − dp/dt (here + 800 mm Hg/sec during contraction and −700 mm Hg/sec during relaxation); left atrial pressure (here 3 cm H_2O); venous return flow (here 41 ml/min); cardiac output (40.5 ml/min). Cardiac power at the beginning is $40 \times 40.5 = 1620$ mm Hg × ml/min, and intraventricular pressure development (dP/dt) is 800 mm Hg/sec.

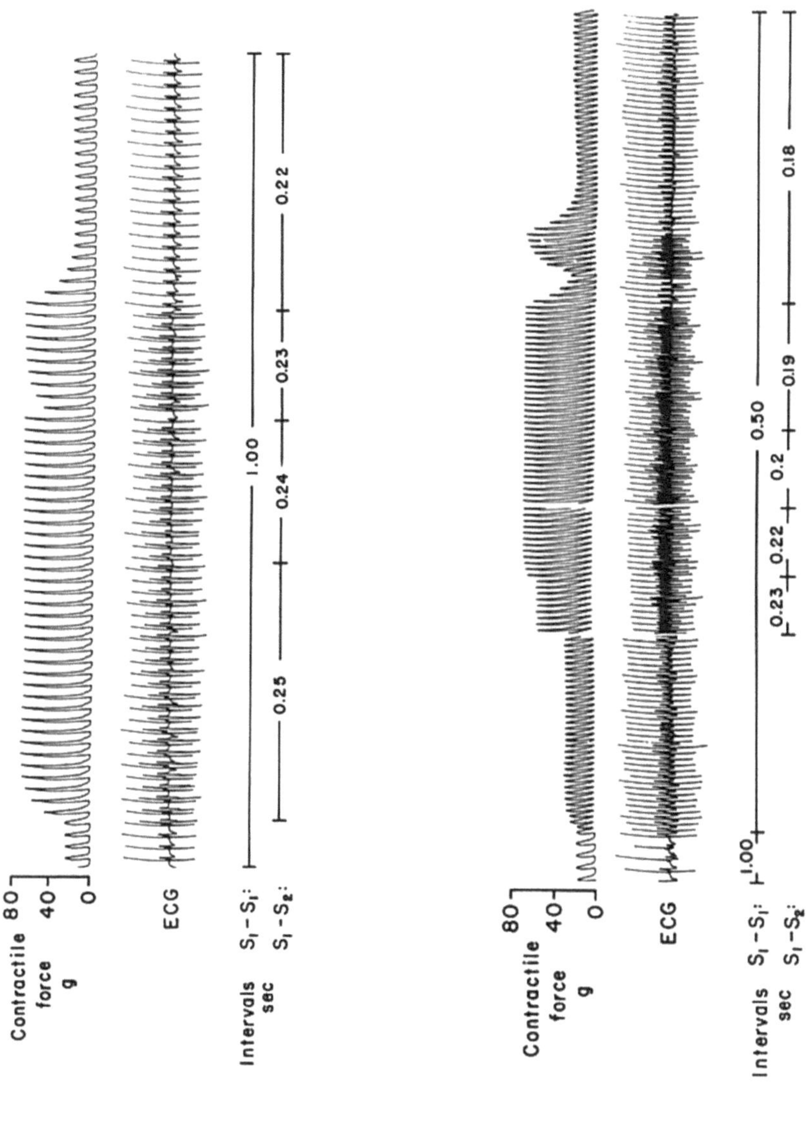

Figure 3. Same arrangement as Figure 2. Basal interval in lower record changed from 1.0 to 0.5 sec.

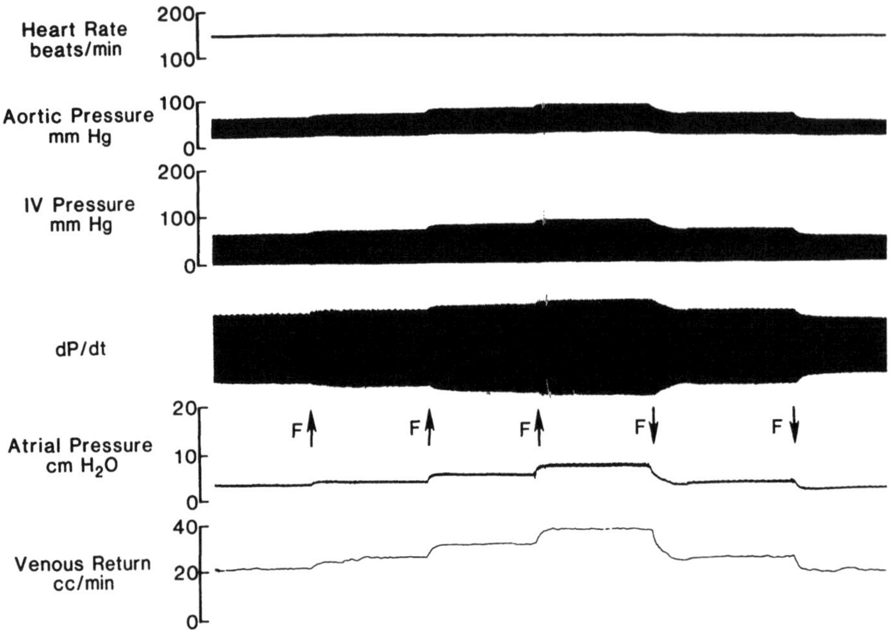

Figure 4. Original record of a volume-load experiment in an isolated work-performing rabbit heart. Record from top: EKG or heart rate tachograph; time; aortic pressure; intraventricular *P*; left ventricular d*P*/d*t*; left atrial *P*; venous return flow.

Also recorded (but not shown here) are left and right ventricular contractile force from two strain gauge arches and the force developments during contraction and relaxation (d*f*/d*t*).

The range of volume work the heart is able to perform is now tested with manipulations of the venous return adjuster, increasing and decreasing the volume stepwise for 1 min each as shown in Figure 4. After reequilibration for 10 min, the pressure load capability of the heart is tested: venous return is kept constant, but the aortic resistance (afterload) is now manipulated (Figure 5). Resistance is increased stepwise until aortic flow becomes zero and is then decreased to the original resistance.

Heart rate was constant in our examples (Figures 4 and 5) during both load experiments (145 bpm); therefore, stroke volume changed with venous return in the volume experiment but did not change in the pressure experiment. Aortic flow rose in the volume experiment from 23 to 38 ml/min, and coronary flow from 18 to 47 ml/min. In the pressure experiment, aortic flow fell from 23 to 0, whereas coronary flow rose from 18 to 40 ml/min.

The power developed in the volume experiment ranged from 1620 to 5600 mm Hg × ml/min, and in the pressure experiment from 1620 to 2800 mm Hg × ml/min. The possible power range in the example heart was 4100 mm Hg × ml/min in volume load and only 1300 mm Hg × ml/min in pressure load. However, the left ventricular rate of pressure development was about equal for both loads: 1150 to 2000 mm Hg/sec in volume load and 1150 to 1900 mm Hg/sec in pressure load.

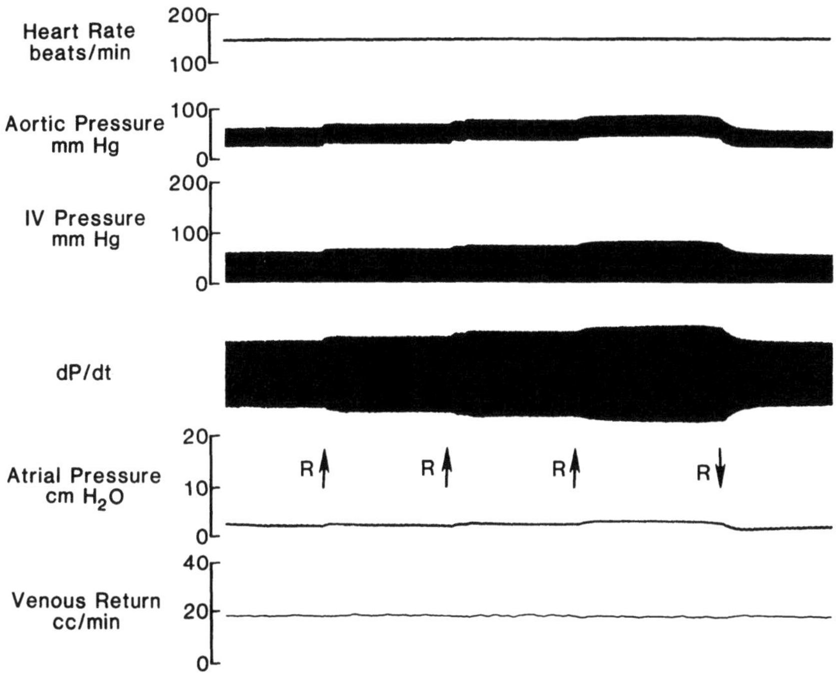

Figure 5. Same as Figure 4 but pressure-load experiment.

In other words, this rabbit heart handled an increment of work of 4100 mm Hg × ml/min produced by volume load with a increment of 850 d*P*/d*t* mm Hg/sec or a rate of 20.73 d*P*/d*t* per power [mm Hg/sec/(mm Hg × ml/min) × 100]. The heart handled the pressure load with a d*P*/d*t* per power rate of 57.7. To move the same load required, therefore, 2.8 times more power in pressure than in volume load.

In Figure 6,the dp/dt_{max} during contraction and during relaxation are plotted against the power developed in a volume-load experiment. Load was changed from 600 to 5400 mm Hg × ml/min. It is clear that in this heart only the power between 1400 and 3800 mm Hg × ml/min showed a linear relationship to d*p*/d*t*; below 1400 there was a steep falloff of power, probably caused by a compromise of coronary flow (systolic aortic pressure was below 50 mm Hg), and above 3800 the isolated heart could no longer increase power: it became overloaded (high left atrial pressure). The linear volume power increment was 2400 mm Hg × ml/min, achieved at a d*P*/d*t* increment of 460 mm Hg/sec, giving a d*P*/d*t* per power rate of 19.09 during contraction. It is of interest to see that the rate of relaxation changed by a similar order of magnitude as the rate of contraction.

Figure 7 depicts the linear part of the d*P*/d*t* per power relationship in still another rabbit heart. The pressure work load was terminated when aortic flow ceased; the volume load was only extended to the work load performed during pressure load. The d*P*/d*t* rate per power developed by this heart during volume load was 16.7 and during pressure load 33.6, indicating that twice the d*P*/d*t* per power rate was required to do pressure work than volume work.

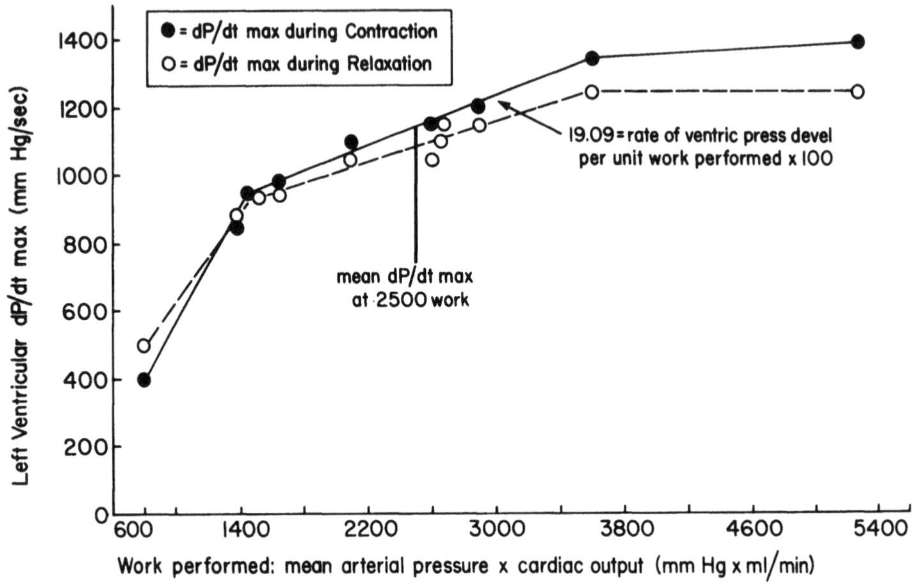

Figure 6. d*P*/d*t* per relationship during contraction (filled symbols) and relaxation (open symbols) in a volume-load experiment in an isolated work-performing rabbit heart.

There are many other ways to estimate or quantitate or semiquantitate the quality of myocardial function. Most methods select a static moment during cardiac action to "freeze" that state to represent myocardial function. Starling function curves, although taking several of the "moments" into consideration, do not have reference points allowing heart-to-heart comparison. In asking for the quality

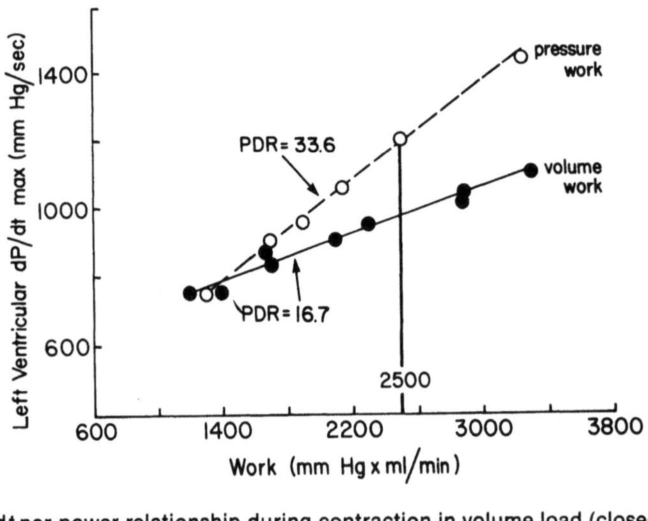

Figure 7. d*P*/d*t* per power relationship during contraction in volume load (closed symbols) and pressure load (open symbols).

of myocardial function, one asks for the complete range of work performance a heart can go through. This information is amplified when two, instead of one, load types can be obtained. The numerical expression of the rate of ventricular power development per rate of work performed during volume work and during pressure work gives a simple but reliable measure of the actual functional state a heart is in and allows a heart-to-heart comparison of their ability to do two different kinds of work.

ACKNOWLEDGMENTS

Original work of the author cited in this survey was supported in part by grants from the American Heart Association, Southwestern Ohio Chapter, and by NIH Program Project Grant PO1 HL 22619. Appreciation is expressed to Mr. Tim Hickerson for valuable suggestions.

REFERENCE

Sonnenblick, E. H., and Strobeck, J. E. 1977. Current concepts in cardiology. *N. Engl. J. Med.*, *296*:978–982.

Chapter 11

Isolation and Characterization of Plasma Lipoproteins and Apolipoproteins

Alan D. Cardin, George Holdsworth, and Richard L. Jackson

Division of Lipoprotein Research
Department of Pharmacology and Cell Biophysics
University of Cincinnati College of Medicine
Cincinnati, Ohio

I. INTRODUCTION

The plasma lipoproteins are the major carriers of lipid in the circulation. Structurally, these particles represent a microemulsion of triglyceride and cholesteryl ester stabilized by a polar surface of phospholipid, cholesterol, and protein (Bradley and Gotto, 1978; Morrisett *et al.*, 1977). Four major classes of plasma lipoproteins have been designated on the basis of their ultracentrifugal flotation properties in salt solutions. These are the chylomicrons, very-low-density lipoproteins (VLDL), low-density lipoproteins (LDL), and high-density lipoproteins (HDL). Chylomicrons and VLDL float at $d < 1.006$ g/ml. The LDL are isolated between $d = 1.02$ and 1.063 g/ml, and HDL between $d = 1.063$ to 1.210 g/ml. Although the classification based on ultracentrifugation in salt solutions has proven to be a useful nomenclature, each of these density ranges actually contains a complex mixture of lipoproteins of varying protein and lipid composition. The physical and chemical properties of human plasma lipoproteins are summarized in Table I. Chylomicrons and VLDL contain primarily triglycerides as their neutral lipid, whereas LDL and HDL are the major carriers of cholesteryl esters and phospholipids.

Present address for George Holdsworth: Oak Ridge Research Institute, Oak Ridge, Tennessee.

Table I. Physical Chemical Properties of the Human Plasma Lipoproteins

Properties	Chylomicrons	VLDL	LDL	HDL
Electrophoretic mobility	Origin	Pre-β	β	α
Solvent density isolation	1.006	1.006	1.019–1.063	1.063–1.210
Flotation rate				
S_f (1.063 g/ml)	400	20–400	0–12	—
S_f (1.21 g/ml)	—	—	—	4–9, 0–4
Molecular weight	>4 × 10^8	5 × 10^6	2.7 × 10^6	1.8–3.9 × 10^5
Diameter (Å)	750–2000	250–750	200–225	40–140

The metabolism of plasma lipoproteins has been summarized in several recent reviews (Jackson *et al.*, 1976; Smith *et al.*, 1978). Chylomicrons are synthesized in the intestine, whereas VLDL are of hepatic origin. Most plasma LDL are derived from the metabolism of VLDL; HDL are synthesized in both the liver and the intestine. Each lipoprotein class contains specific proteins, termed apoproteins (apo). The major apoproteins of each class are given in Table II. Apoprotein B and apoA-I are the major protein constituents of chylomicrons. The major protein in VLDL and LDL is also apoB. Recent information suggests that chylomicrons have a different form of apoB than VLDL and LDL. As described by Kane *et al.* (1980), the approximate molecular weight of the apoB in chylomicrons is 264,000, whereas that in VLDL and LDL is 549,000. In addition to apoB, chylomicrons and VLDL contain the C apoproteins (apoC-I, apoC-II, apoC-III).

Table II. The Chemical Compositions of the Human Plasma Lipoproteins

Composition (weight %)	Chylomicrons	VLDL	LDL	HDL
Lipid				
Triglyceride	84	50	11	4
Cholesterol, unesterified	2	7	8	4
Cholesterol, esterified	7	12	37	14
Phospholipid	7	18	22	25
Protein	2	8	21	48
Major apoproteins	ApoB ApoA-I ApoA-II ApoA-IV	ApoB ApoC-I ApoC-II ApoC-III ApoE	ApoB	ApoA-I ApoA-II
Minor apoproteins	ApoC-I ApoC-II ApoC-III ApoE	ApoA-I ApoA-II	ApoE ApoC-I ApoC-II ApoC-III	ApoA-IV ApoC-I ApoC-II ApoC-III ApoD ApoE

The major apoproteins in human HDL are apoA-I and apoA-II; HDL also contain apoE and the C apoproteins as minor constituents. The amino acid sequences of human apoA-I (Brewer *et al.*, 1978), apoA-II (Brewer *et al.*, 1972), apoC-I (Jackson *et al.*, 1974), apoC-II (Jackson *et al.*, 1977), apoC-III (Brewer *et al.*, 1974), and apoE (Rall *et al.*, 1982) are known; the structure of apoB has not been determined to date.

As the apoproteins influence the function and metabolism of the human plasma lipoproteins, it becomes important to understand the structural basis of their actions. However, such an undertaking first requires their purification. The aim of this chapter is to describe the detailed procedures for the isolation of milligram quantities of human plasma apolipoproteins with particular emphasis placed on the isolation of apoA-I, A-II, B, C-I, C-II, and E. The methods used for the isolation of these proteins are, in general, those routinely employed in the authors' laboratory.

II. PLASMA COLLECTION AND STORAGE

There are a number of chemical preservatives that investigators add to plasma during collection and storage to inhibit degradation. In our experience, we have routinely added EDTA, PMSF, aprotinin, and sodium azide to plasma at final concentrations of 1 m*M*, 0.5 m*M*, 50 units/ml, and 0.01%, respectively. The purpose of PMSF and aprotinin is to inhibit proteolysis, whereas the sodium azide inhibits bacterial and fungal growth; EDTA inhibits oxidative bond cleavage of peptide bonds and lipid peroxidation reactions catalyzed by trace metal impurities. Once the purified lipoproteins are isolated from plasma, they are stored in a standard buffer of plasma density (PDB) consisting of 10 m*M* tris-HCl, pH 7.4, 0.9% NaCl, 0.01% NaN_3, and 1 m*M* EDTA.

III. ISOLATION AND CHARACTERIZATION OF PLASMA LIPOPROTEINS

A number of procedures are available for the large-scale isolation of human plasma lipoproteins, including precipitation with heparin, ultracentrifugation in salt solutions, and gel filtration chromatography. The classical method for lipoprotein fractionation is based on the procedure of Havel, Eder, and Bragdon (1955) and involves ultracentrifugation at fixed densities of NaBr or KBr. Chylomicrons and VLDL (triglyceride-rich lipoproteins) are fractionated at plasma density $d <$ 1.006 g/ml, LDL at d = 1.006–1.063 g/ml, and HDL at d = 1.063–1.21 g/ml. The amount of KBr in grams required to adjust plasma of density d_i to a final density d_f for lipoprotein fractionation is given by the formula:

$$g(KBr) = V(d_f - d_i)/[1 - 0.364(d_f)]$$

where V is the total volume of plasma in milliliters, d is the density in grams per milliliter, and the numerical factor 0.364 is the partial specific volume of KBr.

For the isolation of large quantities of lipoproteins, a fixed-angle rotor has proved to be the most convenient method. Typically, a Beckman 45 Ti rotor, which accommodates six tubes holding 60 ml each of plasma (d = 1.006 g/ml), is subjected to ultracentrifugation at 42,000 rpm for 18 hr at 8°C. After centrifugation, the top layer containing chylomicrons and VLDL, which have a cream-like appearance, are removed by aspiration. If the subject is hypertriglyceridemic (plasma triglycerides > 1000 mg/dl), a gel of lipoprotein may form at the top of the tube. A convenient method for removing this gel is first to remove any solution from the top of the gel and then to remove the gel itself by scraping with a spatula. Any chylomicrons and VLDL remaining in the clear zone at the top of the tube are removed by aspiration and saved. The infranatant fraction is then removed along with any pelleted lipoproteins of d > 1.006 g/ml. The infranatant fraction plus pelleted lipoproteins are resuspended at 4°C, and KBr is added to give a final density of 1.063 g/ml.

The LDL are isolated by recentrifugation in a 45 Ti rotor for 20 hr at 42,000 rpm at 8°C. After ultracentrifugation, the LDL form an orange-colored band at the top; these lipoproteins are removed by aspiration. The clear zone between the top fraction and the infranatant fraction is removed by aspiration and may be discarded. Next, the infranatant fraction is removed and adjusted to d = 1.210 with solid KBr. The solution is placed in a Ti 50.2 centrifuge tube (20 ml) and overlaid with 3 ml of PDB previously adjusted to d = 1.21 g/ml with KBr. The HDL are isolated by ultracentrifugation in a Beckman 50.2 Ti rotor for 24 hr at 50,000 rpm at 8°C. After centrifugation, the HDL, which form an orange-colored band at the top, are removed by aspiration and dialyzed against PDB.

In general, the apoCs and apoE are isolated from triglyceride-rich lipoproteins, the high-molecular-weight apoB from LDL, the low-molecular-weight apoB from chylomicrons, and apoA-I and apoA-II from HDL. Prior to the isolation of these apoproteins, each specific lipoprotein class must be refractionated. Typically, the triglyceride-rich lipoproteins are subjected to recentrifugation at plasma density (d = 1.006 g/ml) as described above. The fraction corresponding to d = 1.006–1.063 g/ml is adjusted to d = 1.02 g/ml and subjected again to centrifugation. The LDL are recovered and then isolated by recentrifugation at d = 1.050 g/ml. Similarly, the HDL fraction is reisolated between d = 1.063 and 1.21 g/ml. All lipoproteins should be stored at 4°C in PDB and used within one month of preparation.

IV. PREPARATION AND CHARACTERIZATION OF WATER-SOLUBLE APOLIPOPROTEIN B FROM HUMAN PLASMA LOW-DENSITY LIPOPROTEINS AND CHYLOMICRONS

Currently, little information is available concerning the lipid transport properties of apolipoprotein B (apoB), the major apoprotein of chylomicrons, VLDL, and LDL. Attempts to understand the structural basis of its role in lipoprotein assembly, secretion, and metabolism have been largely unsuccessful because of the poor aqueous solubility and aggregational properties of this apoprotein in the lipid-free state. The presence of detergents, denaturants, or other proteins used to solubilize and disaggregate apoB complicates its sequence analysis. The structural complexity of apoB is further emphasized by the presence of two major forms of this apoprotein in plasma, which have different physiological roles and molecular sizes but closely related chemical compositions and immunologic properties (Kane *et al.*, 1980). In the nomenclature of Kane *et al.* (1980), these apoproteins are the apoB-100 of VLDL and LDL (M_r = 549,000) and the apoB-48 of chylomicrons (M_r = 264,000). The purpose of this section is to describe methods for purifying apoB-100 and apoB-48 from human plasma LDL and chylomicrons, respectively, as intact lipid-free, water-soluble apoproteins.

A. Purification of ApoB-100

Five milliliters of freshly prepared LDL (4 mg protein/ml) are dialyzed 2 hr against 1 m*M* EDTA, pH 8.0, and then lyophilized in 50-ml conical tubes (Kimax). The tubes are then fitted with Teflon® screw caps, and the dried lipoprotein is thrice extracted with 50 ml of diethyl ether : ethanol (3 : 1, v : v). At each step of the extraction, the protein–solvent mixture is allowed to stand at −20°C for 1 hr. The protein is then pelleted by low-speed centrifugation at room temperature, and the solvent removed by aspiration. After the final extraction, the protein is washed once with anhydrous diethyl ether and then pelleted by centrifugation. The solvent is first removed by aspiration and then by gentle evaporation with nitrogen. Care should be taken to leave the protein moist during the evaporation process.

Next, apoB is suspended in 15 ml of 10 m*M* tris-HCl, pH 8.5, 0.01% NaN_3, 1 m*M* EDTA (standard buffer) containing 100 m*M* sodium decyl sulfate (Sigma). This procedure must be performed at room temperature, and the detergent solution filtered (Whatman no. 1) prior to use. Apolipoprotein B will completely dissolve in this solution when the surface layer of residual ether is removed by nitrogen evaporation; gentle vortexing may be necessary to aid dissolution. After solubilization, apoB is dialyzed at 4°C against consecutive 6-liter changes of standard buffer to remove the sodium decyl sulfate. The detergent concentration is monitored using the methylene blue assay for quantitating protein-bound ionic detergent (Hayashi, 1975). After 48 hr of dialysis, the detergent concentration is reduced to <0.1 μg sodium decyl sulfate per milligram protein. Apolipoprotein B remains water soluble at this step with little or no detectable lipids (see Scheme I for quantitative recoveries of apoB at each purification step).

To remove tightly bound residual lipids or possible traces of detergent, apoB is precipitated with ethanol as described previously for glycophorin (Van Zoelen *et al.*, 1978) and Na^+,K^+-ATPase (Jackson *et al.*, 1980); this procedure removes tightly associated lipids, especially acidic phospholipids, from these proteins. To 5.0 ml of apoB (1 mg/ml) in standard buffer, 45 ml of absolute ethanol is added rapidly at room temperature; 5.0 ml of 1 *M* tris-HCl containing 0.01 *M* EDTA, pH 8.5, is then added to precipitate the protein. The precipitate is washed with water and dissolved in standard buffer containing 6 *M* guanidine-HCl. The apoB

Scheme I. Preparation of Water-Soluble ApoB[a]

Step	Procedure	Recovery of protein (percent)
1	20 mg of LDL d = 1.02 − 1.05 g/ml; lyophilization	100
2	3 × ether–ethanol extraction (3:1 v/v); 1 ether extraction; −20°C for 1 hr at each step	N.D.[b]
3	Solubilization in 0.1 *M* sodium decyl sulfate	100
4	Extensive dialysis to remove detergent	75
5	Ethanol precipitation	N.D.
6	Solubilization in standard buffer containing 6 *M* guanidine-HCl	65
7	Dialysis vs. standard buffer	N.D.
8	Resolubilization of apoB in standard buffer containing 6 *M* guanidine-HCl	65
9	Dialysis vs. standard buffer containing 6 *M* urea	N.D.
10	Dialysis vs. standard buffer containing 1 *M* urea	N.D.
11	Dialysis vs. standard buffer	55

[a] Standard buffer is 10 m*M* tris-HCl, 1 m*M* EDTA, and 0.01% NaN_3, pH 8.5.
[b] N.D., not determined.

is then precipitated by dialysis against standard buffer, and the pellet that is obtained by low-speed centrifugation is redissolved in 4 ml of standard buffer containing 6 *M* guanidine-HCl. The completely solubilized apoB is then dialyzed consecutively against three 1-liter changes of standard buffer containing 6 *M* urea followed by 1 *M* urea and finally against standard buffer. The water-soluble apoB prepared in this way (1–2 mg apoB/ml) is optically clear and will not pellet on centrifugation for 30 min at 48,000 × *g*. To prevent carbamylation of apoB, fresh solutions of 8 *M* urea (analytical grade) should be prepared, deionized on a column of Rexyn I-300 (Fisher Scientific Co.), and then used immediately.

During the lipid extraction with organic solvents (steps 1–3, Scheme I), apoB will undergo intermolecular disulfide exchange to yield high-molecular-weight aggregates that will not enter 3% polyacrylamide gels unless a reducing agent is included (Cardin *et al.*, 1982). Several procedures may be used to inhibit or reverse this covalent aggregation. The inclusion of thiodiglycol (TDG) to 0.02% (v/v) in the sample can be used to reduce all disulfide bonds. Alternatively, the two free sulfhydryls on LDL that catalyze the exchange reaction may be blocked with iodoacetamide prior to lipid extraction. This latter procedure is efficacious as long as none of the intramolecular disulfide bonds in apoB becomes reduced at later stages of handling to yield free sulfhydryls capable of catalyzing exchange. Finally, apoB can be fully reduced and alkylated at step 8 of the purification procedure (see Scheme I) using the method of Haeberli *et al.* (1975).

To alkylate apoB fully, reduction of disulfide bonds is performed at room temperature for 4 hr at a protein concentration of 2 mg/ml in 6 *M* guanidine-HCl, 0.5 *M* tris-HCl, 30 m*M* EDTA, pH 8.6. A 100-fold molar excess of 2-mercaptoethanol per protein disulfide bond is employed. Alkylation is carried out in the dark at 24°C for 30 min using a molar ratio of iodoacetamide to 2-mercaptoethanol

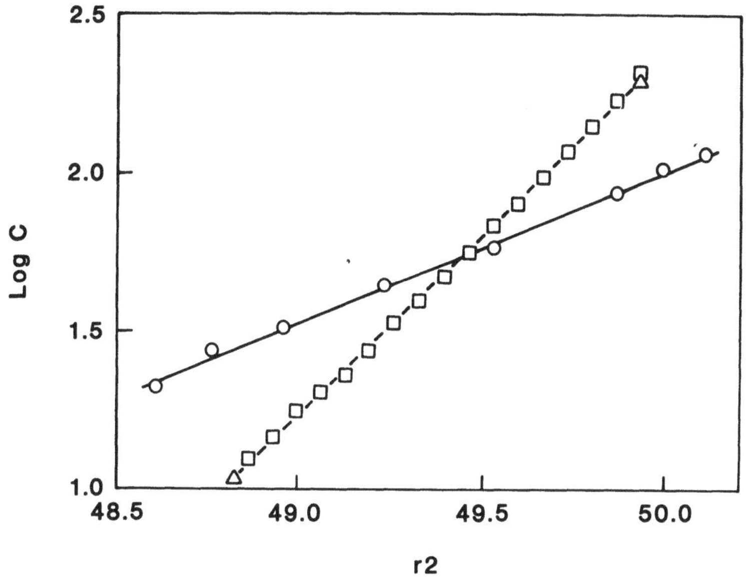

Figure 1. Analytical sedimentation equilibrium of water-soluble apoB-100 (100 μg/ml) in standard buffer containing 0.02% TDG (□) and in standard buffer containing 7 *M* guanidine-HCl, 0.02% TDG (○).

of 2.5. The fully reduced and carboxamidomethylated apoB (RCAM-apoB) is then precipitated by dialysis against three 2-liter changes of standard buffer. The pellet is then dissolved in standard buffer containing 6 *M* guanidine-HCl and dialyzed against two 1-liter changes of standard buffer containing 6 *M* urea followed by 1 *M* urea and, finally, standard buffer to yield water-soluble RCAM-apoB. The optimal concentration of RCAM-apoB in standard buffer is typically 1.9–2.5 mg/ml.

B. Characterization of Water-Soluble ApoB-100

Analytical ultracentrifugation experiments (Figure 1) show that apoB-100 in standard buffer has a $M_r \simeq 640{,}000$; in 7 *M* guanidine-HCl or 7 *M* urea, the M_r of apoB-100 $\simeq 320{,}000$. These data suggest that the total mass of apoB-100 in LDL (640,000 g-atoms/LDL particle) may exist as a dimer of two 320,000-M_r protein units. Circular dichroism (CD) studies suggest that the secondary structural composition of this water-soluble apoB-100 is similar to the structure of apoB-100 in LDL (Cardin *et al.*, 1982). Together, these physical studies indicate that the quaternary and secondary structure of apoB-100 in LDL may reflect a water-soluble conformation. This conformation may play an important role in determining the solubility of VLDL and LDL in the circulation.

Figure 2 shows a 3–20% polyacrylamide pore-gradient gel of water-soluble apoB-100 from the LDL of three normal volunteers (lanes a–c). When compared to the mobilities of protein standards of known M_r, the mobility of apoB corresponds to a M_r >500,000 (Cardin *et al.*, 1982). These findings are consistent with

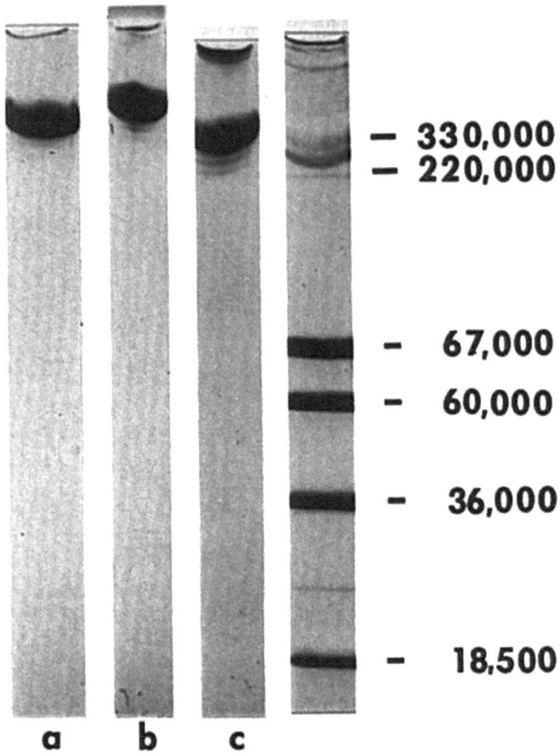

Figure 2. Polyacrylamide gel electrophoresis of apoB-100 prepared from the LDL of three normal volunteers (lanes a–c). Electrophoresis was conducted on a 3–20% pore-gradient gel containing 0.1% SDS and 6 *M* urea; 15 μg of water-soluble apoB-100 containing 1% 2-mercaptoethanol was loaded in each well. The samples were then electrophoresed for 5 hr at 10 mA. The gel was fixed overnight in isopropanol : acetic acid : water (25 : 10 : 65, v/v), stained for 2 hr in 0.2% Coomasie brilliant blue R (Pierce Chemicals) dissolved in methanol : acetic acid : water (50 : 10 : 40, v/v) and then destained in isopropanol : acetic acid : water (10 : 10 : 80, v/v).

the large size of apoB-100 as determined by the analytical ultracentrifugation experiments. However, the measurement of the M_r for apoB-100 by the gel method is less accurate, as apoB-100 migrates in the nonlinear region of the gradient.

The amino acid composition of water-soluble apoB-100 is shown in Table III. Apolipoprotein B-100 prepared as outlined in Scheme I shows complete immunologic identity with LDL in immunodiffusion tests when tested with anti-apoB-100 (Figure 3). Rabbit antisera prepared against human apoE, C-I, C-II, C-III, and A-I did not give an observable reaction over a range of apoB concentrations.

C. Purification of ApoB-48

Recently, Kane *et al.* (1980) showed that chylomicrons obtained from human lymph contain an apoB with approximately half the M_r of apoB-100 of VLDL and LDL. This apoprotein has been designated apoB-48. Apolipoprotein B-48 is produced in the gut for the assembly of dietary fat into chylomicron particles. The rat also has both a high-M_r apoB of hepatic origin and a low-M_r apoB of alimentary origin. These apoproteins correspond exactly in M_r to the apoB-100 and apoB-48 of human plasma LDL and chylomicrons, respectively (Elovson *et al.*, 1981), as determined by gel electrophoresis. This section describes the purification of apoB-48 from rat lymph chylomicrons. The methods presented here can be applied in principle to the purification of apoB-48 from human lymph chylomicrons. The

Table III. Amino Acid Compositions of the Major Apolipoproteins of Human Plasma Very-Low-Density, Low-Density, and High-Density Lipoproteins[a]

AA	ApoA-I	ApoA-II	ApoB-100	ApoC-I	ApoC-II	ApoC-III	ApoE
ASP	21	3	27	5	5	7	12
THR	10	6	14	3	9	5	11
SER	15	6	24	7	8	11	14
GLU	46	16	27	9	14	5	71
PRO	10	4	8	1	4	2	8
GLY	10	3	12	1	2	3	17
ALA	19	5	15	3	6	10	35
CYS	—	1	1	—	—	—	2
VAL	13	6	8	2	4	6	22
MET	3	1	3	1	2	2	7
ILEU	—	1	8	3	1	—	2
LEU	37	8	23	6	8	5	37
TYR	7	4	6	—	5	2	4
PHE	6	4	12	3	2	4	3
HIS	5	—	6	—	—	1	2
LYS	21	9	14	9	6	6	12
ARG	16	—	6	3	1	2	33
TRP	4	—	1	1	1	3	7

[a] The compositions of apoA-I, A-II, C-I, C-II, C-III, and E are based on their primary sequences; the data are expressed on a per-mole basis using molecular weights of 28,300, 8690, 6500, 10,000, 10,000, and 34,145, respectively, for these apoproteins. The data for apoB-100 represent a total of nine determinations of 24-hr hydrolysates and are expressed in moles of amino acid per 25,000 g of polypeptide, excluding weight contributions attributable to carbohydrate (5–7%).

purification of apoB-48 is more problematic than the purification of apoB-100. As chylomicrons contain several different apoprotein species, the purification of apoB-48 requires a chromatographic step. The method used to prepare pure water-soluble apoB-48 is a modification of the procedure described originally by Sparks and Marsh (1981).

Twenty milligrams of rat lymph chylomicrons (0.5 mg of protein/ml) are dialyzed 2 hr against 1 m*M* EDTA, pH 8.0, and lyophilized. The dried lipoprotein is extracted with 50 ml diethyl ether:ethanol (3:1, v/v) by vigorous vortexing, and the mixture is incubated at −20°C for 1 hr. The protein is then pelleted by low-speed centrifugation, and the solvent removed by aspiration. After the extraction is repeated twice more, the protein is washed twice with anhydrous diethyl ether and pelleted, and the ether is removed by aspiration followed by evaporation with nitrogen. Care should be taken to leave the protein moist with ether. The protein is extracted with 10 ml of 4.2 *M* tetramethylurea (TMU) in 50 m*M* tris-HCl, pH 8.5, 0.02% TDG, for 30 min at 37°C. The TMU-soluble apoproteins are then removed by aspiration. This step improves the chromatographic separation of apoB from the TMU-soluble lower-molecular-weight apoproteins and is a modification of a procedure described originally by Kane *et al.* (1975).

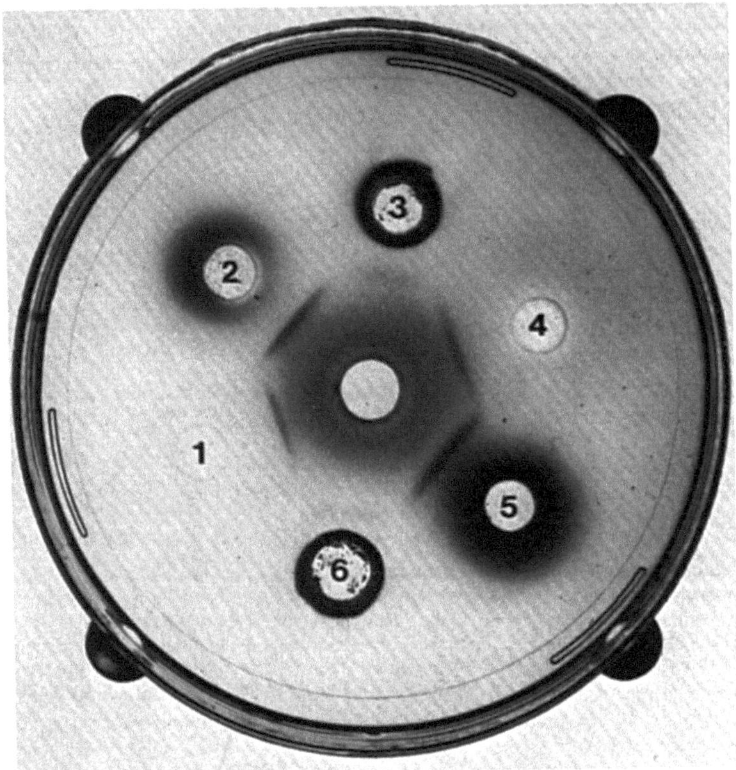

Figure 3. Immunodiffusion of apoB. The center well contained 10 μl of goat antihuman apoB (step 4). The outer wells contained 10 μl of the following: 1 and 4, LDL, 1 mg/ml; 2 and 5, apoB step 4, 1 mg/ml; 3 and 6, apoB step 11, 1 mg/ml. Immunodiffusion was carried out in premade Ouchterlony plates (ICN Pharmaceuticals). The plates were developed overnight at room temperature and then at 4°C for 48–72 hr. The gels were extensively washed with 0.9% NaCl and then stained with a solution of 0.02% Coomassie blue containing 2-propanol–acetic acid–water (10 : 10 : 80, v/v); the gels were destained in a solution of 2-propanol–acetic acid–water (10 : 10 : 80, v/v).

The TMU-insoluble apoproteins are washed twice with 5 ml of standard buffer containing 0.02% TDG, and the supernatants are removed by aspiration. The protein pellet is then suspended in 3 ml of standard buffer containing 100 m*M* sodium decyl sulfate, 0.02% TDG and gently swirled to aid dissolution. The sample is incubated at room temperature with nitrogen evaporation until the sample completely dissolves. The sample is then chromatographed on a column (1.5 × 60 cm) of Sepharose CL-6B equilibrated in standard buffer containing 50 m*M* sodium decyl sulfate, 0.02% TDG; 2 ml fractions are collected. The first peak contains mostly apoB-48 and a small amount of apoB-100 (Figure 4). Fractions are analyzed

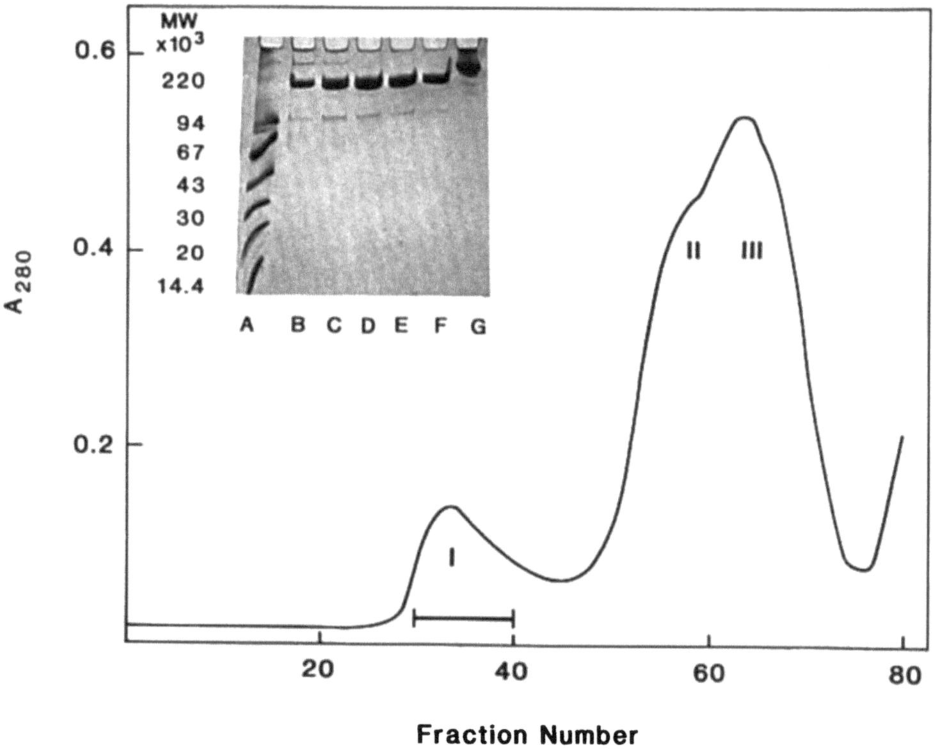

Figure 4. Gel filtration chromatography on Sepharose CL-6B of total rat lymph chylomicron apoproteins. The apoproteins obtained from the organic solvent extraction of rat lymph chylomicrons were dissolved directly in standard buffer containing 100 m*M* sodium decyl sulfate, 0.02% TDG and then applied to a column (1.5 × 60 cm) equilibrated in standard buffer containing 50 m*M* sodium decyl sulfate, 0.02% TDG. Two-milliliter fractions were collected, and 100-μl aliquots from zone I were assayed by pore-gradient gel electrophoresis (inset). Lane A of the inset corresponds to the molecular weight markers (from top to bottom): ferritin half unit (220,000); phosphorylase *b* (94,000); bovine serum albumin (67,000); ovalbumin (43,000); carbonic anhydrase (30,000); soybean trypsin inhibitor (20,000); α-lactalbumin (14,400). Lanes B–F correspond to 100-μl aliquots of the Sepharose CL-6B fractions numbers 30, 32, 34, 36, and 38, respectively (zone I). Lane G represents 15 μg of apoB-100 of human plasma LDL. The gels were fixed and stained as described in Figure 2.

on 3–20% pore-gradient polyacrylamide gels (Figure 4, inset), and the fractions corresponding to the apoB-48 species are pooled and dialyzed extensively against standard buffer to remove the last traces of sodium decyl sulfate. The apoprotein prepared in this way is ≃200 μg/ml and is completely water soluble.

D. Characterization of ApoB-48

Figure 4 shows the elution profile of total rat lymph chylomicron apoproteins from Sepharose CL-6B. Zone I represents the area of the chromatogram containing the total apoB (apoB-48 + apoB-100), whereas zones II and III contain the E, A, and C apoproteins. Fractions 30, 32, 34, 36, and 38 were analyzed by

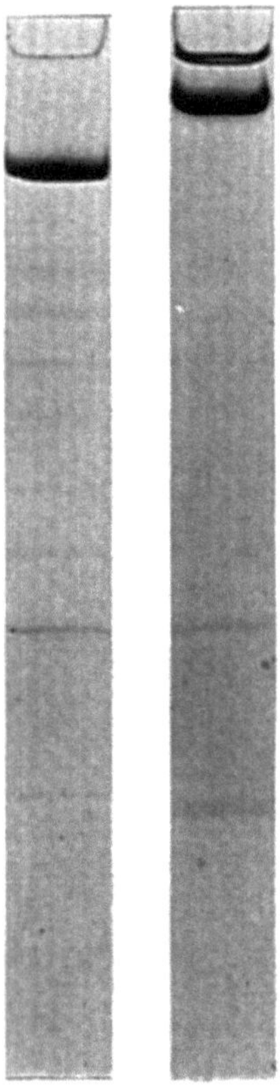

Figure 5. A 3–20% pore-gradient polyacrylamide gel of water-soluble apoB-48 of rat lymph chylomicrons (lane a) and of water-soluble apoB-100 of human plasma LDL (lane b). Each lane received 10 μg of protein. The gels were fixed and stained as described in Figure 2.

pore-gradient gel electrophoresis (Figure 4, inset), and the results are shown in lanes b–f of the gel, respectively. Lane A contains standard proteins of known molecular weights, and lane G contains apoB-100 of human plasma LDL. Fractions 30 and 32 (lanes B and C) contain a trace amount of apoB-100, whereas fractions 34-38 contain only apoB-48. Fractions 34–38 were pooled and extensively dialyzed against standard buffer to yield water-soluble apoB-48. A 3–20% pore-gradient polyacrylamide gel of the pooled sample is shown in Figure 5 (lane a). The M_r of apoB-48 is 170,000 by polyacrylamide gel electrophoresis in SDS; its M_r is ≃167,000 in standard buffer as determined by analytical ultracentrifugation. Circular dichroism analysis (data not shown) shows that water-soluble apoB-48 contains a high degree of ordered structure but less than human apoB-100.

V. PURIFICATION OF APOLIPOPROTEINS A-I AND A-II FROM HIGH-DENSITY LIPOPROTEINS

Five milliliters of d = 1.063–1.210 g/ml HDL (≃150 mg protein) in PDB are extracted with 45 ml of acetone : ethanol (1 : 1, v/v) that was prechilled to −20°C.

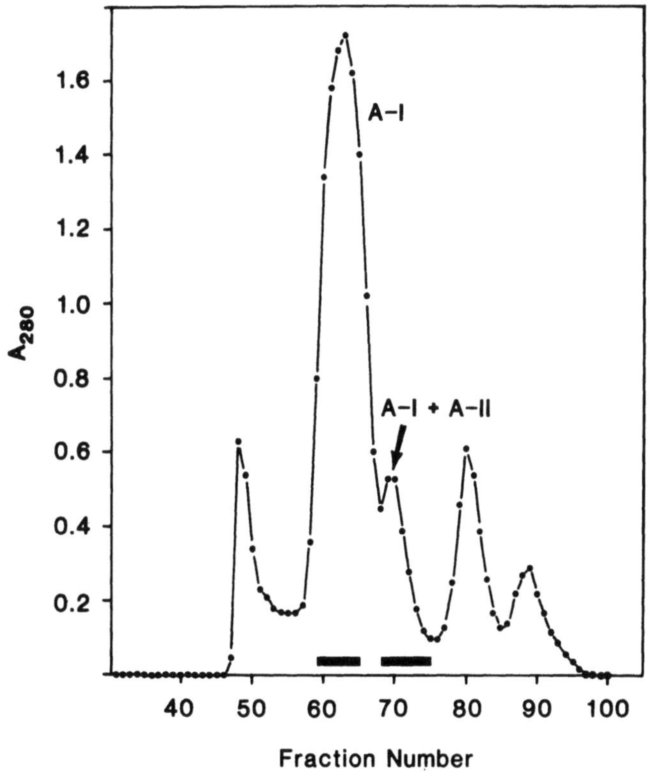

Figure 6. Sephacryl S-200 column chromatography of apoHDL. The HDL lipids were extracted with acetone:ethanol (1:1, v/v), the apoproteins solubilized in 10 ml of column buffer (50 m*M* tris-HCl, pH 8.0, 6 *M* urea), and the resulting apoHDL (150 mg protein) applied to a column (2.5 × 200 cm) of Sephacryl S-200; 9-ml fractions were collected. Bars indicate the fractions that were pooled and subsequently rechromatographed.

The extraction is performed by vigorous vortexing in 50-ml conical tubes (Kimax) sealed with Teflon® caps; the mixture is left to stand at −20°C for 1 hr. Following the extraction, the apoproteins are pelleted by low-speed centrifugation, and the supernatant removed by aspiration. The extraction is performed twice more, and after the final extraction, the apoproteins are dispersed by vortexing in 45 ml of anhydrous diethyl ether prechilled to −20°C. The apoproteins are then recovered by low-speed centrifugation, and the diethyl ether is removed first by aspiration and then by nitrogen evaporation. Care should be taken to leave the protein moist. The apoproteins are then dissolved in 10 ml of 50 m*M* tris-HCl, pH 8.0, containing 6 *M* urea, and insoluble material is removed by ultracentrifugation in a J-20 rotor at 16,000 rpm for 15 min at 8°C. Then, 10 ml of the supernatant fraction (≃15 mg/ml based on an $\epsilon_{280}^{0.1\%} = 1.0$) are applied to a column (2.5 × 200 cm) of Sephacryl S-200 equilibrated in 50 m*M* tris-HCl, pH 8.0, 6 *M* urea; 9.0-ml fractions are collected, and the absorbance at 280 nm is monitored continuously. Figure 6 shows a typical Sephacryl S-200 column elution profile of HDL apoproteins.

Tubes corresponding to apoA-I and apoA-II as shown in Figure 6 are pooled, dialyzed against 10 m*M* NH_4HCO_3, and lyophilized. The apoproteins are then

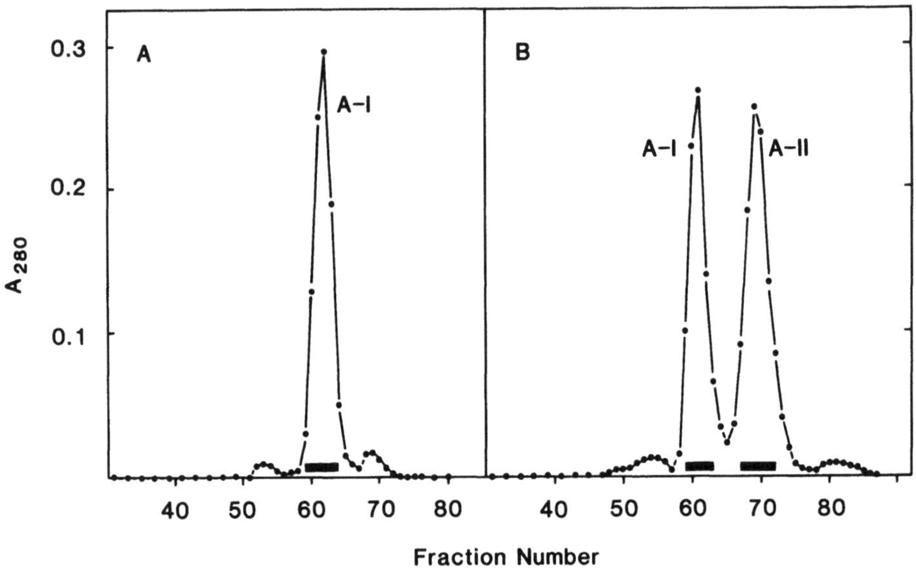

Figure 7. The rechromatography of apoA-I and apoA-II on Sephacryl S-200. The peak fractions of Figure 6 corresponding to apoA-I and apoA-II were pooled, lyophilized, resolubilized in column buffer, and rechromatographed on a column (2.5 × 200 cm) of Sephacryl S-200. The rechromatography of the apoA-I fractions of Figure 6 are shown in A; the rechromatography of the apoA-I + apoA-II fractions are shown in B. After rechromatography, fractions containing apoA-I and apoA-II were identified by electrophoresis on 7.5% polyacrylamide gels and by amino acid analysis (Table III).

redissolved to a final concentration of 15 mg/ml in 50 m*M* tris-HCl, pH 8.0, containing 6 *M* urea; 10 ml of each apoprotein are then rechromatographed on Sephacryl S-200. Figure 7, A and B, show, respectively, the rechromatography of the apoA-I and apoA-I plus apoA-II peaks of Figure 6. Fractions containing either pure apoA-I or apoA-II are identified by electrophoresis on 7.5% polyacrylamide gels containing SDS. Figure 8 shows purified apoA-II, its reduced monomer, and apoA-I on 7.5% polyacrylamide gels in SDS. The purified apoproteins are dialyzed against 10 m*M* NH_4HCO_3, lyophilized, and stored at −20°C. The amino acid compositions of apoA-I and apoA-II are shown in Table III.

VI. PURIFICATION OF THE E AND C APOLIPOPROTEINS

The solvent extraction of freshly isolated triglyceride-rich lipoproteins followed by the solubilization of the apolipoproteins and their subsequent separation by gel filtration and ion exchange chromatography have been described by Jackson *et al.* (1974, 1977). In this section, we provide a detailed account of these procedures, incorporating some later modifications.

A. Solubilization and Separation of the Apolipoproteins

Five milliliters of freshly isolated triglyceride-rich lipoprotein (150 mg protein) are mixed with 45 ml of acetone:ethanol (1:1, v/v). The sample is vortexed in

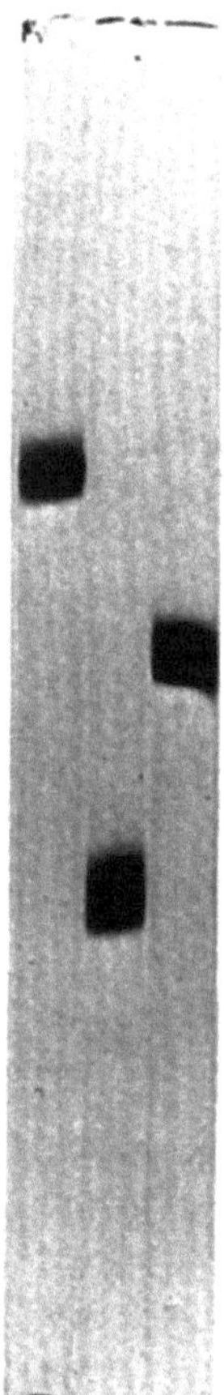

Figure 8. Polyacrylamide gel electrophoresis of purified apoA-I and apoA-II. Gel 1, apoA-I electrophoresed in the absence of 2-mercaptoethanol; gel 2, apoA-II electrophoresed in the presence of 2-mercaptoethanol; gel 3, apoA-II electrophoresed in the absence of 2-mercaptoethanol.

50-ml conical tubes (Kimax) sealed with Teflon® caps and then stored for at least 1 hr at −20°C. The apoproteins are sedimented by low-speed centrifugation for 30 min at 1000–2000 rpm using a table-top centrifuge, and the solvent phase is removed by aspiration. The apoproteins are then redispersed in 45 ml of solvent by gentle vortexing, and the extraction procedure is repeated until the solvent phase is colorless, indicating that most of the lipid has been removed. Finally, the sedimented apoproteins are dispersed in anhydrous diethyl ether by gentle vortexing at room temperature, pelleted by low-speed centrifugation, and the solvent removed by aspiration. The sedimented apoproteins are partially dried under a stream of nitrogen. Before the last of the ether has evaporated, the apoproteins are suspended in 10 ml of solubilization buffer composed of 50 m*M* tris-HCl, pH 8.6, and 6 *M* urea. The mixture is then subjected to vigorous stirring at 4°C overnight. Nitrogen evaporation may be used to remove the last traces of ether and thus aid dissolution. The mixture is then centrifuged in a J-20 rotor at

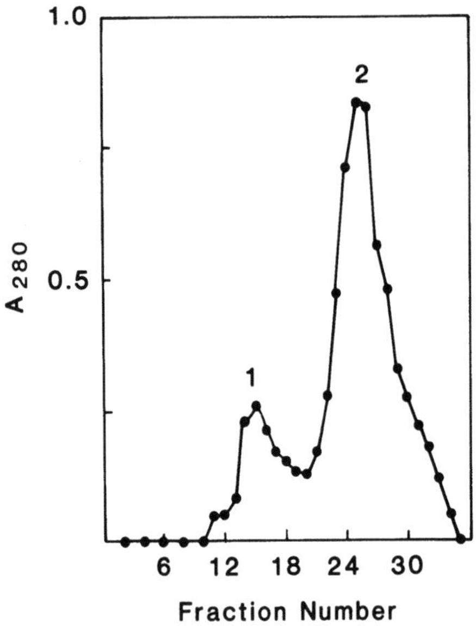

Figure 9. Elution of urea-soluble apolipoproteins from Sephadex G-75. Samples of 150 mg of urea-soluble apolipoproteins were eluted from Sephadex G-75 in 50 m*M* tris-HCl, pH 8.6, 6 *M* urea; 40 × 8 ml fractions were collected. Peak 1: apoproteins B and E. Peak 2: apoproteins C.

18,000 rpm for 30 min, and the aqueous supernatant containing the E and C apolipoproteins is carefully removed by aspiration and stored at 4°C. The sedimented pellet is then resuspended in 5 ml of solubilization buffer and stirred for 1 hr at 4°C, and the supernatant fraction obtained after centrifugation is removed by aspiration and stored at 4°C. The insoluble residue contains mainly apolipoprotein B.

Gel filtration chromatography of the urea-soluble apoproteins is performed on a column (2.5 × 90 cm) of Sephadex G-75 (Pharmacia, Inc.) equilibrated at 4°C with solubilization buffer. The maximum column load is 15 ml or 150 mg of protein. The protein concentration of the urea-soluble apoproteins is determined by assuming an $\epsilon_{280\ \mathrm{nm}}^{0.1\%} = 1$. The apoprotein sample is then loaded onto the column and eluted with solubilization buffer; 8-ml fractions are collected. The $A_{280\ \mathrm{nm}}$ of each fraction is then recorded.

Figure 9 shows a typical G-75 elution profile of the urea-soluble apoproteins. The first peak to elute (void peak) contains mostly apoE, whereas the second peak contains the C apoproteins. In order to purify apoE, the void fractions from the G-75 column are pooled, equilibrated by dialysis in PDB, and subjected to affinity chromatography on heparin-Sepharose. The preparation of heparin-Sepharose is described in the Appendix (Section VII.A). Thirty milliliters of heparin-Sepharose in PDB are left to stir gently overnight at room temperature with the sample containing apoE. The slurry is poured into a column (4 × 15 cm) and eluted with PDB until the $A_{280\ \mathrm{nm}}$ of the eluate reaches base-line absorbance. The column is then eluted with PDB containing 0.4 *M* NaCl; 4-ml fractions are collected. The $A_{280\ \mathrm{nm}}$ of each fraction is recorded, and the fractions containing absorbance are pooled.

Figure 10 shows a typical elution profile of apoE from heparin-Sepharose. The apoE pools are dialyzed against 10 m*M* NH_4HCO_3 and lyophilized. Figure

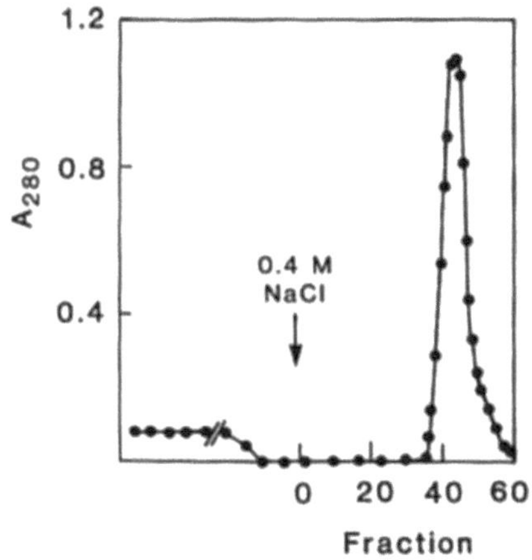

Figure 10. Elution of apolipoprotein E from heparin-Sepharose. The void peak (peak 1) from the G-75 column was dialyzed against PDB and then incubated overnight with heparin-Sepharose. The slurry was then poured into a column and eluted with PDB until the A_{280} achieved a background value. The elution buffer was then made 0.4 *M* with sodium chloride (arrow), and 60 × 4 ml fractions were collected.

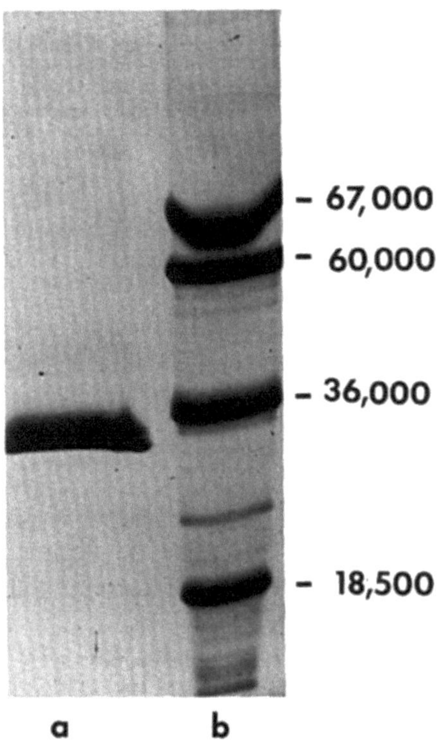

Figure 11. Gradient gel electrophoresis of apolipoprotein E. Twenty micrograms of apoE in 10 m*M* tris-HCl, pH 8.0, 6 *M* urea, and 1% 2-mercaptoethanol were electrophoresed on a 3–20% polyacrylamide gradient gel containing 0.1% SDS and 6 *M* urea. Lane a, apoE; lane b, standard proteins.

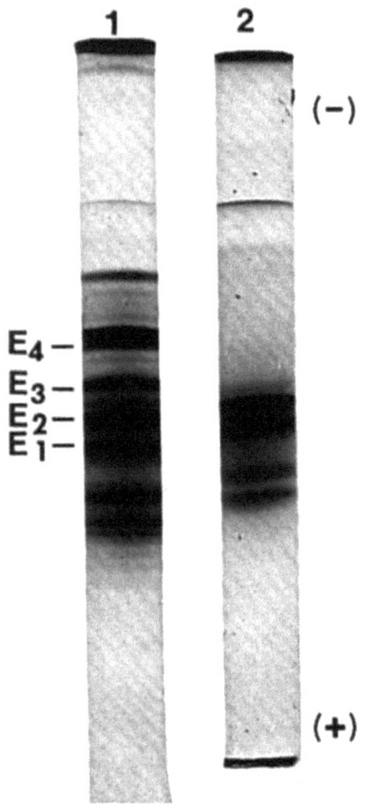

Figure 12. Analytical isoelectric focusing of apoprotein E. Apoprotein E pools from heparin-Sepharose columns were dialyzed against 10 m*M* NH_4HCO_3, pH 8.0, and freeze-dried. For IEF, 40-μg aliquots were solubilized in 10 m*M* tris-HCl, pH 8.0, and then focused between pH 4.0 and 8.0. Gel 1: type V hypertriglyceridemic patient. Gel 2: type III hypertriglyceridemic patient.

11 shows a 3–20% pore-gradient polyacrylamide gel of apoE obtained by heparin-Sepharose chromatography. Figure 12 shows the analytical isoelectric focusing (IEF) pattern of apoE; the gel has a pH gradient between 4.0 and 8.0. The major isoform designations are shown in the figure. Table III lists the amino acid composition of apoE. The method for analytical IEF described in detail by Kashyap *et al.* (1981) is summarized in the Appendix (Section VII.B).

B. Preparation of the C Apolipoproteins

The total C apoproteins obtained by G-75 gel filtration chromatography are desalted by dialysis against 10 m*M* NH_4HCO_3 or chromatographed on a column (5 × 48 cm) of BioGel® P-2 equilibrated in 10 m*M* NH_4HCO_3; the fractions containing the C peptides are lyophilized and stored at −20°C.

The apoC peptides are separated by ion-exchange chromatography on a DEAE-Sephacel column (2.5 × 35 cm) equilibrated with 10 m*M* tris-HCl, pH 8.0, containing 6 *M* urea. The lyophilized peptides (approximately 250 mg protein) are dissolved in 10–15 ml of the equilibrating buffer. The conductivity of the sample must be <0.5 mmho before chromatography is initiated. Should the sample have

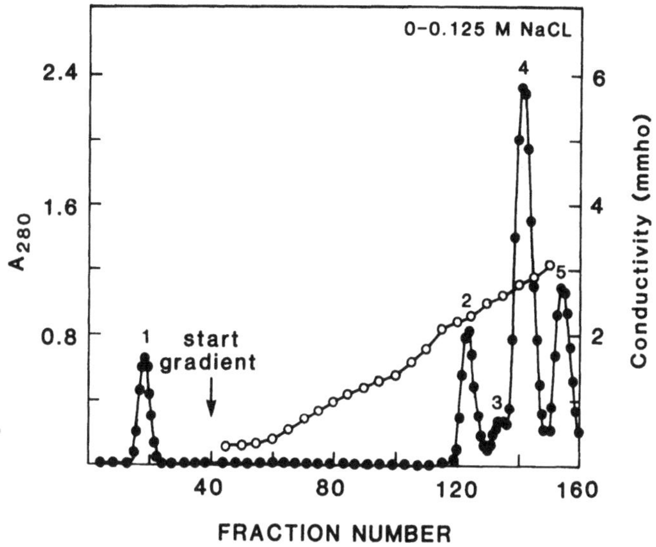

Figure 13. Ion-exchange chromatography of the C apoproteins: 250 mg of apoprotein C were loaded onto a DEAE-Sephacel column, equilibrated in 6 *M* urea–10 m*M* tris, pH 8.0, and eluted with a 0–0.125 *M* NaCl gradient, as described in the text. Each peak is labeled with its major apoC peptide component. Peak 1, apoC-I; peak 2, apoC-II; peak 3, apoC-III_0; peak 4, apoC-III_1; peak 5, apoC-III_2.

a higher conductivity, it must be dialyzed against the equilibrating buffer until the conductivity is within the acceptable limits.

After the sample has entered the resin, the column is washed with equilibrating buffer; elution is performed at 4°C, and 8-ml fractions are collected. Apolipoprotein C-I does not bind to the resin and appears in the void peak. In order to obtain the remaining apoC peptides, a 1-liter gradient of 0–0.125 *M* NaCl in equilibrating buffer is used to elute sequentially apoC-II and apoC-III from the column; 8-ml fractions are collected. A typical elution profile of the apoCs from DEAE-Sephacel is shown in Figure 13. The various apoC peptides are then pooled, and their purity is established by IEF and amino acid analyses (Table III).

C. Preparative Isoelectric Focusing of Apolipoprotein C-II

Figure 14 shows the analytical IEF pattern of two apoC-II preparations obtained from DEAE-Sephacel column chromatography. The pH gradient of the IEF gels was 4.0 to 6.0. As can be seen, the DEAE-Sephacel apoC-II peak contains more than one peptide band in the IEF gels. The peptide focusing between apoC-III_1 and apoC-III_2 is apoC-II_2. This peptide was first described by Catapano *et al.* (1979) and in more detail by Havel *et al.* (1979). Havel *et al.* (1979) separated this peptide from the other apoC peptides by preparative isoelectric focusing and showed that it has lipoprotein lipase-activating properties and an identical amino

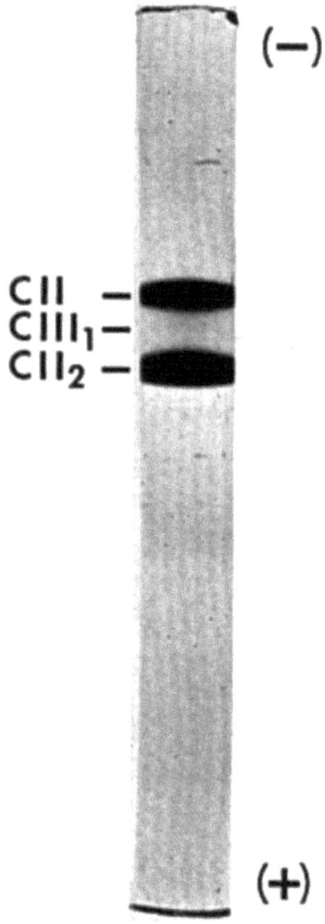

Figure 14. Analytical isoelectric focusing of apoprotein C-II. The apoC-II peak obtained from the DEAE-Sephacel column (peak 2, Figure 13) was loaded (75- to 150-μl aliquots) onto IEF gel and focused between pH 4 and 6.

acid composition to apoC-II. We have verified these results using preparative isoelectric focusing to separate these peptides.

Preparative isoelectric focusing of apolipoprotein C-II is carried out essentially as described in LKB Application Note 198 (1975) with some modifications as described by Havel *et al.* (1979) and is detailed in the Appendix (Section VII.C). The total apoC-II obtained from the DEAE-Sephacel is equilibrated in 3 ml of 10 m*M* tris-HCl, pH 8.2, containing 0.5% sodium decyl sulphate (Eastman Kodak).

To load the sample, an 8-cm section of gel is removed 4 cm from the cathode end with the aid of a section cutter. The sample is then mixed with the Ultrodex® cut from the gel, and the mixture is poured back into the section cutter. The cutter is then carefully removed from the gel. Air bubbles should be removed carefully with a Pasteur pipette. Electrofocusing is performed for 16 hr at 6 W.

After focusing is complete, the pH gradient may be determined by cutting small cubes of Ultrodex® from the gel at 1-cm intervals, dispersing them in water, and measuring their pH. Alternatively, a surface electrode may be used to measure directly the pH of the Ultrodex® surface at 1 cm intervals.

It is not a standard practice in this laboratory to make a paper print of the gel to visualize the proteins, as this leads to high protein losses. Figure 15, however, shows such a replica. If a paper print is required, the protocol given in the LKB Application Note (1975) should be followed.

As the focused peptides are highly concentrated in the gel, the bands can be visualized directly using a dark background and side lighting. The positions of

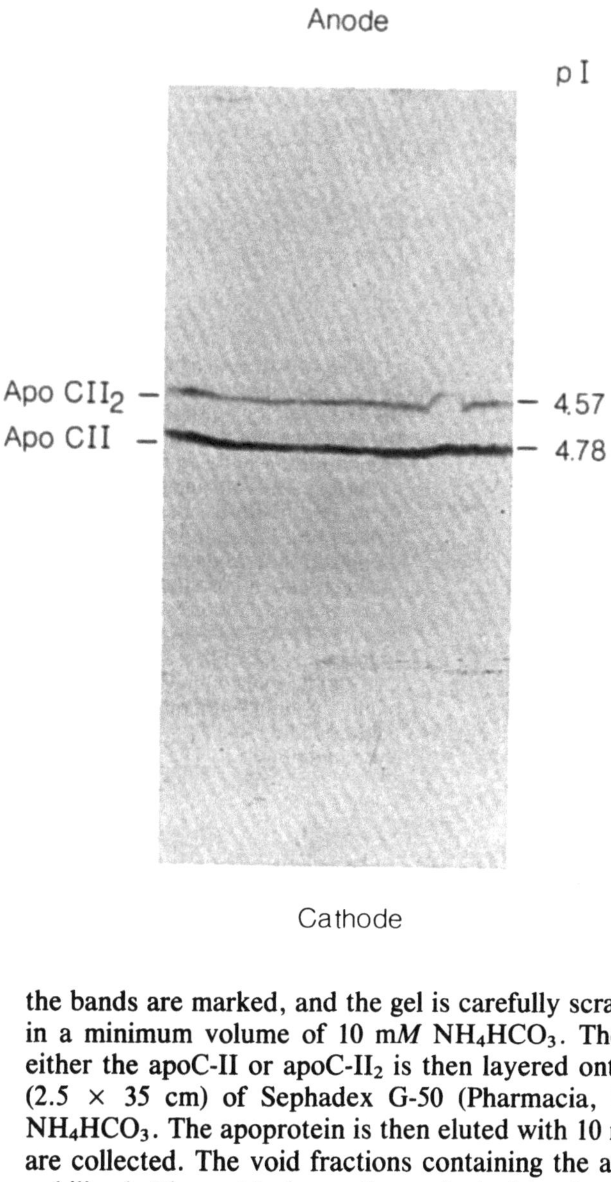

Figure 15. Preparative isoelectric focusing of apoprotein C-II. A paper print of a preparative IEF gel of apoproteins C-II was made as described in the text and stained in Coomassie brilliant blue R in 50% methanol and 10% acetic acid. The pH gradient had been measured following the excision of small cubes of gel at successive 1-cm distances from the anode and dispersing the gel cubes in 1 ml of H_2O.

the bands are marked, and the gel is carefully scraped off the tray and dispersed in a minimum volume of 10 m*M* NH_4HCO_3. The Ultrodex® slurry containing either the apoC-II or apoC-II_2 is then layered onto the gel surface of a column (2.5 × 35 cm) of Sephadex G-50 (Pharmacia, Inc.), equilibrated in 10 m*M* NH_4HCO_3. The apoprotein is then eluted with 10 m*M* NH_4HCO_3; 4-ml fractions are collected. The void fractions containing the apopeptides are pooled and lyophilized. Figure 16 shows the analytical isoelectric focusing gels (pH interval 4.0 to 6.0) of the DEAE-Sephacel acquired apoC-II/apoC-II_2 (1) and of apoC-II (2) and apoC-II_2 (3) isolated by preparative isoelectric focusing in Ultrodex®.

VII. APPENDIX

A. Preparation of Heparin-Sepharose

Heparin may be covalently linked to cyanogen bromide-activated Sepharose 4B by a modification of the method of Iverius (1971). Preswollen Sepharose 4B-

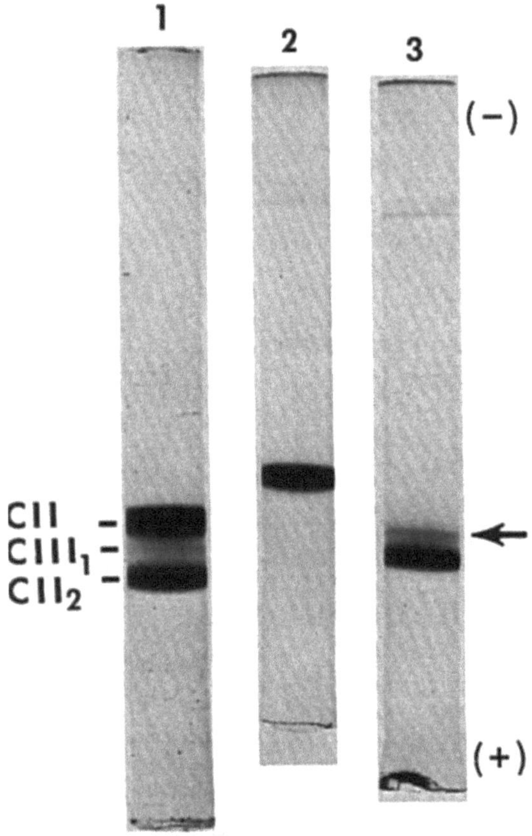

Figure 16. Analytical isoelectric focusing of apoprotein C-II and C-II_2. The focused C-II apoproteins obtained by preparative isoelectric focusing were cut from the gel tray and eluted from a Sephadex G-50 column as described in the text. The void peaks were freeze-dried, and 50-μg fractions were resolubilized in 6 *M* urea–10 m*M* tris, pH 8.0 (50 μl) and loaded onto the gels. The gels were focused between pH 4.0 and 6.0. Gel 1, apoprotein C-II + C-II_2 isolated by DEAE-Sephacel chromatography (Figure 13). Gel 2, apoprotein C-II. Gel 3, apoprotein C-II_2; arrow indicates a small amount of apoC-III_1 contamination.

CL (500 g) is washed with 6 liters of H_2O by suction filtration (filter washed); a large sintered glass funnel and a 4-liter side-arm conical flask attached to a vacuum port are required. Under a well-ventilated fume hood, 30 g of cyanogen bromide in 500 ml of H_2O are added to the Sepharose in a 2-liter beaker. The pH is immediately adjusted to 11.0 with 2 *N* NaOH and maintained at that pH for at least 12 min. The activated Sepharose is then filter washed with 4 liters of 0.1 *M* $NaHCO_3$. During filtration, care should be taken to leave the activated gel moist. Finally, the gel is resuspended in 500 ml of 0.1 *M* $NaHCO_3$ and incubated with 2.5 g of heparin (Sigma) at 4°C overnight with gentle end-over-end rotation. The heparin-substituted Sepharose is recovered by suction filtration, and the wet gel incubated with 1 liter of 0.1 *M* glycine at room temperature for 3 hr with gentle stirring. The resin is then filter washed consecutively with 2 liters H_2O, 1 liter 1.0 *M* NaCl, 2 liters 0.1 *M* $NaHCO_3$, and, finally, 2 liters H_2O. The heparin-Sepharose is then stored in PDB at 4°C.

B. Analytical Isoelectric Focusing

Glass gel tubes, 5 mm × 10 mm, are washed with detergent, rinsed in distilled water, then air dried. Care should be taken not to chip the ends of the gel tubes.

The gel tubes are then sealed at one end with Parafilm® and placed upright in a level gel stand holder. The ingredients used to prepare either 12 or 18 tube gels for electrofocusing are presented in tabular form below.

The acrylamide–bisacrylamide solution consists of 30 g acrylamide and 0.8 g bisacrylamide dissolved to a final volume of 100 ml with distilled water.

	12 gels	18 gels
Acrylamide/bisacrylamide solution	6.0 ml	9.0 ml
T.E.M.E.D.	20 μl	30 μl
Urea	10.24 g	15.36 g
Distilled water	7.8 ml	11.7 ml
Ampholine pH 3.5–5.0	0.8 ml	1.2 ml
Ampholine pH 4–6	0.2 ml	0.3 ml
Ampholine pH 5–8	0.2 ml	0.3 ml

The mixture is degassed for 15 min, and then 0.8 ml (for 12 gels) or 1.2 ml (for 18 gels) of a 14 mg/ml ammonium persulfate solution is added to the mixture. Exactly 1 ml of the gel solution is poured into each tube. The top surface of the gel is overlayered with about 0.2 ml of distilled water to prevent drying of the gel.

After polymerization, the gels are put into an electrophoresis chamber (Buchler), and the Parafilm® at the bottom of the gels is removed; 0.1 *M* phosphoric acid is placed in the anode reservoir, and 0.02 *M* sodium hydroxide is placed in the cathode reservoir. The gels are prefocused at 100 V for 1 hr or until the current drops to a stable low level, typically <3 mA.

After prefocusing, the current is shut off, the leads are disconnected, and the samples (30–100 μg of protein) are loaded onto the gel surface with a Pasteur pipette. The sample solution should be of low conductivity but contain urea or sucrose to raise the sample density to facilitate layering of sample on the gel surface. Electrofocusing is first conducted at 100 V for 1 hr and then at 400 V for 2 to 4 hr. When the current drops to a low stable level, focusing is assumed complete. The gels are then removed from the tubes and stained for 16 to 48 hr in 0.04% Coomassie brilliant blue G250 dissolved in 3.5% perchloric acid; gels are stored in 7% acetic acid.

C. Preparative Isoelectric Focusing

To prepare the gel, 27 g of ultrapure urea (Schwartz/Mann) are dissolved in 80 ml of water, 2.5 ml each of ampholines, pH 3.5–5.5 and pH 4.0–6.0, are added, and the final volume is adjusted to 104 ml. To this solution is slowly added 4 g of Ultrodex® (LKB, Inc.), and the mixture is stirred briefly until homogeneous.

The electrophoresis tray is carefully washed and dried, and three 0.3 × 10.8 cm paper strips previously soaked in an aqueous solution of ampholines at the same concentration as the Ultrodex® slurry are layered at each end.

The following weighings are then carried out: (1) beaker + slurry; (2) tray + strips. After the slurry is poured into the tray and set on a leveled table, the

Table IV. Summary of Calculations to Determine the Degree of Weight Loss of Water Required to Prepare the Ultrodex® Gels for Electrofocusing

(*a*) Wt. of beaker + slurry
(*b*) Wt. of beaker
(*c*) Initial wt. of slurry = $a - b$
(*d*) Required water loss from slurry = $c \times 0.27$
(*e*) Wt. of tray + strips
(*f*) Initial wt. of tray, strips, and slurry = $e + c$
(*g*) Final wt. of tray, strips, and slurry = $f - d$

beaker is reweighed. This gives the weight of the Ultrodex® slurry transferred to the tray. This weight is then multiplied by 0.27 to give the weight of water that must be lost by evaporation before the gel is suitable for electrofocusing. This value, subtracted from the sum of the initial slurry weight and the weight of the tray plus strips, gives the final weight of the tray plus slurry required for the preparative IEF (Table IV provides a summary of these calculations).

To facilitate evaporation, a fan is set sufficiently high above the gel so as not to cause turbulence across the surface. Evaporation is then effected to the predetermined weight point (Table IV). The ampholine-soaked strips at each end of the tray are now replaced by strips of the same dimension soaked in either 1.0 *M* phosphoric acid (anode) or 1.0 *M* sodium hydroxide (cathode). The tray is then placed onto the cold plate of the Multiphor apparatus, which has a thin layer of 0.1% Triton X-100. The detergent acts as a seal between the cold plate and tray to efficiently dissipate heat during electrofocusing. The apparatus is precooled to 10°C, the gel is prefocused for 1 hr at 6 W, and the sample is electrofocused as described above.

D. Pore-Gradient Gel Electrophoresis

Polyacrylamide gel electrophoresis is performed as described by Socorro and Camejo (1979). Electrophoresis is performed on a gel (3 mm thick) in a verticle slab cell unit (Bio-Rad Model 220) at a constant current of 10 mA/gel. The ratio of acrylamide to bisacrylamide is 30:1; polymerization is induced by the addition of 1.5 μl of N,N,N′,N′-tetramethylethylenediamine and 2.5 mg of ammonium persulfate per 10 ml of gel. A 0–20% (w/v) sucrose gradient is superimposed over the acrylamide gradient (3–20% w/v) to improve gradient linearity. The gel contains 0.25 *M* tris-HCl, 0.1% sodium dodecyl sulfate, and 6 *M* urea, pH 9.0. The electrophoresis buffer contains 25 m*M* tris-HCl, 0.2 *M* glycine, and 0.1% sodium dodecyl sulfate, pH 8.4. The samples are adjusted to 0.5 mg/ml in a buffer containing 10 m*M* tris-HCl, pH 6.8, 1% sodium dodecyl sulfate, 20% sucrose, 1 m*M* EDTA, 6 *M* urea, and 0.03% bromophenol blue and then heated at 60°C for 15 min in the presence of 1% 2-mercaptoethanol. Following electrophoresis, gels are fixed overnight in 2-propanol–acetic acid–water (25:10:65 v/v), stained for 2 hr in 0.2% Coomassie brilliant blue R (Pierce Chemicals), dissolved in methanol–acetic acid–water (50:10:40 v/v), and destained in 2-propanol–acetic acid–water (10:10:80 v/v).

ACKNOWLEDGMENTS

This work was supported in part by United States Public Health Service grant P01-HL-22619. We gratefully acknowledge Janet Simons for preparing the manuscript for publication and Gwen Kraft for preparing the figures.

REFERENCES

Bradley, W. A., and Gotto, A. M., Jr. 1978. Structure of intact plasma lipoproteins. In: *Disturbances in Lipid and Lipoprotein Metabolism*, pp. 111–137 Ed. by Dietschy, J. M. Gotto, A. M., Jr., and Ontko, J. A. Williams & Wilkins, Baltimore.

Brewer, H. B., Jr., Lux, S. E., Ronan, R., and John, K. M. 1972. Amino acid sequence of human apo Lp-Gln-II (apoA-II), an apolipoprotein isolated from the high density lipoprotein complex. *Proc. Natl. Acad. Sci. U.S.A., 69:*1304–1308.

Brewer, H. B., Shulman, R., Herbert, P., Ronan, R., and Wehrly, K. 1974. The complete amino acid sequence of alanine apolipoprotein (apoC-III), an apolipoprotein from human plasma very low density lipoproteins. *J. Biol. Chem., 249:*4975–4984.

Brewer, H. B., Jr., Fairwell, T., LaRue, A., Ronan, R., Houser, A., and Bronzert, T. J. 1978. The amino acid sequence of human apoA-I, an apolipoprotein isolated from high density lipoproteins. *Biochem. Biophys. Res. Commun., 80:*623–630.

Cardin, A. D., Witt, K. R., Barnhart, C. L., and Jackson, R. L. 1982. Sulfhydryl chemistry and solubility properties of human plasma apolipoprotein B. *Biochemistry, 21:*4503–4511.

Catapano, A. L., Jackson, R. L., Gilliam, E. G., Gotto, A. M., Jr., and Smith, L. C. 1979. Quantification of apoC-II and apoC-III of human very low density lipoproteins by analytical isoelectric focusing. *J. Lipid Res., 19:*1047–1052.

Elovson, J., Huang, Y. O., Baker, N., and Kannan, R. 1981. Apolipoprotein B is structurally and metabolically heterogeneous in the rat. *Proc. Natl. Acad. Sci. U.S.A., 78:*157–161.

Haeberli, A., Bilstad, J., Edlehoch, H., and Rall, J. E. 1975. Elementary chain composition of guinea pig thyroglobulin. *J. Biol. Chem., 250:*7294–7299.

Havel, R. J., Eder, H., and Bragdon, J. 1955. The distribution and chemical composition of ultracentrifugally separated lipoproteins in human serum. *J. Clin. Invest., 34:*1345–1353.

Havel, R. J., Kotite, L., and Kane, J. P. 1979. Isoelectric heterogeneity of the cofactor protein for lipoprotein lipase in human blood plasma. *Biochem. Med., 21:*121–128.

Hayashi, K. 1975. A rapid determination of sodium dodecyl sulfate with methylene blue. *Anal. Biochem., 67:*503–506.

Iverius, P. H. 1971. Coupling of glycosaminoglycans to agarose beads (Sepharose 4B), *Biochem. J., 124:*677–683.

Jackson, R. L., Sparrow, J. T., Baker, H. N., Morrisett, J. D., Taunton, O. D., and Gotto, A. M., Jr. 1974. The primary structure of apolipoprotein-serine. *J. Biol. Chem., 249:*5308–5313.

Jackson, R. L., Morrisett, J. D., and Gotto, A. M., Jr. 1976. Lipoprotein structure and metabolism. *Physiol. Rev., 56:*259–299.

Jackson, R. L., Baker, H. N., Gilliam, E. B., and Gotto, A. M., Jr. 1977. Primary structure of very low density apolipoprotein C-II of human plasma. *Proc. Natl. Acad. Sci. U.S.A., 74:*1942–1945.

Jackson, R. L., Verkleij, A. J., van Zoelen, E. J. J., Lane, L. K., Schwartz, A., and van Deenen, L. L. M. 1980. Asymmetric incorporation of Na^+,K^+-ATPase into phospholipid vesicles. *Arch. Biochem. Biophys., 200:*269–278.

Kane, J. P., Sata, T., Hamilton, R. L., and Havel, R. J. 1975. Apoprotein composition of very low density lipoproteins of human serum. *J. Clin. Invest.*, *56*:1622–1634.

Kane, J. P., Hardman, D. A., and Paulus, H. E. 1980. Heterogeneity of apolipoprotein B: Isolation of a new species from human chylomicrons. *Proc. Natl. Acad. Sci. U.S.A.*, *77*:2465–2469.

Kashyap, M. L., Hynd, B. A., Robinson, K., and Gartside, P. S. 1981. Abnormal preponderance of sialylated apolipoprotein C-III in triglyceride-rich lipoproteins in type V hyperlipoproteinemia. *Metabolism*, *30*:111–117.

LKB Application Note No. 198. 1975. Preparative flat-bed electrofocusing in a granulated gel with the LKB 2117 Multiphor. LKB, Stockholm, Sweden.

Morrisett, J. D., Jackson, R. L., and Gotto, A. M., Jr. 1977. Lipid-protein interactions in the plasma lipoproteins. *Biochim. Biophys. Acta*, *472*:93–133.

Rall, S. C., Jr., Weisgraber, K. H., and Mahley, R. B. 1982. Human apolipoprotein E. The complete amino acid sequence. *J. Biol. Chem.*, *257*:4171–4178.

Smith, L. C., Pownall, H. J., and Gotto, A. M., Jr. 1978. The plasma lipoproteins: Structure and metabolism. *Annu. Rev. Biochem.*, *47*:751–777.

Socorro, L., and Camejo, G. 1979. Preparation and properties of soluble, immunoreactive apoLDL. *J. Lipid Res.*, *20*:631–638.

Sparks, C. E., and Marsh, J. B. 1981. Analysis of lipoprotein apoproteins by SDS-gel filtration column chromatography. *J. Lipid Res.*, *22*:514–518.

Van Zoelen, E. J. J., Verkliej, A. J., Zwool, R. F. A., and van Deenen, L. L. M. 1978. Incorporation and asymmetric orientation of glycophorin in reconstituted protein-containing vesicles. *Eur. J. Biochem.*, *86*:539–546.

Chapter **12**

Cardiac and Vascular Measurements in Conscious and Anesthetized Animals

R. W. Millard

Department of Pharmacology and Cell Biophysics
University of Cincinnati College of Medicine
Cincinnati, Ohio

I. INTRODUCTION

The intent of the following discussion is to provide instructional diagrams, typical recordings, practical applications, and references to methods used to evaluate changes in cardiac size (i.e., mechanics) and in the coronary circulation. Transit-time ultrasound technique and electromagnetic and ultrasonic flow techniques are described. Other methods and approaches to obtain similar measurements are available but have not been described.

II. CARDIAC DIMENSION ANALYSIS

A. Analysis of Global Cardiac Mechanics

Sonicrometry methods introduced by Rushmer *et al.* (1956) have been applied in the analysis of dynamic cardiac shape changes and in the derivation of indices of cardiac inotropic state. These devices have been used in many experimental studies including those in the fetal sheep heart of lambs *in vitro* (Kirkpatrick *et al.*, 1973), in dog hearts for modeling ventricular dynamic geometry (Rankin *et al.*, 1976), and in the analysis of new cardiotonic drugs (Nakaya *et al.*, 1983). Piezoelectric crystal transducers are typically located either at the opposing endocardial surfaces of the left ventricle or sewn to the epicardial surfaces (Figure 1). Orientation of the transducer crystal pair is most commonly in the left ventricle

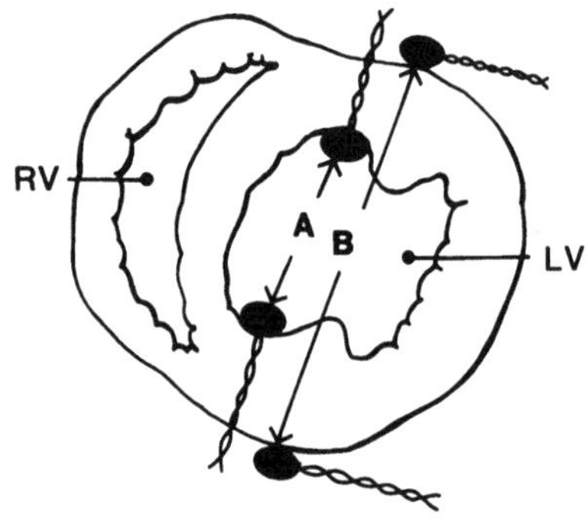

Figure 1. Implantation sites of sonomicrometer transducers in minor-axis orientation for monitoring global left ventricular mechanics (diameter) at either endocardial (A) or epicardial (B) surfaces.

minor axis, although occasionally major-axis applications have been made. Sasayama *et al.* (1979) have also applied these devices to the atria in attempts to study the distending forces on atrial proprioceptive receptors.

The data from continuous tracings are measurements of dimensions (D) at end diastole (ED) and systole (ES), the extent of shortening during systole ($ED - ES$), the fractional shortening during systole [$(ED - ES)/ED$], and the rate of systolic shortening ($\mathrm{d}D/\mathrm{d}t$). The rate of shortening is reflective of cardiac inotropic responses to experimental interventions but is somewhat different from the more traditional inotropic index, the first derivative of left ventricular pressure ($\mathrm{d}P/\mathrm{d}t$). The difference is that $\mathrm{d}P/\mathrm{d}t$ peak values occur during the preejection phase of the cardiac cycle prior to opening of the aortic valves, whereas peak $\mathrm{d}D/\mathrm{d}t$ values occur during ejection of blood from the ventricle into the aorta (Figure 2).

B. Analysis of Regional Cardiac Mechanics

Dimensions of regions of the heart can be monitored easily with sonomicrometer transducers implanted in subepicardial or subendocardial locations (Figure 3). These measurements are solely reflective of length changes (Sabbah *et al.*, 1981) and do not directly yield myocardial force data. It is clear that regional myocardial ischemia produces locally abnormal mechanical motion (Figure 4). Myocardial regional mechanics are affected by subendocardial ischemia (Gallagher *et al.*, 1980), progressive coronary artery stenosis (Millard, 1981), and by abrupt coronary artery occlusion in dog (Vatner *et al.*, 1976) and pig hearts (Millard, 1980) (Figure 5).

The measurements that are routinely obtained from regional sonomicrometer transducers include end-diastolic segment length (EDL) and end-systolic segment length (ESL), which allow the derivation of extent of shortening ($\Delta L = EDL - ESL$), regional shortening fraction ($\%SS = \Delta L/EDL$), and velocity of shortening ($\mathrm{d}L/\mathrm{d}t$) during ventricular ejection.

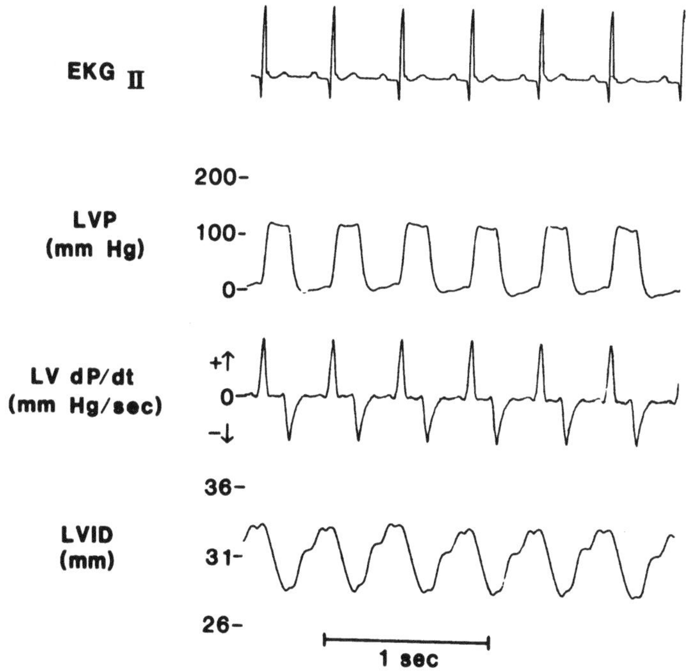

Figure 2. Tracings from a conscious dog or left ventricular minor-axis diameter (LVD) from an endocardial sonomicrometer transducer and left ventricular pressure (LVP) from a miniature transducer implanted chronically.

III. VASCULAR DYNAMICS ANALYSIS

A. Blood Volume and Velocity Flow Rates

The measurement of blood flow in the regional circulations can be made using one of two major principles: electromagnetic and ultrasonic. Electromagnetic flow transducers require that the fluid (blood) contain ions. The ions in the blood produce a current when they flow through the magnetic field of the transducer.

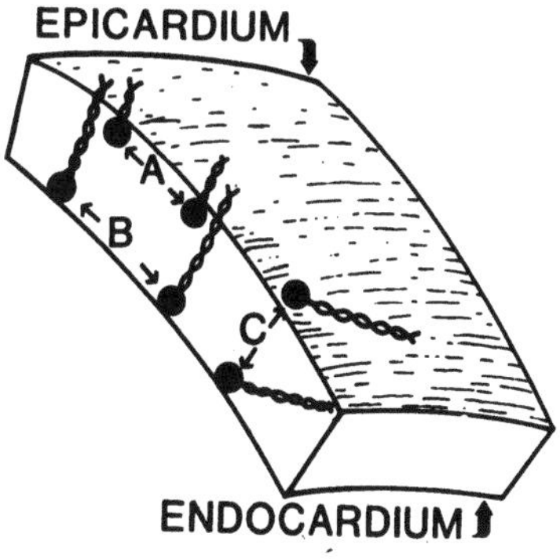

Figure 3. Implantation sites for regional myocardial mechanics measurement with sonomicrometer transducers. Subepicardial (A) and subendocardial (B) segments and wall thickness (C) can be continuously monitored.

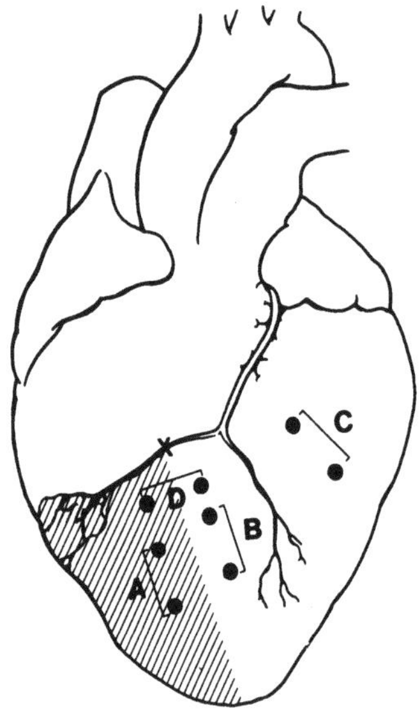

Figure 4. Myocardial mechanics in the pig heart with induced ischemia (shaded area) are monitored with sonomicrometer transducers in homogeneous blood flow regions called ischemic (A), border (B), and normal (C). A second border orientation (D) includes myocardium that is partly ischemic and partly normally perfused.

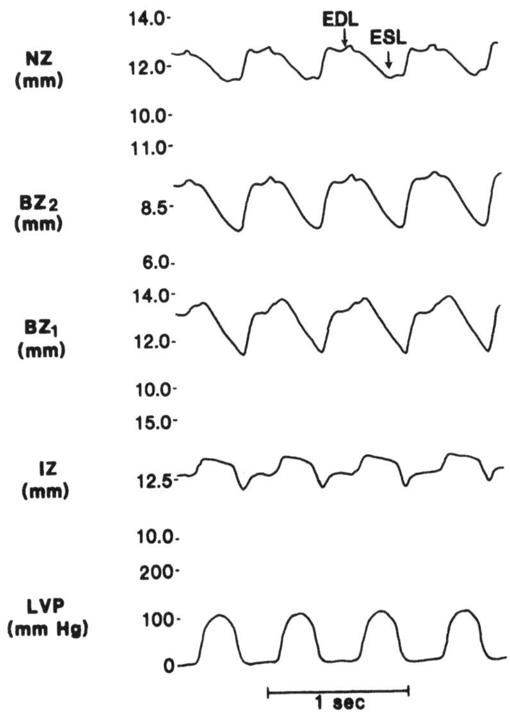

Figure 5. Simultaneous tracings from four sonomicrometer transducers and a miniature left ventricular (LVP) transducer in an open-chest anesthetized pig after a coronary artery was abruptly ligated to produce transmural myocardial ischemia. The transducer pairs are located parallel with and at 2 cm (normal zone, NZ), 1 cm (border zone 2, BZ2), and 0.5 cm (border zone 1, BZ1) from the sharp ischemic margin and within the center of the ischemic zone (IZ).

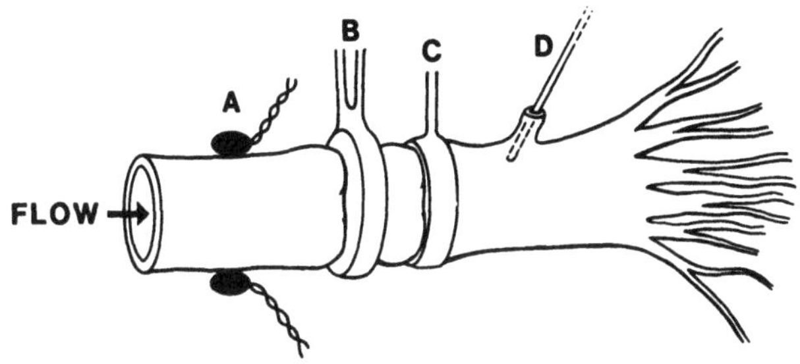

Figure 6. Relative location of sonomicrometer artery diameter transducer (A), flow transducer (B), hydraulic occlusive cuff (C), and intraarterial catheter for injection and pressure monitoring (D) for evaluation of conduit and resistance arterial responses to vasoactive interventions.

The final result is a voltage proportional to the volume blood flow. A reliable zero flow level is obtained only through the inflation of an hydraulic cuff distal to the flow transducer (Figure 6). Ultrasonic flow transducers require that the fluid (blood) contain reflectors. These reflectors are the blood cells, and the flow measurement depends on the difference between the sound frequency transmitted into the artery and that reflected from the moving cells in the artery. Thus, this approach truly measures velocity of blood and not volume blood flow. Zero flow is zero frequency difference and, thus, is easily obtained and is reliably and electronically stable. If an assumption that the blood vessel diameter does not decrease inside the transducer applies, then the output voltage signal, which is proportional to flow velocity, is also proportional to blood flow.

B. Vascular Dimensions

The external diameter of blood vessels, particularly arteries, can be dynamically recorded using transit-time principle ultrasound transducers secured to opposing adventitial surfaces (Figure 6). Two methods of affixing the transducers to the arterial adventitia have been found effective: securing by 5-0 sutures through an attached woven medical Dacron® patch or bonding with cyanomethacrylate medical-grade tissue adhesive. Piezoelectric transducer material with a resonance frequency of 5 or 10 MHz is used. Distance resolution is smaller than 0.05 mm at these frequencies. Sound is transmitted at a rate of 1.56 mm/μsec. The vessel diameter, which is measured by the sound transit time between the two piezoelectric transducers, is determined 800 times each second, so that the amplifier output becomes a continuous voltage proportional to external vessel diameter. These devices have been applied to the aorta (Pagani *et al.*, 1975) and coronary arteries (Vatner *et al.*, 1980; Tomoike *et al.*, 1981).

C. Analysis of Conductance and Resistance Vessel Responses

When the methods for blood flow and artery diameter measurement are combined and complemented by simultaneous blood pressure measurement, the large conduit artery responses can be separated from the responses of the arteriolar

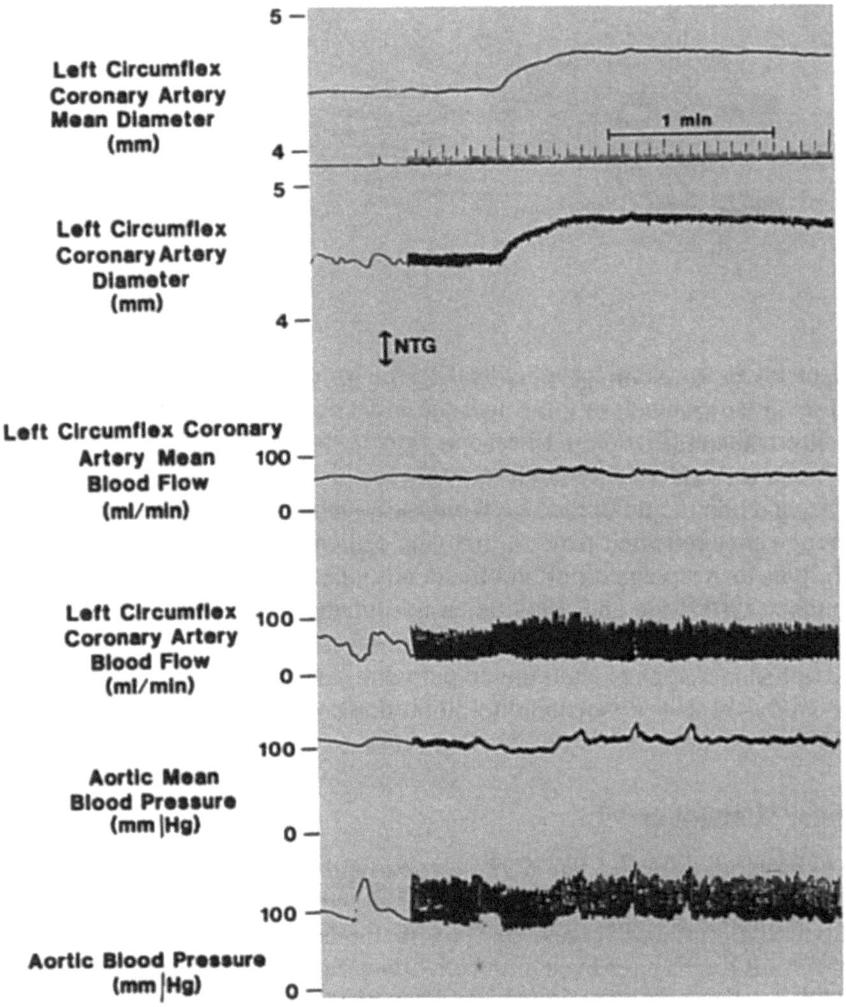

Figure 7. Representative coronary artery response to an intravenous nitroglycerin dose (3 μg/kg) that dilates proximal coronary artery but fails to significantly affect either coronary blood flow or coronary vascular resistance.

resistance vessels. The approach is straightforward, and for any intervention (e.g., nitroglycerin), the response of these anatomically distinct segments of the arterial circulation to any organ (e.g., heart) can be quantified (Figure 7). The proximal conduit artery diameter is directly read from the precalibrated oscillograph, but the average vascular resistance must be calculated as the quotient of average arterial blood pressure and average arterial blood flow. In this way, a comparative assessment between the effects of two putatively distinct vasodilators on the coronary circulation can be made by the dose–response studies to intravenous or close intraarterial injections (Figure 8).

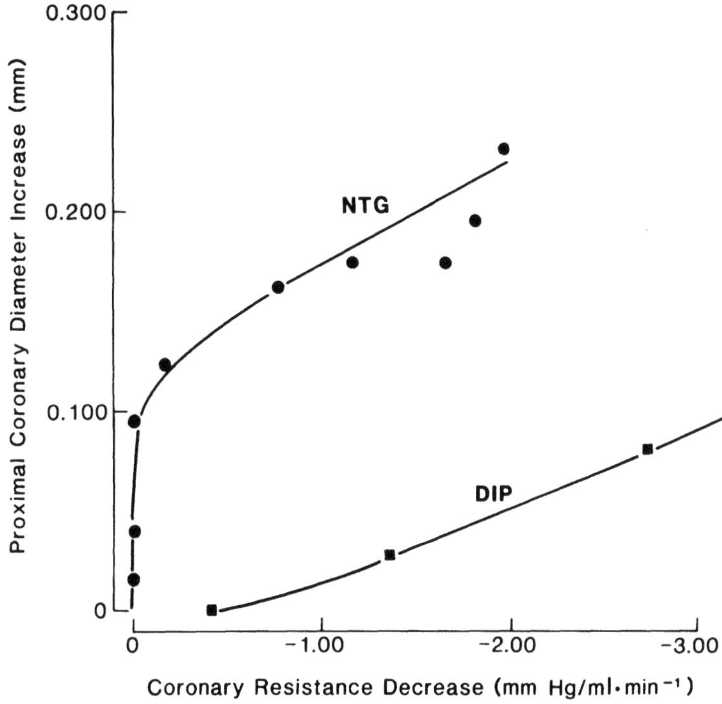

Figure 8. Responses to all doses of nitroglycerin (NTG) and dipyridamole (DIP) given intravenously are plotted on coronary artery diameter—mean coronary vascular resistance axes. Clearly, nitroglycerin dilates large vessels at the lower dose levels without significant effect on resistance vessels. Only when diameter is nearly maximum do doses begin to reduce vascular resistance. The converse is seen with dipyridamole.

REFERENCES

Gallagher, K. P., Kumada, T., Koziol, J. A., McKown, M., Kemper, W. S., and Ross, J., Jr. 1980. Significance of regional wall thickening abnormalities relative to transmural myocardial perfusion. *Circulation, 62:*1266–1274.

Kirkpatrick, S. E., Covell, J. W., and Friedman, W. F. 1973. A new technique for the continuous assessment of fetal and neonatal cardiac performance. *Am. J. Obstet. Bynecol., 116:*963–972.

Millard, R. W. 1980. Changes in cardiac mechanics and coronary blood flow of regionally ischemic porcine myocardium induced by diltiazem. *Chest, 78*[Suppl.]:193–199.

Millard, R. W. 1981. Induction of functional coronary collaterals in the swine heart. *Basic Res. Cardiol., 76:*486–473.

Nakaya, H., Schwartz, A., and Millard, R. W. 1983. Reflex chronotropic and inotropic effects of calcium channel-blocking agents in conscious dogs. *Circ. Res., 52:*302–311.

Pagani, M., Schwartz, P., Bishop, V. S., and Malliani, A. 1975. Reflex sympathetic changes in aortic diastolic pressure–diameter relationship. *Am. J. Physiol., 229:*286–290.

Rankin, J. S., McHale, P. A., Arentzen, C. E., Ling, D., Greenfield, J. C., and Anderson, R. W. 1976. The three-dimensional dynamic geometry of the left ventricle in the conscious dog. *Circ. Res., 39:*304–313.

Rushmer, R. F., Franklin, D. L., and Ellis, R. M. 1956. Left ventricular dimensions recorded by sonocardiometry. *Circ. Res., 4:*684–688.

Sabbah, H. N., Marzilli, M., and Stein, P. D. 1981. The relative role of subendocardium and subepicardium in left ventricular mechanics. *Am. J. Physiol., 240:*H920–H926.

Sasayama, S., Takahashi, M., Osakada, G., Hirose, K., Hamashima, H., Nishimura, E., and Kawai, C. 1979. Dynamic geometry of the left atrium and left ventricle in acute mitral regurgitation. *Circulation, 60:*177–186.

Tomoike, H., Ootsubo, H., Sakai, K., Kikuchi, Y., and Nakamura, M. 1981. Continuous measurement of coronary artery diameter *in situ. Am. J. Physiol., 240:*H73–H79.

Vatner, S. F., Millard, R. W., Patrick, T. A., and Heyndrick, G. R. 1976. Effects of isoproterenol on regional myocardial function, electrogram, and blood flow in conscious dogs with myocardial ischemia. *J. Clin. Invest., 57:*1261–1271.

Vatner, S. F., Pagani, M., Manders, W. T., and Pasipoularides, A. D. 1980. Alpha adrenergic vasoconstriction and nitroglycerin vasodilation of large coronary arteries in conscious dogs. *J. Clin. Invest., 65:*5–14.

Chapter **13**

Applications of Nuclear Magnetic Resonance to the Study of Myocardial Metabolism and Pharmacology

P. M. Matthews and G. K. Radda

Department of Biochemistry
University of Oxford
Oxford, England

I. INTRODUCTION

Since the first volume of this series appeared in 1971 with James Fisher's discussion of the application of nuclear magnetic resonance (NMR) relaxation measurements to the investigation of the binding of small molecules to proteins, instrumental sensitivity and experimental techniques have improved tremendously. In 1974, high-resolution NMR spectra were obtained from phosphate-containing metabolites in whole muscle (Hoult *et al.*, 1974). In subsequent years, many reports of metabolic studies using perfused organs and whole animals appeared. The area has been extensively reviewed (Gadian, 1982; Gadian and Radda, 1981; Gadian *et al.*, 1980; Radda and Seeley, 1979; Garlick and Radda, 1979; Shulman *et al.*, 1979; Burt et al., 1979; Hollis, 1979).

Nuclear magnetic resonance has been shown to provide a noninvasive and dynamic method for determining intracellular pH and probing intracellular metabolite concentrations, interactions, and reaction rates. One may develop an impression of the scope of the method by considering examples of recent applications of ^{31}P NMR:

Present address for P. M. Matthews: Department of Pharmacology, Stanford University School of Medicine, Stanford, California.

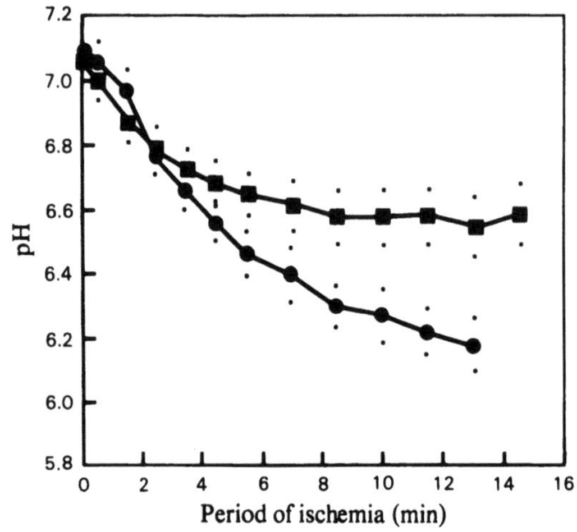

Figure 1. Time course of changes in intracellular pH in total global ischemia. Symbols: ●, control hearts (n = 7); ■, glycogen-depleted hearts (n = 6). The small symbols represent S.E.M. values.

1. In an elegant series of experiments, Dawson, Gadian, and Wilkie have used ^{31}P NMR to measure the concentrations of high-energy phosphate compounds while simultaneously controlling tension development to directly relate chemical energetics to mechanical function in skeletal muscle (Dawson *et al.*, 1977, 1978, 1980).
2. Relying on the pH dependence of the NMR signal from intracellular orthophosphate, Garlick *et al.* (1979) have defined the acidosis during ischemia in the isolated, perfused rat heart, quantitatively related it to postulated mechanisms of proton production, and demonstrated that cardioplegic solutions having high buffering capacity can greatly reduce the decrease in pH (Figure 1).
3. The intracellular concentration of Mg^{2+} has been calculated from nuclear magnetic resonance characteristics of intracellular phosphocreatine and ATP (Cohen and Burt, 1977; Wu *et al.*, 1981).
4. Determination of the kinetic parameters and the steady-state fluxes through specific enzymes in the intact tissue has become possible using saturation transfer NMR techniques (Gadian *et al.*, 1980), and measurement of the steady-state of ATP synthesis allows direct evaluation of mitochondrial function *in situ* (Matthews *et al.*, 1981).

Perhaps a more direct relevance to readers of this volume is that the effects of pharmacological interventions in the isolated, perfused heart are beginning to be explored using ^{31}P NMR to measure concentrations of high-energy phosphate compounds and intracellular pH. Early results suggest that NMR could play a significant role in explaining the metabolic consequences of administration of a broad range of drugs.

Recent studies in this laboratory correlated biochemical and functional changes following administration of the positive inotropic agents epinephrine, ouabain, or the ionophore R02-2985 (X537A) (Matthews *et al.*, 1982a). Two advantages of using NMR for metabolite assay were exploited: the ability to simultaneously collect data on the biochemistry and the physiological function and the ability to observe the dynamics of metabolic changes in a single preparation over the full time course of the experiment. Thus, it was immediately apparent that, despite constant levels of mechanical function, high-energy metabolite concentrations changed throughout the observation period under some conditions, reflecting aspects of the short-term adaptation to the increased energy demands. As an important addition to information on relative changes, absolute concentrations were determined. Of particular interest were concentrations of free intracellular orthophosphate, which is difficult even to estimate by chemical assay because of nonspecific orthophosphate binding to intracellular structures (Gergely and Maruyama, 1960).

In total global ischemia, the extent of intracellular acidosis is a good index of lactate production, the control of which could be an important focus of efforts to prolong the viability of ischemic tissue. The ease with which NMR determines intracellular pH therefore has considerable potential in studies of ischemic protection. For example, Pieper and his colleagues (1980) have demonstrated that prior propranolol administration reduces the extent of acidosis in the totally globally ischemic guinea pig heart. Observation of a reduced rate of net phosphocreatine hydrolysis demonstrated immediately that the treatment lowered energy demand during the ischemic period in addition to lowering the rate of glycolytic energy production.

These results mark just the first crude beginning of NMR applications to cardiac pharmacology. A remarkably wide range of parameters that can define metabolite concentrations, fluxes, and the nature of the intracellular environmental are able to be measured, and a rapidly growing range of experimental models can be used. As is discussed in more detail below, it is now possible to make such measurements on hearts *in situ* in whole animals, and technological advances may soon make it possible to study hearts in live humans (see Section V.F).

However, although considerable information is available from a well-designed NMR measurement on whole tissue, it is important to emphasize that NMR provides information that is to a large degree complementary to that obtained from standard biochemical procedures. The fundamental problem is the inherent insensitivity of the method. It is unlikely that it will ever prove convenient (or even possible) to perform a broad range of assays for compounds other than those in concentrations that give at least about 1.0 μmoles of identical nuclei in the sample volume. Thus, direct study of compounds in very low concentrations (such as cAMP) will probably never be possible.

Nonetheless, the noninvasive and dynamic character of the measurement offers advantages that can outweigh the lack of sensitivity, particularly in pharmacodynamic studies. It is hoped that this chapter will provide a simple, general description of these types of NMR experiments that is more practically biased than the discussions currently available. For more sophisticated introductions to the theory and practice of NMR, the reader is referred to some of the many texts now available (for example, Gadian, 1982; Shaw, 1976; Farrer and Becker, 1971) and the comprehensive review by Campbell and Dobson (1979).

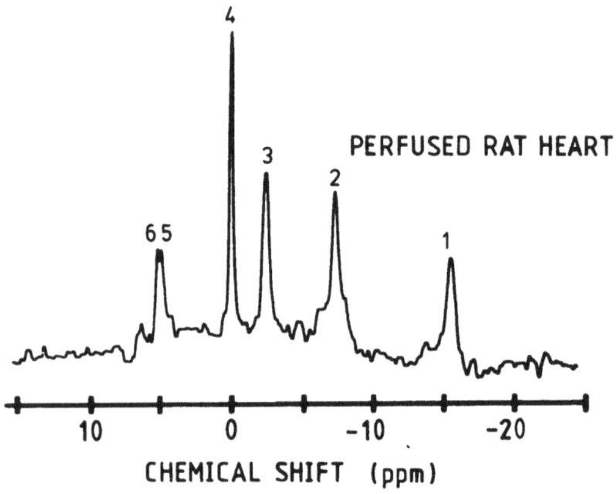

Figure 2. 73.84 MHz ^{31}P NMR spectrum of Langendorff perfused rat heart; 408 sampling pulses were applied, requiring a total of 8 min for collection. Sweep width was 3 kHz. Peak assignments: 1, β-ATP; 2, α-ATP + α-ADP + phosphodiesters; 3, γ-ATP + β-ADP; 4, phosphocreatine; 5, intracellular inorganic phosphate; 6, extracellular phosphate in Krebs–Henseleit buffer.

This chapter should provide some basis for the nonspectroscopist to assess the suitability of NMR for investigation of a new range of problems in cardiac biochemistry and pharmacology. More ambitiously, it represents an attempt to describe some of the technical aspects of the experiment in a way that might help physiologists or pharmacologists working in collaboration with spectroscopists to understand better the nature of the data available from the measurement.

II. THE BASIC QUESTION

A. What Is Nuclear Magnetic Resonance?

The high-resolution ^{31}P NMR spectrum of a perfused rat heart is reproduced in Figure 2. It may be considered simply as a plot of frequency of energy absorption (abscissa) as a function of the absorption intensity (ordinate) (see Section II.C). The frequency of each peak is characteristic of the nucleus, the type of compound the nucleus is in, its position within the molecule, and even the environment of the molecule. The intensity is proportional to the number of identical nuclei giving rise to that peak. The spectrum is said to be of "high resolution" because differences in absorption frequencies on the order of fractions of a part per million are able to be discerned, allowing the very specific information about the origin of the signal noted above to be inferred.

Only nuclei that have magnetic moments may be observed using NMR. Fortunately, most elements in the periodic table have isotopes that possess magnetic moments, including the biologically important nuclei phosphorus (^{31}P), hydrogen (^{1}H), and carbon (^{13}C) (Table I). When placed in a magnetic field, the nuclear magnets in a sample will align either with or against the field, rather as a compass needle is oriented by the earth's magnetic field (Figure 3). Nuclei aligned with the field have a lower energy and may absorb energy in the radio frequency range to "flip" to the higher energy state of the opposed alignment (Figure 4). The frequency of absorption is primarily a function of the type of nucleus but is also

Table I. Magnetic Isotopes of Biologically Important Elements

Mass number	Nucleus	Freq. (MHz)	Spin quantum number	Natural isotopic abundance (%)	Relative sensitivity[a]
1	H	180.00	$\frac{1}{2}$	99.985	1
2	H	27.63	1	1.5×10^{-2}	9.6×10^{-3}
3	H	191.99	$\frac{1}{2}$	—	1.21
13	C	45.26	$\frac{1}{2}$	1.108	1.6×10^{-2}
14	N	13.00	1	99.63	1.0×10^{-3}
15	N	18.24	$\frac{1}{2}$	0.37	1.0×10^{-3}
17	O	24.40	$\frac{5}{2}$	0.037	2.9×10^{-2}
19	F	169.34	$\frac{1}{2}$	100	0.83
23	Na	47.61	$\frac{3}{2}$	100	9.1×10^{-2}
25	Mg	11.01	$\frac{5}{2}$	10.13	2.7×10^{-3}
31	P	72.87	$\frac{1}{2}$	100	6.7×10^{-2}
33	S	13.81	$\frac{3}{2}$	0.76	2.2×10^{-3}
35	Cl	17.64	$\frac{3}{2}$	75.53	4.7×10^{-3}
37	Cl	14.68	$\frac{3}{2}$	24.47	2.7×10^{-3}
39	K	8.40	$\frac{3}{2}$	93.10	5.1×10^{-4}
43	Ca	12.11	$\frac{7}{2}$	0.145	6.3×10^{-2}
203	Tl	102.87	$\frac{1}{2}$	29.50	0.18
205	Tl	103.88	$\frac{1}{2}$	70.50	0.19

[a] Sensitivity relative to ^{1}H.

affected by the many factors determining the electron density about the nucleus, e.g., the nature of the bonds to the atom and intermolecular interactions.

The magnetic moments of nuclei are a consequence of a quantum mechanical property known as spin. As its name suggests, nuclear spin may be conveniently visualized, and most consequences important to the NMR experiment predicted,

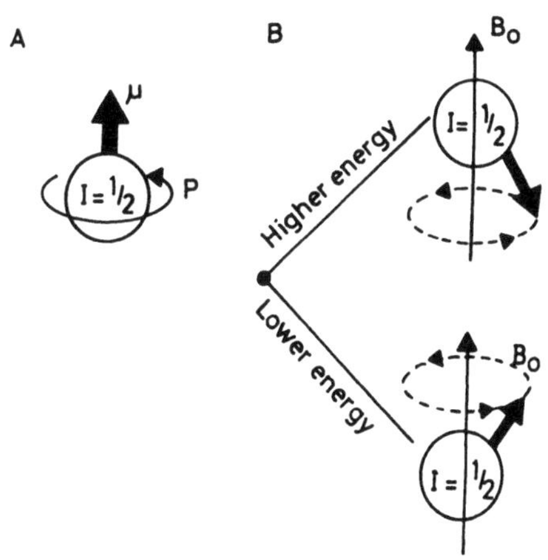

Figure 3. (a) A representation of nuclear spin. The nuclear spin angular momentum $p = h[I(I + 1)]^{1/2}$ gives rise to a magnetic moment $\mu = \gamma p$, where γ is a constant known as the gyromagnetic ratio that is directed along the axis of rotation. (b) A representation of nuclear spins orientated in an applied magnetic field. The nuclear magnetic moments of spin-$\frac{1}{2}$ nuclei can assume one of two orientations relative to an applied static magnetic field, B_0. The directions of the nuclear magnetic moments are not precisely defined; they precess along the surface of cones around the applied field vector.

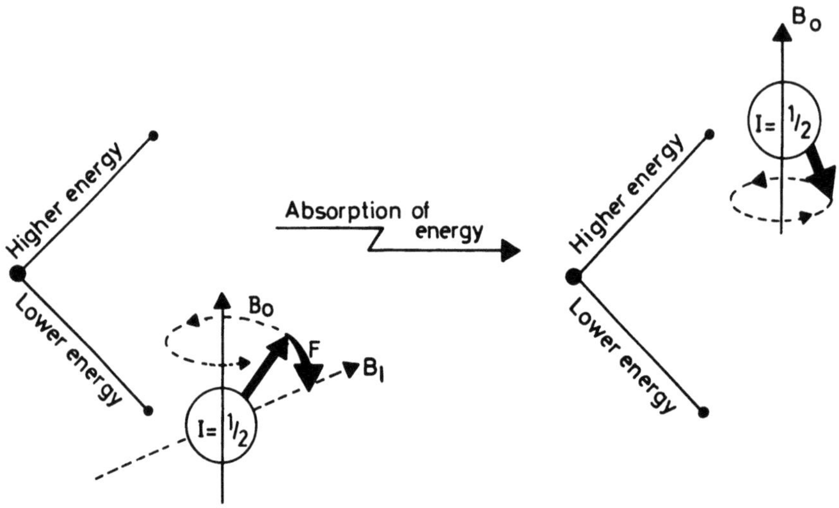

Figure 4. A representation of a nuclear spin transition. An oscillating RF field, B_1, applied at a right angle to the direction of the static B_0 field will induce a force F on the nuclear magnetic moment, μ. If B_1 and μ are precessing at the same rate, then F acts consistently and can induce an energy transition, i.e., a change in the orientation of the nuclear magnetic moments with respect to B_0.

using the model of a charged sphere spinning about its axis. To facilitate communication with the more theoretically minded, however, it should be noted that spin is defined by a quantum number, I, which, depending on the nucleus, may assume values $I = \frac{1}{2}, 1, \frac{3}{2}, 2, \ldots$. This chapter is primarily concerned with ^{31}P and other nuclei for which $I = \frac{1}{2}$. Applications of nuclei having $I > \frac{1}{2}$ (quadrupolar nuclei) to cardiac studies have yet to be made, partly because these nuclei are technically more difficult to observe.

The magnetic moment of a nucleus having spin is directed along its axis of rotation. It may be considered to arise in much the same way that an electromagnet generates a magnetic field. In an electromagnet, a current is made to flow along a circular path, creating a field directed according to the "right-hand rule" of elementary physics courses. The spinning of a charged nucleus gives it the properties of a circulating current. The magnitude of the field produced by an electromagnet increases with the current flowing through the circular coils. Similarly, the magnetic moment of a nucleus is proportional to its angular momentum. The exact constant of proportionality (the "gyromagnetic" or "magnetogyric" ratio) is different for each nucleus, however, This is fortuitous, for it will be seen below (eq. 1) that this is the basis of the distinction among different types of nuclei in NMR.

When a nuclear magnetic moment interacts with an applied static magnetic field (B_0), it acquires an energy determined by its relative orientation in the field. Quantum mechanics predicts that only $2I + 1$ defined orientations are possible and, consequently, that the nuclear energy levels are split into $(2I + 1)$ discrete states by application of the field. Thus, for a spin-$\frac{1}{2}$ nucleus, the levels are split into two states: a low-energy state for nuclei with a magnetic moment parallel to the field and a high-energy state for the antiparallel orientation.

But, because the nuclei possess angular momentum, they are not statically orientated in the applied field. The angular momentum of a spinning gyroscope, for example, results in its precession about the vector of the "applied" gravitational field. The magnetic moments of nuclei similarity precess about the direction of B_0 with an angular frequency, ω_0, determined by the angular momentum characteristic of the nucleus and the strength of the applied field:

$$\omega_0 = 2\pi\nu = \gamma B_0 \tag{1}$$

(where γ is the gyromagnetic ratio).

In the NMR experiment, transitions between adjacent energy states are induced by the application of an oscillating magnetic field, B_1, at a right angle to the direction of the static B_0. For B_1 to interact with the nuclear magnetic moments, it must be oscillating at precisely the frequency of precession, ω_0. In practice, an electromagnetic wave in the radio frequency range is applied, so B_1 is commonly referred to as the radio frequency (RF) field. Only the magnetic component interacts with the spins to induce transitions.

It is important to note that transitions both from high to low and from low to high states are induced with equal probability. Net absorption of energy occurs only when there is a population difference between adjacent states: if the populations are equal, there are an equal number of transitions in both directions, and there is no absorption of energy by the nuclei. At equilibrium, the populations of nuclei in the various energy states are determined by the ratio of the relative energies of these states to the thermal energy of the sample. The greater the thermal energy, the smaller the population difference. The ratio is usually quite small, so populations differ by less than 1 part in 10^4 even at temperatures far lower than those practical with biological systems. In consequence, there is only a very weak absorption of energy. It is for this reason that NMR is an inherently insensitive analytical technique.

Note that an increase in the B_0 field increases the energy difference between adjacent states and hence their population difference, thereby enhancing the net absorption of energy. As a result, it is ideal that experiments with small samples of living tissue (~1 g wet wt.), in which most metabolites are at concentrations that give less than 10 μmoles of identical nuclei, be done at high field strengths. Most of the types of experiments described in this chapter are more easily done at field strengths of 3 Tesla (in which ω_0 is about 130 MHz for protons) or more.

The absorption frequency of a given nucleus depends on its gyromagnetic ratio and the magnitude of the applied field, B_0, at the nucleus, as given by eq. 1. As noted above, the gyromagnetic ratios vary, so different nuclei absorb, or resonate, at widely different frequencies. For example, in a 4.2-Tesla field, ^{31}P nuclei resonate at roughly 73.84 MHz, ^{13}C at 45.869 MHz, and ^{1}H at 182.4 MHz. As the spectrometer electronics are tuned to respond maximally to frequencies in a narrow range, nuclei of only one type are conventionally observed in a single experiment.

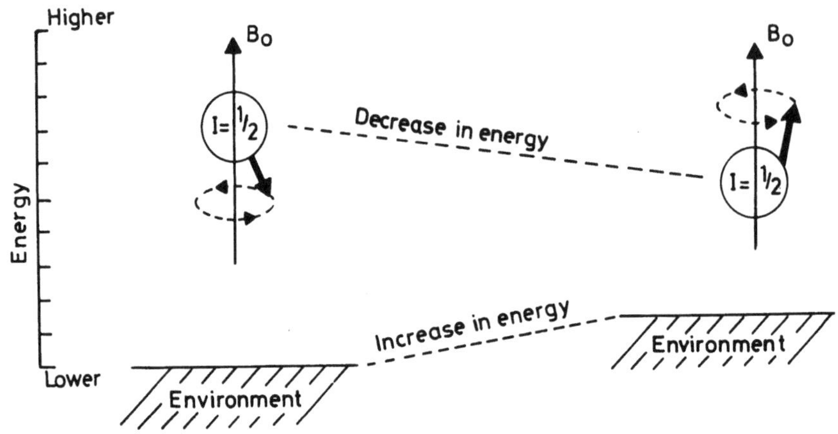

Figure 5. A representation of T_1 relaxation processes. Spin–lattice relaxation (described by a reciprocal first-order rate constant, T_1) occurs when there is a net transfer of energy from the spin system to its environment.

But NMR provides more than simply a qualitative guide to the types of nuclei present in a sample. The applied magnetic field, B_0, induces orbital motions in the electrons surrounding the nuclei, which, in turn, produce very small magnetic fields proportional in magnitude to B_0 but opposed in direction. Hence, a particular nucleus experiences a field that is the sum of the applied field and the small local fields (the "shielding" resulting from the circulation of neighboring electrons). As the electron density about each nucleus is characteristic of the molecule in which it is found and, in fact, of its position within that molecule, the frequency of precession in an applied field, ω_0, will vary for nuclei in different molecules and at different positions within a molecule. Resonance frequencies can also change in response to environmental factors such as the solvent, pH, ionic strength, temperature, and even molecular conformation.

The absorption of energy by a spin system in a static field will decrease the population difference between adjacent states and can eventually eliminate it, preventing further absorption. As the spins interact with the oscillating B_1, they assume states of higher energetics than those at equilibrium. They can maintain such nonequilibrium states only with the continued input of energy. When B_1 is off, the spins spontaneously relax towards equilibrium by means of various processes that depend on the action of fluctuating magnetic fields at the nucleus. The return of the spins from a higher to a lower energy state is described by a reciprocal first-order rate constant known as the longitudinal relaxation time, T_1 (Figure 5). The energy that the spin system loses during this process is returned to the environment, commonly called the lattice, as thermal energy. A second relaxation process, characterized by the transverse relaxation time, T_2, is responsible for randomizing the phases of precession of the spins, which are ordered by interaction with the oscillating B_1. T_2 establishes the inherent line width of a signal at half-height ($\nu_{1/2} = 1/\pi \cdot T_2$).

To summarize, nuclei having magnetic moments can assume different energy states in a static magnetic field, B_0. The NMR phenomenon arises with the absorption of energy from an oscillating magnetic field, B_1, applied at a right angle to B_0, that can promote transitions between these states. Thus, the minimum requirements for the NMR experiment are (1) a sample, (2) a strong magnet to polarize the magnetic spins, (3) a sensitive antenna surrounding the sample to transmit the radio frequency and detect its absorption, and (4) appropriate equipment to generate the frequency, amplify the absorption signal, and display it.

B. How Is It Observed?

The experiment is prepared by placing the sample within the field of a radio frequency transmitter/receiver coil (sometimes two coils, a transmitter and a receiver, are used in a "crossed-coil" arrangement) tuned to resonate at the precession frequency of the nucleus being observed, e.g., 73.84 MHz for ^{31}P in a 4.2-Tesla field (see eq. 1). Tuning the coil makes it a particularly powerful antenna for electromagnetic oscillations at the precession frequency. During an experiment, the probe, which includes the RF coil, is positioned in the bore of the magnet so that the sample is in the most homogeneous part of the field.

Differences in the magnitude of the B_0 field over the sample volume cause the same nuclei to resonate at different frequencies depending on the exact value of the field at the different points within the sample. In severe cases, this can give rise to a broad, low-intensity signal from which all high-resolution information has been lost. In high-resolution NMR, when frequency shifts of the order of 0.1 part per million (ppm) are to be observed, the homogeneity of the static B_0 field over the sample volume must be maintained to at least the same precision. Because introduction of the probe assembly into the field can seriously disturb the homogeneity within these tolerances, field correction coils (commonly referred to as shim coils) must be adjusted to create small magnetic fields that oppose and compensate for these inhomogeneities. The shim coils are fitted into the bore of the magnet, and each one is designed so that the passage of an electrical current through it generates a different, well-defined field gradient. The shim coils are adjusted until the resonance of some clearly observable signal, e.g., from the protons in water (Ackerman *et al.,* 1981), is sufficiently narrow for the desired resolution. The sample is often spun to average out field inhomogeneities and further narrow the line widths, but this is generally impossible with whole-tissue preparations.

The conventional continuous wave experiment in which the B_1 field is slowly swept through a range of radio frequencies is highly inefficient for the collection of signals from samples containing many resonances. Whole-tissue studies (a notable exception being ^1H NMR studies of tissue water) generally demand the use of Fourier transform NMR (FT NMR), a method first discussed by Ernst and Anderson (1966). In FT NMR, the signal is collected following perturbation of the spins from the equilibrium state by a short, intense RF pulse (B_1), the magnetic component of which is directed at a right angle to the B_0 field. It may be shown that application of an RF pulse, typically lasting about 1–100 μsec, can simultaneously excite all of the nuclei that one wishes to observe in the sample. Immediately after the pulse, the coil begins to function as a receiving antenna and has small voltage changes induced in it (~5 nV) by magnetization changes of the excited nuclei (Hoult and Richards, 1975). Data collection follows the decay of transverse magnetization for a period of several T_2 (often around 50–100 msec), where T_2 is the time constant for decay of the signal and a function of both spin–spin relaxation processes and inhomogeneities in the magnetic field.

When one is observing metabolites in living tissue, the pulse–data collection cycle generally must be repeated many times and the results summed to yield a sufficient ratio of signal to noise in the final spectrum. Because the noise is random, it increases in amplitude more slowly than a resonance signal as the transients following the pulses are summed. The pulses are repeated after waiting periods during which the perturbed nuclei return at least partially to their equilibrium states.

Aside from considerations of spectrometer and probe design, the experimental parameters most critical in determining the signal-to-noise ratio available from a given sample are the pulse length and waiting period between pulses. The optimal combinations are governed by the spin–lattice relaxation times of the resonances of interest. Becker *et al.* (1979) discusses the selection of optimal parameters in a particularly useful manner.

In FT NMR, the signal collected is known as the free induction decay (FID). The FID is the superposition of decaying wave patterns, one corresponding to each of the resonant nuclei, oscillating at rates determined by their resonance frequencies. The initial intensity of each decay is proportional to the concentration of nuclei resonating with that frequency in a given sample volume. The amplitude-*vs.*-time data in the FID include all of the information necessary for the more conventional amplitude-*vs.*-frequency spectrum. The latter may be obtained from the FID by means of a Fourier transformation that can be rapidly performed by an on-line computer. Spectra are usually stored as the FIDs on magnetic disks to allow later Fourier transformation and analysis.

C. What Is an NMR Spectrum?

The NMR spectrum is a representation of the intensity of absorption as a function of frequency. A plot of signal amplitude against frequency is ideally a lorentzian curve, as illustrated in Figure 6.

1. The Chemical Shift and Spin–Spin Coupling

As discussed in the previous section, the exact resonance frequency of a given nucleus varies with its chemical environment because of local magnetic fields produced by circulating electrons. However, shielding effects are so small relative to the applied field (B_0) that differences between resonance frequencies are only on the order of a few parts in 10^6. The differences also vary with the strength of the applied field. To facilitate representation of the resonance frequencies measured in different magnets, they are expressed as a "chemical shift"

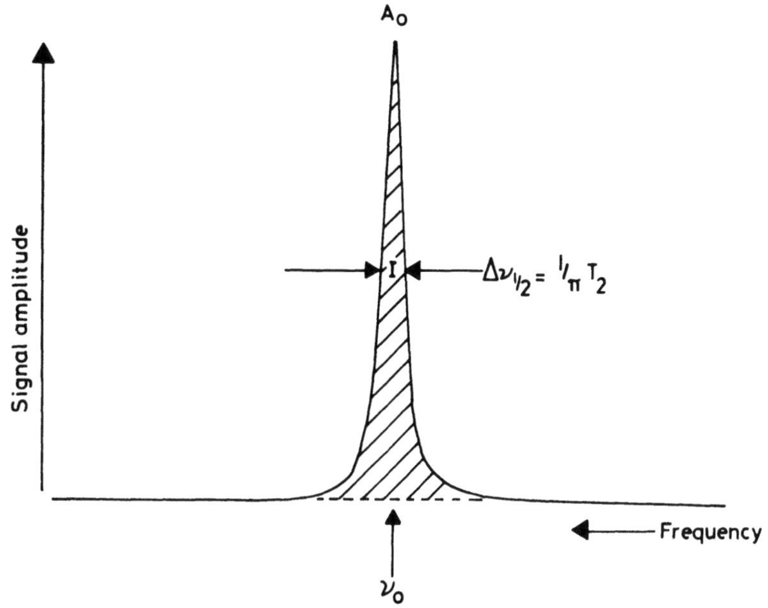

Figure 6. Parameters of the nuclear magnetic resonance signal. The nuclear magnetic resonance signal is characterized by its intensity (*I*), amplitude (*A*), central frequency (ν_0), and line width ($\nu_{1/2}$). The resonances generally have a Lorentzian shape, $g(\nu)$, described mathematically as $g(\nu) = T_2/2^{-2}[1 + 4^{-2}T_2^2(V_0 - \nu)^2]$.

in terms of parts per million (ppm) relative to the frequency of some standard compound:

$$\text{ppm} = (\nu_{\text{std}} - \nu_{\text{obs}}) \times 10^6/\nu_{\text{std}}$$

(where ν_{std} and ν_{obs} are the frequencies of the standard and observed peaks, respectively). Thus, the chemical shift is independent of field strength. It is a generally accepted convention that the chemical shift of a resonance is positive if the sample nucleus is more shielded than the reference. Unfortunately, as not all spectroscopists are conventional, some ^{31}P NMR spectra have been published with the reverse orientation.

The ^{31}P NMR resonances of, for example, the α and β phosphates of ATP are split into two and three main peaks, respectively. This splitting arises from the interaction of neighboring magnetic nuclei and is transmitted through the bonding electrons. The magnitude of the splitting is independent of the applied B_0 field strength. In general, a resonance is split into $2nI + 1$ peaks by n neighboring nuclei of spin I. This effect, known as spin–spin coupling, is rapidly attenuated as the number of bonds between the interacting nuclei increases. Although spin–spin coupling has not been of much importance in whole-organ studies to date because resolution of ^{31}P spin coupling has been poor, with the advent of ^{13}C NMR, it may become quite important, as it allows quantitation of relative isotopic enrichment at adjacent sites (Cohen *et al.*, 1979a; Bailey *et al.*, 1981). This splitting can also provide important information concerning molecular interactions or the molecular architecture about a nucleus (Gupta *et al.*, 1978; Karplus, 1959).

2. *Reference Compounds*

In order to get reproducible chemical shifts, the choice of a reference compound must be made carefully. It is essential that the reference frequency can be measured at any time throughout an experiment without disturbing the experimental configuration, as even small changes in coil position, for example, can lead to significant shifts in the field strength. Ideally, the reference should give a narrow resonance that is well removed from those expected from the sample. It should be chemically inert, and, as far as possible, its resonance frequency should be independent of the nature of the sample. If it does shift with changes in pH, temperature, or solvent conditions encountered during the course of an experiment, it is essential that the extent and direction of the shift be well characterized. The reference compound may be internal to the sample, or it may be put in a closed capillary tube within the sample chamber or perhaps in an annulus around it, as an external reference.

In the early studies of muscle, chemical shifts were expressed relative to 85% phosphoric acid as an external standard. However, this proved not to be an ideal standard: its line width is large, and because it perturbs magnetic lines of force in a significantly different way than does a saline solution or whole tissue, chemical shifts measured relative to it change slightly with orientation of the sample in the applied field (Gadian *et al.*, 1980; Burt *et al.*, 1979).

For heart and muscle, the phosphocreatine naturally present may be used as a reference compound in ^{31}P NMR (Dawson *et al.*, 1977). When one is observing other nuclei, it has been suggested that the water resonance may be used as a general, internal frequency standard (Ackerman *et al.*, 1981). Because its concentration in any biological sample is very high, it can be observed even with spectrometers tuned for other nuclei simply by an appropriate adjustment of the B_1 transmitter frequency. Its frequency variation over the range of pH and temperature encountered in a biological study is easily determined.

3. *Spectral Assignment*

Fortunately, enough work has already been done with the relatively simple ^{31}P spectrum to propose unambiguous assignments for most observable metabolites (Table II), but in unusual circumstances or when ^{1}H or ^{13}C NMR is used, the crucial problem of assigning resonances to specific nuclear sites in metabolites may not be trivial. A tentative assignment may be based on the chemical shifts by comparison with those observed in previous experiments or with those observed for pure compounds in solution. As the chemical shift may change significantly with solvent, pH, the counterions present, the nature of specific intermolecular interactions, and temperature, studies with pure compounds are best done over a broad range of the conditions likely to be encountered. For example, the β resonance of ATP shifts by 2.8 ppm to lower frequency on binding to Mg^{2+}

Table II. ^{31}P Chemical Shifts of Some Biologically Important Compounds

Compound	Chemical shift (ppm)[a,b]	Comment	Reference[c]
Nucleotides			
ATP·Mg		5 m*M* ATP + 10 m*M* $MgCl_2$	
γ	−2.5	+ 180 m*M* KCl, pH 7.16	a
α	−7.6		
β	−16.1		
ATP			
γ	−3.8	5 m*M* ATP, pH 7.26	a
α	−8.0		
β	−18.9		
ADP·Mg			
β	−3.0	5 m*M* ADP, pH 7.26	a
α	−7.0		
ADP			
β	−4.4	5 m*M* ADP + 10 m*M* $MgCl_2$,	a
α	−7.9	pH 7.12	
AMP/IMP	6.3	pH 7.01	a
Pyridines and flavins			
NAD	−8.3	Negligible pH dependence	a
NADH	−8.1	Negligible pH dependence	a
FAD	−6.1	Conditions not reported	a
Sugar phosphates			
Glucose-1-phosphate	5.0	pH 7.01	a
Glucose-6-phosphate			
β	7.1	pH 7.01	a
α	7.4	160 m*M* KCl, pH 7.42	a
Fructose-6-phosphate	6.4	pH 7.01	a
Fructose-1,6-diphosphate			
α	7.7, 6.6	pH 7.32	a
β	6.8, 6.6		
Deoxyglucose-6-phosphate	7.1	Rat heart (enriched), pH 7.08	d
Further glycolytic intermediates			
2-Phosphoglycerate	5.8	pH 7.13	a
3-Phosphoglycerate	6.5	pH 7.12	a
Glycerol-1-phosphate	7.0	pH 7.23	a
Glycerol-2-phosphate	6.6	pH 7.23	a
Glyceraldehyde-3-phosphate	7.0	pH 7.22	a
Dihydroxyacetone phosphate (hydrate-free)	7.6	pH 7.22	a
Phosphoenolpyruvate	2.0	pH 7.12	a
Phosphodiesters			
Phosphorylcholine	6.1	Ehrlich ascites cell extract	b
Glycerol-3-phosphorylcholine	2.8	Ehrlich ascites cell extract	b
Glycerol-3-phosphorylethanolamine	3.3	Ehrlich ascites cell extract	b

(continued)

Table II. (*Continued*)

Compound	Chemical shift (ppm)[a,b]	Comment	Reference[c]
Miscellaneous compounds			
Pyrophosphates (nonterminal)	−15.1 to −20.2	Yeast cell, pH 6.3	c
Inorganic phosphate	5.0	pH 7.10	d
Adenosine diphosphoglucose			
β	−9.8	Conditions not reported	e
α	−8.3		

[a] Values referenced to phosphocreatine assuming it to be 2.32 ppm upfield of an 85% phosphoric acid standard (Gadian *et al.*, 1980).
[b] Downfield shifts are recorded as positive.
[c] References are as follows: (a) Gadian *et al.* (1980); (b) Navon *et al.* (1977); (c) Salhany *et al.* (1975); (d) Bailey *et al.* (1981a); (e) Navon *et al.* (1978).

(see Table II), and the orthophosphate resonance shifts by 3.5 ppm as the relative amounts of HPO_4^{2-} and PO_4^{3-} change (Figure 7). Consideration must also be given to possible effects of binding to macromolecules in the whole tissue (Roberts *et al.*, 1981).

Proposed assignments based on chemical shifts should be assessed in the light of metabolite concentrations determined by classical methods. Caution must be exercised in assigning resonances solely on the basis of chemical shift, for the relatively broad lines in whole-tissue NMR may preclude the resolution of metabolites with similar chemical shifts; e.g., in ^{31}P NMR of rat hearts, the NAD^+ resonance often cannot be distinguished from the α-phosphate resonance of ATP. The line widths may also provide a clue; as a general statement, resonances will be sharp enough to be observed only if the molecules from which they arise possess considerable freedom of movement. This will occur for species in free

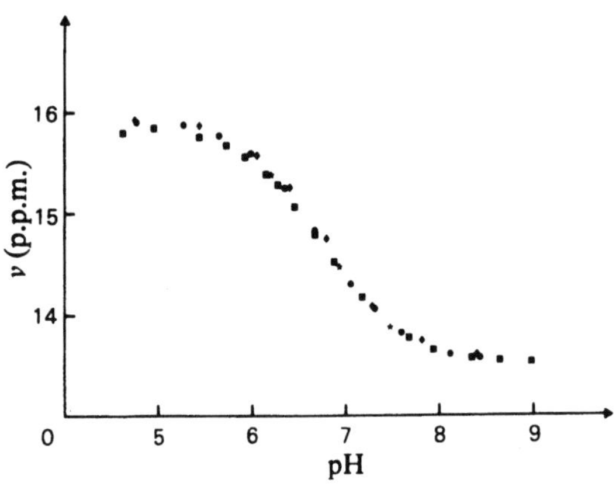

Figure 7. Variation of inorganic phosphate (P_i) chemical shift with solution pH. Solutions containing 10 m*M* P_i were adjusted to various ionic strengths by addition of KCl or NaCl and titrated at 37°C by addition of HCl and KOH or NaOH. Symbols: ◆, 0.12 *M* KC1; ■, 0.16 *M* KCl; ●, 0.2 *M* KCl; μ = 0.16 *M* NaCl. The chemical shift is expressed with respect to an internal standard (methylenediphosphonate), 19.2 ppm from PCr.

solution (e.g., in the cytosol) rather than, for example, those bound to membranes or to large proteins.

The spectra of extracts of freeze-clamped tissue can provide information useful in assignment. Because smaller volumes may be used and they can be spun, broadening of the resonances caused by slight variations in the B_0 field strength across the sample (inhomogeneity broadening) will be much less than with whole tissue, and, in consequence, resolution can be expected to increase significantly. Initially, this will increase the discernment of assignment on the basis of chemical shift. Spin–spin coupling constants, often obscured by inhomogeneity broadening in whole tissue, can provide some information on the number and type of atoms bonded to a nucleus. More important, however, is that the experimenter is free to modify the environment of the molecules to affect metabolites or their environment in specific ways. A general technique is to alter the pH of the extract solution, observing changes in the chemical shifts as the titration progresses to determine the p*K*s of the molecules associated with each resonance. Another is to add small amounts of known compounds to the extract to see if their resonances superimpose on those already observed from the sample. Ugurbil *et al.* (1978a) have confirmed ^{13}C spectral assignments by the specific enzymic transformation of one of the metabolites in the extract.

Spin–lattice relaxation times of metabolites are generally appreciably shorter in whole tissue than in an extract solution. Thus, it may take longer to accumulate spectra from identical amounts of compound in an extract than when the whole organ is used. This may be particularly important in ^{13}C NMR, where the relaxation times of unprotonated carbons can be as long as several tens of seconds. Of course, if solubility is not a problem, extracts from a number of organs may be pooled to increase the concentrations in the sample.

Another approach is to reduce relaxation times in extracts. Relying on the reduction in relaxation times that occurs with decreasing mobility for small molecules in solution, Sternlicht and co-workers (1971) were able to greatly reduce the ^{13}C relaxation times of amino acids by adding an ion-exchange resin to partially immobilize them. Alternatively, paramagnetic ions may be added to achieve any desired reduction in relaxation time. A drawback is that it may be difficult to choose a concentration that lowers the spin–lattice relaxation times of compounds in the extract sufficiently without broadening resonances to the extent that the signal-to-noise ratio is degraded. Gadolinium triethylenetetraamine hexaacetate has been suggested as a useful relaxation agent that causes minimal undesirable resonance broadening (Lettvin and Sherry, 1977).

III. KEY ELEMENTS OF THE SPECTROMETER

A. The Probe

The NMR receiver is discussed thoroughly by Hoult (1978) and Gadian (1982). The probe is a main component of the receiver and of particular importance in physiological experiments, where it is generally essential to maximize the sensitivity of the experiment. A fundamental way in which this can be achieved is

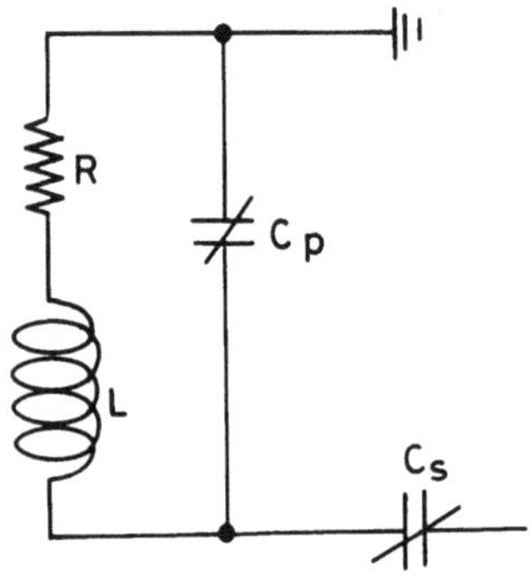

Figure 8. A resonant circuit. The circuit is tuned to resonate at a particular frequency by an appropriate choice of coil inductance, *L*, and adjustment of the parallel capacitance, C_p. The variable capacitor in series with the resonant circuit, C_s, allows it to be *"matched" to 50 Ω*. It is important to minimize the resistance, *R*, of the tuned circuit to obtain an optimal signal-to-noise ratio.

by completely filling the active volume of the coil with sample. With biological preparations of fixed dimensions, it is therefore ideal to be able to design the probe specifically for particular applications. This is much easier than might be suspected, for the probe is basically just a radio frequency transmitter/detector coil on an appropriate support. Biological applications often demand that it also include systems for perfusion of the tissue, electrical stimulation, and so on. The support may be made of nonferromagnetic aluminum and should surround the coil (perhaps with a detachable section to permit ready access) to shield it from extraneous radio frequency radiation. Its dimensions are adjusted to position the coil in the most homogeneous region of the magnetic field when in place. An example of the sort of probe employed in this laboratory is illustrated in Figure 10.

Although an enormous variety of coil designs is possible, they must all produce an RF B_1 field in a plane perpendicular to the direction of the applied magnetic field B_0. Two classical coil designs fulfilling this criterion are in common use: the Helmholtz and the solenoid. Hoult and Richards (1976) have predicted that a solenoidal coil should produce three times the signal-to-noise ratio of a Helmholtz coil for a fixed sample volume. In practice, the sensitivity of a solenoid can be expected to be better only by a factor of about 1.5–2.0, but even this corresponds to a reduction in accumulation time for a spectrum of 2–4. It should also be noted that samples must be placed "sideways" when using a solenoid in a superconducting magnet. This generally limits the use of a solenoid to wide-bore magnets.

The coil detects a signal by means of a magnetic coupling with the spin dipoles after the latter are perturbed by a radio frequency pulse (Hoult and Richards, 1976). In this context, coupling means that an electromotive force (EMF) is induced in the coil by the changing magnetic field of the perturbed spins, a consequence of Faraday's law of electromagnetic induction. The magnitude of the EMF oscillates with the precession frequency of the spins. By making the coil part of a tuned circuit that can be adjusted to resonate in the frequency region of interest, one can enormously enhance the sensitivity of the coil to weak oscillations in the sample.

Figure 8 is a diagram of the simple tuned circuit commonly used in NMR probes designed for detection of a single nucleus. For a solenoidal coil, the fre-

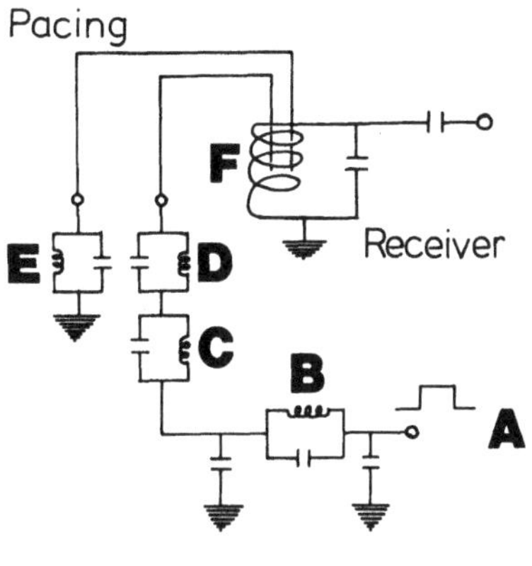

Figure 9. Radio frequency isolation circuit for heart pacing during an NMR experiment. A, rectangular DC pulses from pacing unit; B, RF filter on pacing wire; C–E, RF chokes on pacing wire; F, NMR receiving coil.

quency at which the circuit resonates is determined by the number of turns in the coil (or, more technically, the inductance of the coil) and the value of the capacitance in parallel with the coil.

The final signal-to-noise ratio of a spectrum is proportional to the ratio of the EMFs generated by the signal and the noise in the tuned circuit. The EMF of the signal can be optimized at a given field strength for a given sample volume by maximizing the coil inductance. Important gains can be realized by minimizing contributions from factors that can increase noise EMF at the same time. The most obvious source of noise is the same random, thermal motion of electrons in the coil that is responsible for the electrical resistance. It is therefore advisable to wind the coil from large-diameter wire (as current flows on the outside "skin") having high conductivity, e.g., 10-gauge copper wire for a 10-ml sample volume. The wire cannot be too thick, however, as fewer turns can be used for the sample volume (lowering B_1) as the wire diameter increases. In addition, the turns should not be too closely juxtaposed in the coil because this can significantly increase the resistance of the wire by the so-called "proximity effect." An optimal winding geometry has been proposed in which adjacent turns are separated by three times the radius of the wire (Hoult, 1978).

A further contribution to the noise arises in biological samples because tissue water is electrically conducting. In consequence, when an EMF is generated in the receiving coil, eddy currents that dissipate power are introduced into the sample. This adds an additional term to the effective resistance of the tuned circuit. If this term dominates the total resistance of the circuit, then little or no improvement in signal-to-noise ratio can be expected by further optimization of the coil design. Reaching this condition should therefore be regarded as a desirable goal in coil design for biological systems. Furthermore, relative gains in signal-to-noise ratio with increased sample volume will decrease as this condition is approached. Differences in the signal-to-noise ratio achieved for a given sample volume using Helmholtz and solenoidal coils will also decrease.

In practice, contributions to the total signal from broad resonance lines are considerably more difficult to discern than those from narrow lines. Thus, the signal-to-noise ratio depends on the homogeneity of the B_1 and B_0 fields as well

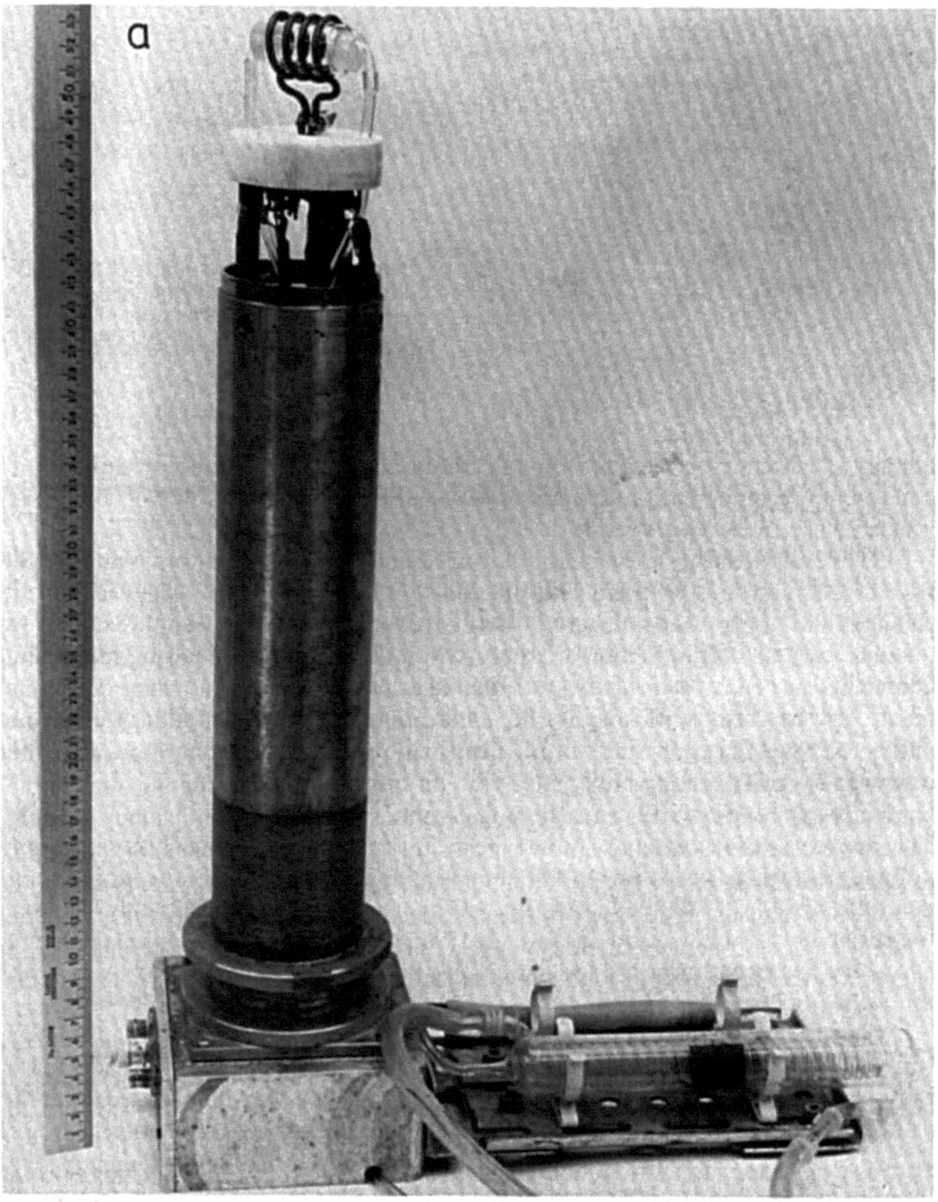

Figure 10. A probe used in the Oxford laboratory for ^{31}P NMR studies of perfused rat hearts. In a, the full probe is shown with a heat exchanger mounted to warm the perfusion buffer. Connections at the back of the probe base are for the thermocouple sensor, the detected signal, and DC pulses for pacing the heart. In b a detailed view of the top of the probe is shown (covered by a removable aluminum top when in the magnet): 1, solenoidal RF coil; 2, the "parallel" tuning capacitor; 3, perfusion fluid inflow; 4, fluid outflow; 5, thermostating air jets; 6, sample chamber.

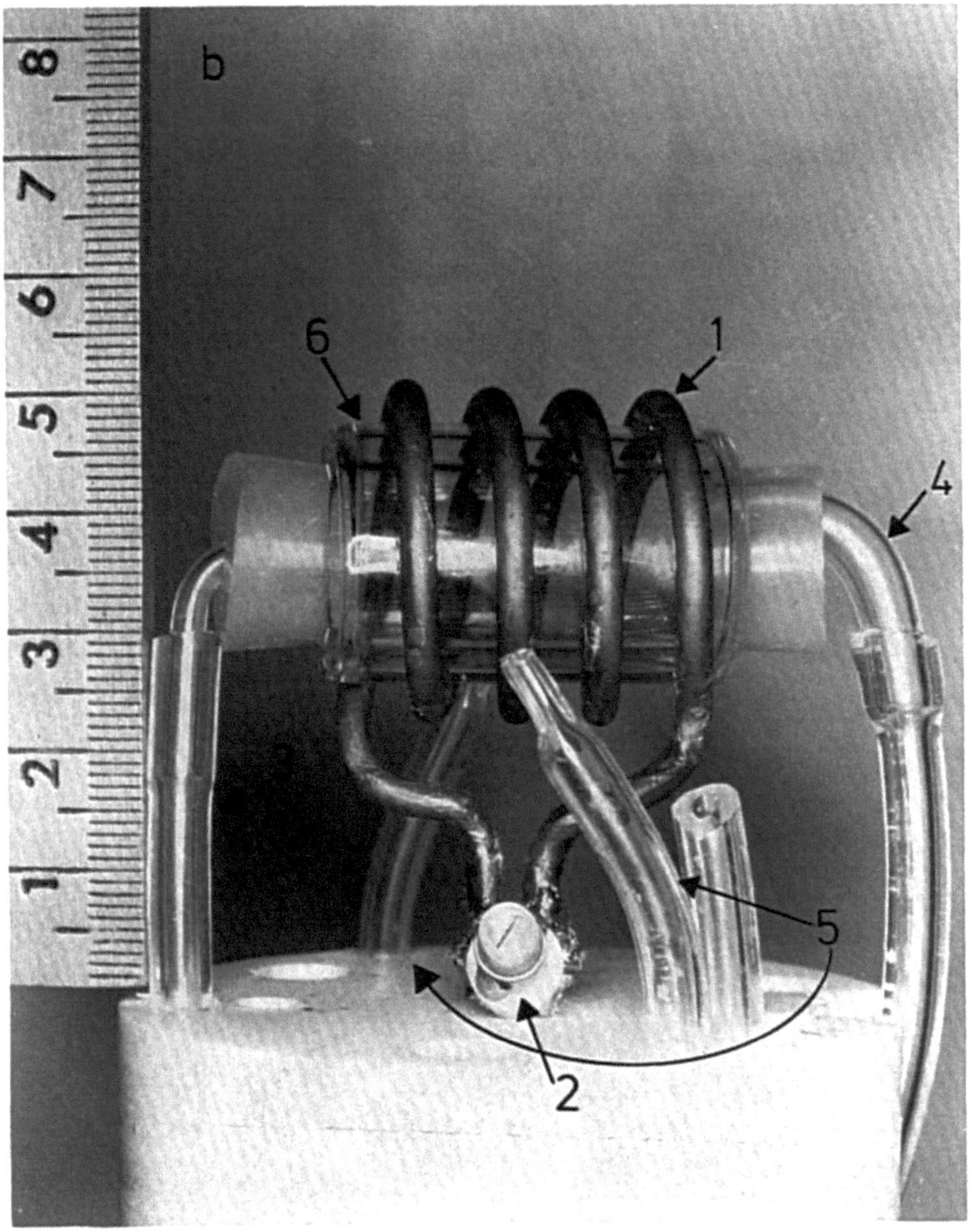

Figure 10. (*Continued*)

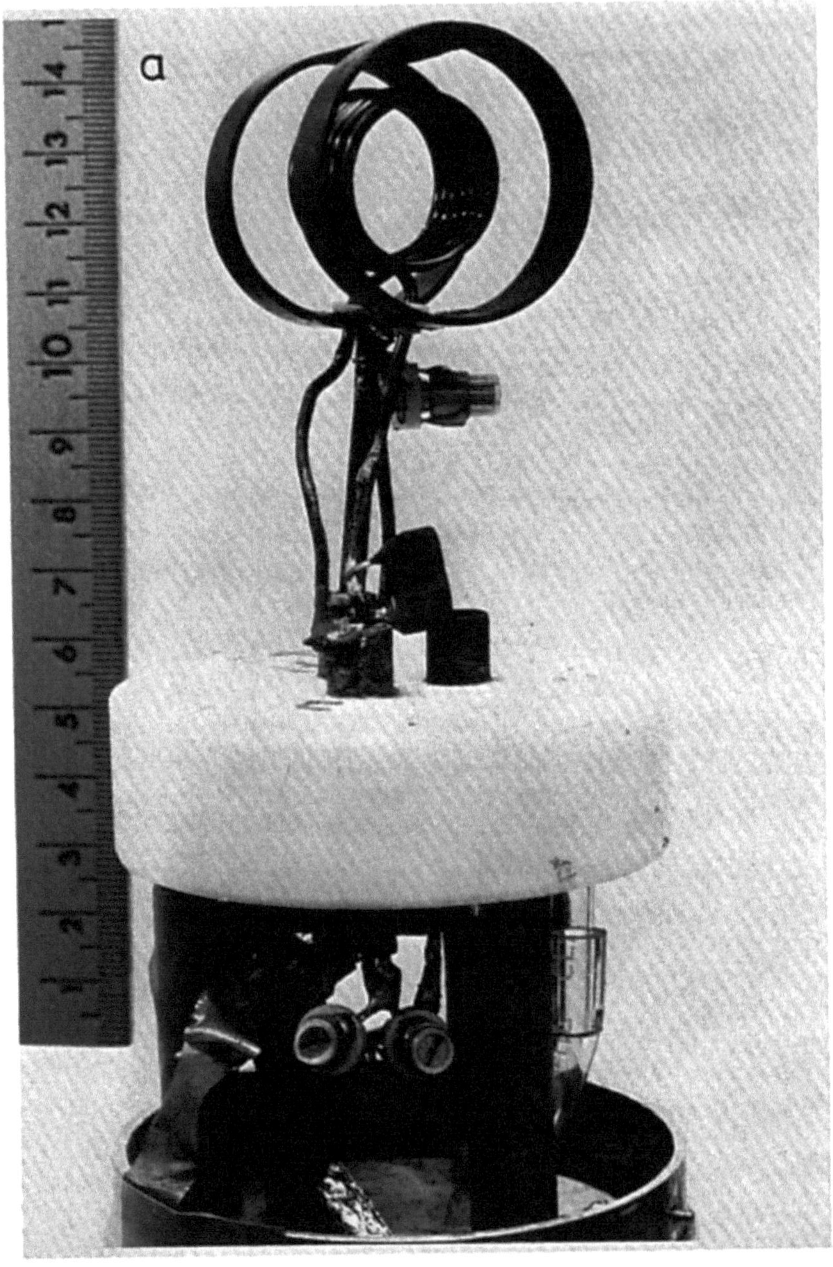

Figure 11. A selection of RF coils used in the Oxford laboratory for whole-tissue NMR studies: (a) ^{13}C coil mounted inside a tuned ^{1}H decoupling coil for ^{13}C studies of perfused rat hearts; (b) ^{31}P coil to accomodate single barnacle muscle fibers; (c) ^{31}P coil (covered with a protective tape) for placement around rat kidneys *in vivo*; (d) ^{31}P surface coil for observation of metabolites from a localized disk approximately 5 mm $\times$ 5 mm. Scale given in centimeters.

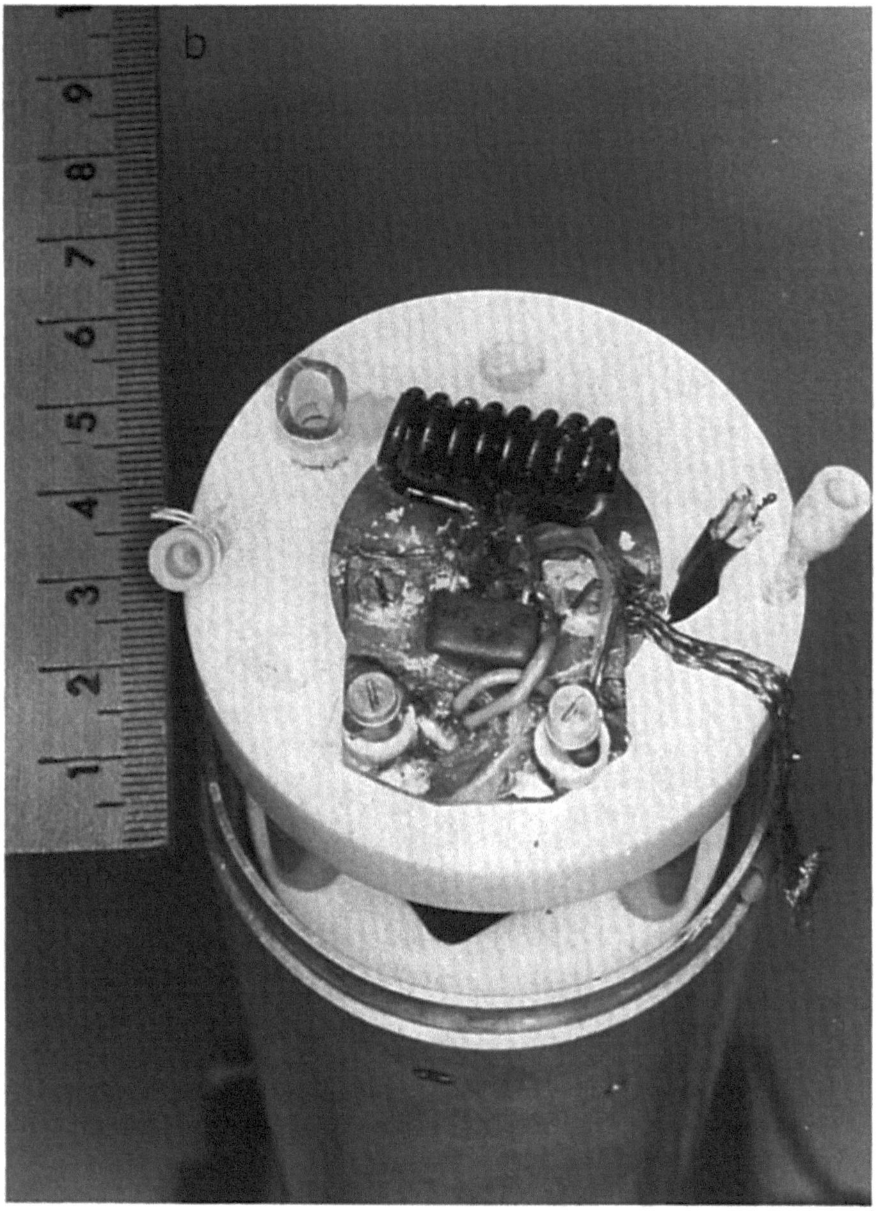

Figure 11. (*Continued*)

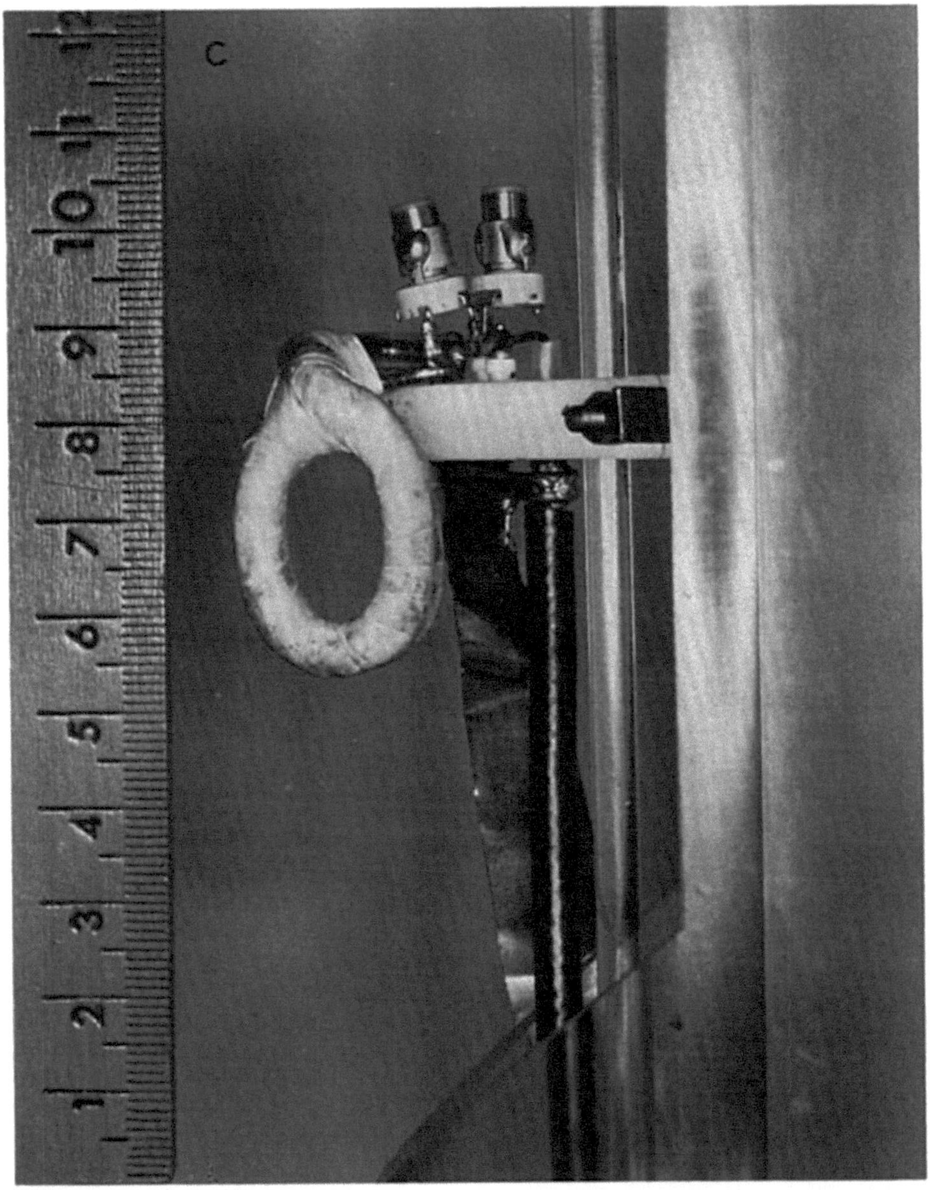

Figure 11. (*Continued*)

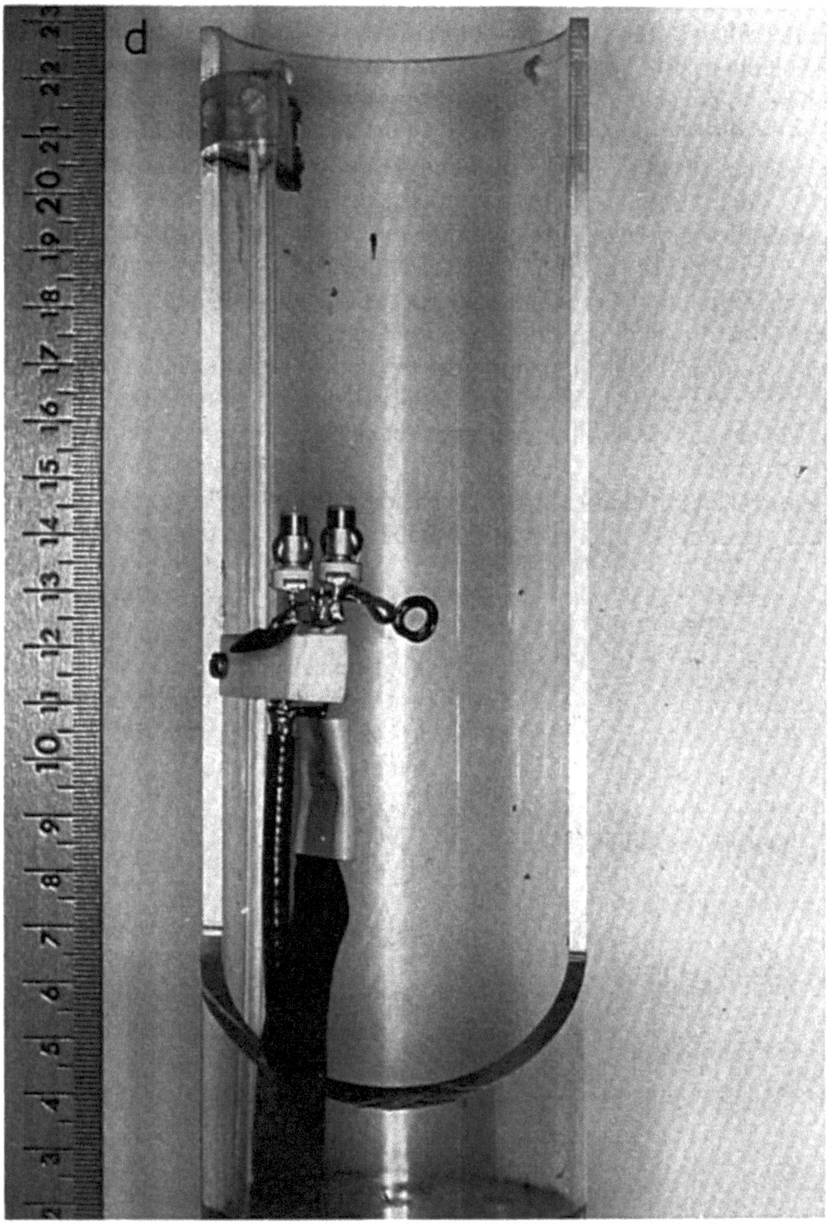

Figure 11. (*Continued*)

as the characteristics of the tuned circuit. The B_1 field is most homogeneous in the center of a solenoidal coil, and so it is best to confine the sample to this region. It has been observed that B_1 field homogeneity in a superconducting magnet is often better when a Helmholtz coil rather than a solenoid is used around the same sample volume. Use of thinner wire or even metal strips for coil construction may increase field homogeneity but, depending on sample size, perhaps only at the cost of increasing the resistance of the tuned circuit. In general, with the relatively large sample volumes used in studies of living tissue, the field inhomogeneity is large enough to greatly minimize any potential gains in signal-to-noise ratio resulting from use of the very small diameter wire found in most commercial probes.

The homogeneity of the B_0 field is dependent on many factors, including magnet construction, the proximity of large ferromagnetic materials to the magnet, and the skill with which the shim coils have been used. It is critically dependent on the nature of materials in and around the coil. It is particularly important that ferromagnetic materials be excluded. In practice, this means that metal used for the coil should be free of impurities and that circuit elements, such as capacitors, be nonferromagnetic.

Electrical circuit elements such as pacing wires or thermistors may be placed in or near the radio frequency coil if suitable isolation circuits are provided. Isolation in this instance means prevention of electrical interaction between the pacing wires or thermistors and the tuned RF resonance circuit. Perfused hearts are paced within the RF coil in this laboratory using the circuit diagrammed in Figure 9. This design allows the passage of DC current from an external square-wave generator but prevents the leak of AC power near the resonance frequency. Both leak of RF away from the coil and pickup of RF from outside the probe by the pacing wires can seriously degrade the signal-to-noise ratio.

In conclusion, it must be emphasized that an optimal signal-to-noise ratio is best insured by designing the probe to suit the specific requirements of the experiment. In the Oxford laboratory, a broad range of coils (some of which are illustrated in Figures 10 and 11) have been constructed for use in different situations. Unfortunately, choosing the most appropriate coil design, beyond applying certain general principles (see Appendix), is very much an empirical process. Hoult (1978) explains how much of the necessary experimentation can be conducted on the bench using equipment no more sophisticated than a frequency generator and an oscilloscope.

In some experiments (e.g., an organ *in vivo*), the shape of the sample precludes use of one of the classical coil designs. In such situations, a "surface coil" (Ackerman *et al.*, 1980) may be of use (see Figure 11d). Unlike the conventional experiment in which a sample is placed within a coil, signals are received by a surface coil that is placed immediately adjacent to the sample area. The circuit for a surface coil is identical to that described above. The unusual design feature is that the inductance coil is flat, so that most of the B_1 field is generated beyond the edges of the coil. The B_1 field contours effectively define the sample volume if the coil is placed on a relatively large sample. An important feature is that as the field profile can be defined either theoretically or experimentally (Ackerman

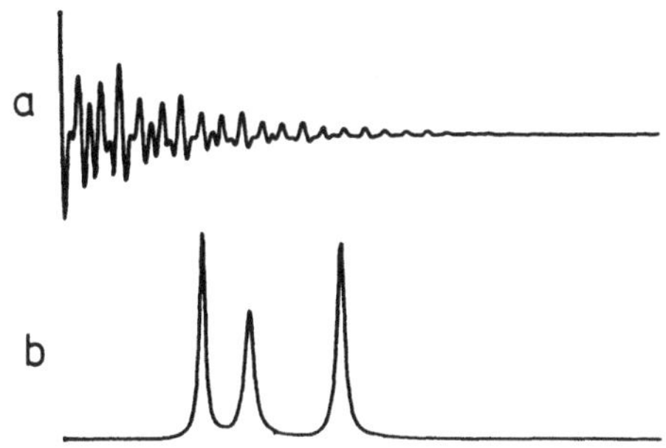

Figure 12. (a) A "free induction decay." Following the RF excitation pulse, a decaying signal composed of the superposition of the sinusoidally oscillating responses from each spin excited in the sample is detected. The components of this so-called "free induction decay" (FID) decrease in magnitude with a time constant $T_2 = 1/\pi \cdot \Delta\nu$, where $\Delta\nu$ is the observed line width of the associated resonance. (b) A fourier transformation of the FID. After Fourier transformation, the amplitude-*vs.*-time information in the FID is expressed as amplitude *vs.* frequency in the resulting spectrum. (Diagram courtesy of Dr. D. G. Gadian.)

et al., 1980), spatially resolved information can be obtained from the sample (see Section IV.C).

B. The Computer

In this section, a brief introduction is given to special considerations concerning the computer in NMR. A more complete discussion is given by Cooper (1976).

Digital computers are invariably used in conjunction with NMR spectrometers. The first stage in accumulation of an FID is therefore done using an analogue-to-digital converter (ADC) that periodically samples the voltage of the input and converts voltages in predetermined ranges to binary numbers. To accurately digitize an FID, the rate at which the digitizer samples the voltage is critical; the so-called sampling theorem states that a waveform must be observed twice in every cycle to uniquely define its frequency. For most modern high-field spectrometers, the rate of sampling must be at least equal to the frequency range of resonances in the FID. If an FID is sampled too slowly, the digitized frequency of the waveform will be less than its true value, and its magnitude will be diminished.

After the FID is accumulated by the computer as a digitized plot of absorption *vs.* time, it is Fourier transformed to convert the time-domain information into the more easily interpreted frequency-domain spectrum (Figure 12) (Bracewell, 1965). An important consequence of the fact that the frequency and time domains are Fourier pairs is that the minimum frequency separation that can be resolved in the Fourier-transformed spectrum is determined by the time for acquisition of the FID: to resolve resonances separated by f hz, it is necessary to sample those frequencies for a time of at least $1/f$ sec.

After Fourier transformation of the FID, the spectrum can appear unusual in that some resonances may have excursions both above and below the base line. This occurs when the different oscillating waveforms in the FID are perceived by the computer to start out of phase. It may be a consequence of electronic artifacts in the receiver or the inevitable delay between the onset of the oscillating voltages of the FID and the first sampling of the waveform. The computer can

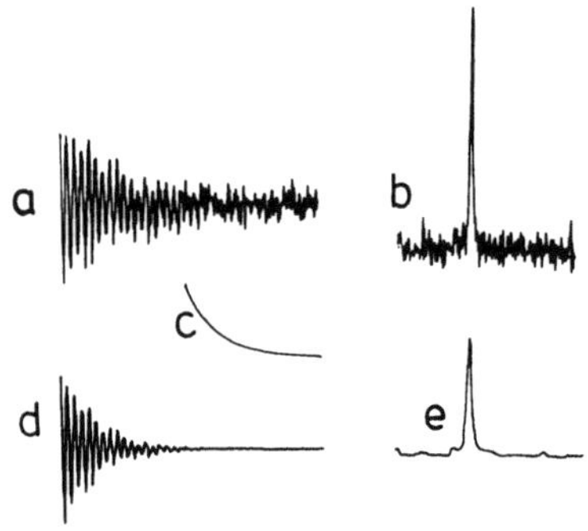

Figure 13. Illustration of signal-to-noise enhancement by exponential multiplication. The Fourier transformation of the FID a yields spectrum b. Convolution of the FID a with an exponentially decaying function (c) gives the FID d. Application of the Fourier transform to d gives spectrum e, in which the signal-to-noise ratio is enhanced relative to b. Note that the resonance line width in e is greater than that in b. (Diagram courtesy of Dr. D. G. Gadian.)

manipulate the spectrum to yield the customary representation by application of phase corrections. Phase corrections can be either zero order and frequency independent, or they may be applied to vary approximately linearly across the spectrum.

As noted above, one of the major advantages of the FT NMR experiment is that the responses after many pulses may be added together to yield a sum having a signal-to-noise ratio sufficient for interpretation in cases in which the signal cannot be observed above the noise in a single scan. The signal intensity builds up more rapidly as successive FIDs are added than does the random noise, so that the signal-to-noise ratio rises as the (number of scans)$^{1/2}$.

To obtain the maximum signal-to-noise ratio possible with a given FID, a digital filter may be applied to the data. This is done by multiplying the total FID by a decaying exponential (Figure 13) (Ernst and Morgan, 1973). The signal-to-noise ratio in the transformed spectrum is enhanced because the exponential weighing preferentially reduces what is detected late in the data acquisition period, when most of the signal has decayed and primarily noise ramains. However, this effectively increases the rate of decay of the signal, which results in a broader line on Fourier transformation. The line broadening introduced by the digital filter may be calculated:

$$\text{line broadening} = \frac{-(\text{time constant of decaying exponential})}{f(\text{acquisition time})} \tag{3}$$

It may be shown that the optimal signal-to-noise ratio results from use of a digital filter that just doubles the line width.

The computer may also be used to enhance the resolution that can be achieved using a given data acquisition routine by zero-filling or the convolution difference procedure. Zero-filling involves doubling the size of the FID in the computer with the addition of an equal number of zeros to the end. Bartholdi and Ernst (1973) have demonstrated that zero-filling maximizes the resolution possible with a given FID in the transformed spectrum by making use of information that otherwise would be discarded. Further addition of zeros, to triple or quadruple the size of the FID, adds no new information but allows interpolation between the points defined by doubling the size of the FID with zeros.

The convolution difference technique (Campbell *et al.*, 1973) may be used to sharpen resonances when they are obscured by superposition of broad resonances. Two copies of the FID are made. One is multiplied by a severely decaying exponential, which leaves behind only the broad line information. The other is multiplied by an exponential that decays much more slowly. The convolution difference spectrum is produced when the two FIDs are transformed and the former is subtracted from the latter. It should be noted that this procedure can distort relative resonance intensities in a spectrum. A variety of other resolution-enhancement procedures have been proposed (Campbell and Dobson, 1979).

In addition to facilitating data analysis, the on-line computer is also commonly used to extend the scope and complexity of experiments. Multipulse sequences controlled by the computer can be used to measure the relaxation times T_1 (Gupta, 1977; Levy and Peat, 1975; Canet *et al.*, 1975) and T_2 (Waugh and Wang, 1967; Meiboom and Gill, 1958; Carr and Purcell, 1954; Hahn, 1950) or to simplify complex spectra (Rabenstein and Nakashima, 1979). Suggestions have been made of ways of using complex pulse sequences to partially correct for imperfections in the B_1 field (Levitt and Freeman, 1979; Van Putte, 1970) that can limit accurate determination of relaxation times. The computer may be used to "gate" data collection in synchrony with a repetitive event in order to increase the time resolution of data collection to as little as 100 msec. Fossel *et al.* (1980) have demonstrated how this approach can be used to define changes in the concentrations of high-energy phosphate compounds through the cardiac contraction cycle.

In principle, gated saturation transfer (see Section V.C) experiments may be performed to define changes in selected reaction rates at specific points in the cycle. Summing spectra accumulated over only a few seconds from different points after repetitive induction of total global ischemia allowed Jacobus and his colleagues (1982) to define with considerable time resolution the pattern of metabolic recovery over the first minute of reflow following a short period of total global ischemia. In a rather different application, Styles *et al.* (1979) have used the computer to switch transmitter frequencies and detection amplifiers on alternate scans to simultaneously accumulate ^{31}P and ^{13}C NMR spectra from red blood cells in a ^{13}C-enriched medium.

C. The Magnet

The millimolar concentrations of metabolites in living tissue are more conveniently observed using spectrometers equipped with superconducting magnets able to operate at high field strengths ($\gtrsim$3 Tesla). As the sensitivity of the experiment rises in proportion to $B_0^{7/5}$ (Hoult and Richards, 1976), it would seem best to work at the highest field strengths available. Theoretical arguments suggest that, at least up to presently available field strengths, this is certainly true for observation of ^{13}C and ^{1}H. The situation is rather less clear for ^{31}P. It has been shown that chemical shift anisotropy (see, for example, Shaw, 1976) contributes significantly to the relaxation of the ^{31}P nucleus in compounds such as those encountered in living systems when they are dissolved in viscous glycerol (Gadian *et al.*, 1980; Berden *et al.*, 1974). In such situations, the resonances may be expected to broaden roughly in proportion to B_0^2, and the signal-to-noise ratio should not improve and may even decrease at higher field strengths. In heart cells, chemical shift anisotropy probably contributes less to relaxation of the molecules observed by NMR, but little work has been done to define ^{31}P relaxation mechanisms in cells. Salhany *et al.* (1975) have reported significant gains in signal-to-noise ratio in ^{31}P NMR studies of yeast cells in comparing of 40.5 MHz with 145.7 MHz spectra. In contrast, Evans (1979) suggests that there is significant broadening of ^{31}P resonances of HeLa cell metabolites at higher frequencies.

Another major consideration is the size of the magnet bore, which ultimately limits the size of the sample. Small rat (Garlick *et al.*, 1977) and mouse (Battersby *et al.*, 1978) hearts can be effectively perfused in a 3.2-cm-bore magnet. Whole rats of 300–350 g may be easily accommodated for *in vivo* (see Section IV.B) experiments in a 7.7-cm bore. In addition to the manipulative advantages, a larger bore allows solenoidal coils to be used, bringing an improvement in signal-to-noise ratio. Recently, a 2 T (82.5 MHz for ^{1}H) magnet with a 20-cm bore has become commercially available (Oxford Research Systems, Oxford, England). This magnet will accommodate experimental animals as large as dogs. It is anticipated that high-field magnets big enough to allow metabolic studies of the internal organs of live humans will soon be manufactured. Already, low field magnets for ^{1}H spin imaging are in use in a number of clinical centers (Pykett, 1982).

In many spectrometers it is necessary to use a field–frequency lock so that the strength of the static B_0 field does not drift during the course of the experiment. The lock constitutes a second channel of the spectrometer, frequently designed to observe the resonance from deuterium within the sample chamber. In whole-tissue experiments, the D_2O is generally contained in a capillary mounted on the probe assembly outside the tissue sample chamber. Once set, the lock continuously monitors the deuterium frequency, compares it to a standard frequency, and provides any slight adjustments to the static field that are necessary to keep the frequency constant by means of a feedback loop.

Field homogeneity is a particular problem in whole-tissue experiments, in which the presence of perfusion tubes and electrical leads precludes sample spinning. In order to minimize field inhomogeneities, the following precautions may be taken:

1. The sample should be positioned as symmetrically as possible in the sample tube.
2. Perfusion lines, stimulation leads, etc should be kept as far from the coil as possible and be as small as is practical.
3. As bubbles in the sample disturb field homogeneity, they should be excluded if possible. This is not a rigid requirement, however; Ugurbil and his colleagues (1980) have continuously oxygenated cell suspensions during accumulation and report that bubbles of less than about 2 mm diameter do not significantly degrade the signal-to-noise ratio.

IV. SOME USEFUL HEART PREPARATIONS

Interfacing a heart preparation with the spectrometer requires a few special considerations. The most obvious is that the isolated organ or whole animal will be in the magnet and unable to be directly observed through the course of the experiment. This demands that extra precautions be taken to insure the long-term viability of the preparation with the minimum need for periodic interventions. It is also desirable to have means of indirectly monitoring its physiological state. Techniques for the latter are complicated by the need to electronically "isolate" electrical monitoring circuitry and to exclude ferromagnetic materials from the region near the coil to preserve magnetic field homogeneity.

A. The Perfused Heart

Most of the cardiac NMR studies reported to date have been collected using some sort of modified Langendorff perfusion apparatus, one example of which is illustrated in Figure 14. Rat (Garlick *et al.*, 1977; Jacobus *et al.*, 1977), guinea pig (Salhany *et al.*, 1979), mouse (Battersby *et al.*, 1978), and rabbit (Hollis *et al.*, 1978) hearts have been studied by ^{31}P NMR in this manner. The requirements of perfusion are quite conventional. The heart needs an uninterrupted supply of oxygenated, buffered, bubble-free perfusion fluid at a controlled temperature. The major problems arise in maintaining these conditions over the long perfusion lines needed to reach into the magnet and in the purely manipulative difficulties associated with positioning a beating heart and any pressure or pacing leads in the sample chamber.

The metal cannulae customarily used for Langendorff perfusion should be replaced by glass to avoid disturbance of the RF field. Dark paint can be fused into the tips of these glass cannulae to allow them to be more easily seen, reducing the risk of damaging the aortic valve during cannulation. Signal-to-noise ratio is optimized by using an RF coil no longer than is necessary to surround the heart. In doing so, it is important that the beating heart be maintained free of the walls of the sample tube; hearts in even light contact with the sample tube develop ischemic patches and may show signs of impaired function (Garlick, 1979). A reference solution, such as methylene diphosphonate in D_2O, may be put into a narrow annulus around the sample chamber.

Studies correlating mechanical and biochemical parameters may perhaps be best performed using a working heart preparation (Neely *et al.*, 1967). A simple version of this system interfaced with the ^{31}P NMR spectrometer has recently been described (Fossel *et al.*, 1980).

B. An *In Vivo* Preparation

Many sorts of experiments, particularly those involving pharmacological interventions, may best be done using a whole animal rather than an isolated heart preparation. It has been demonstrated that spectra having signal-to-noise ratios and resolution only slightly degraded relative to that available with a perfused

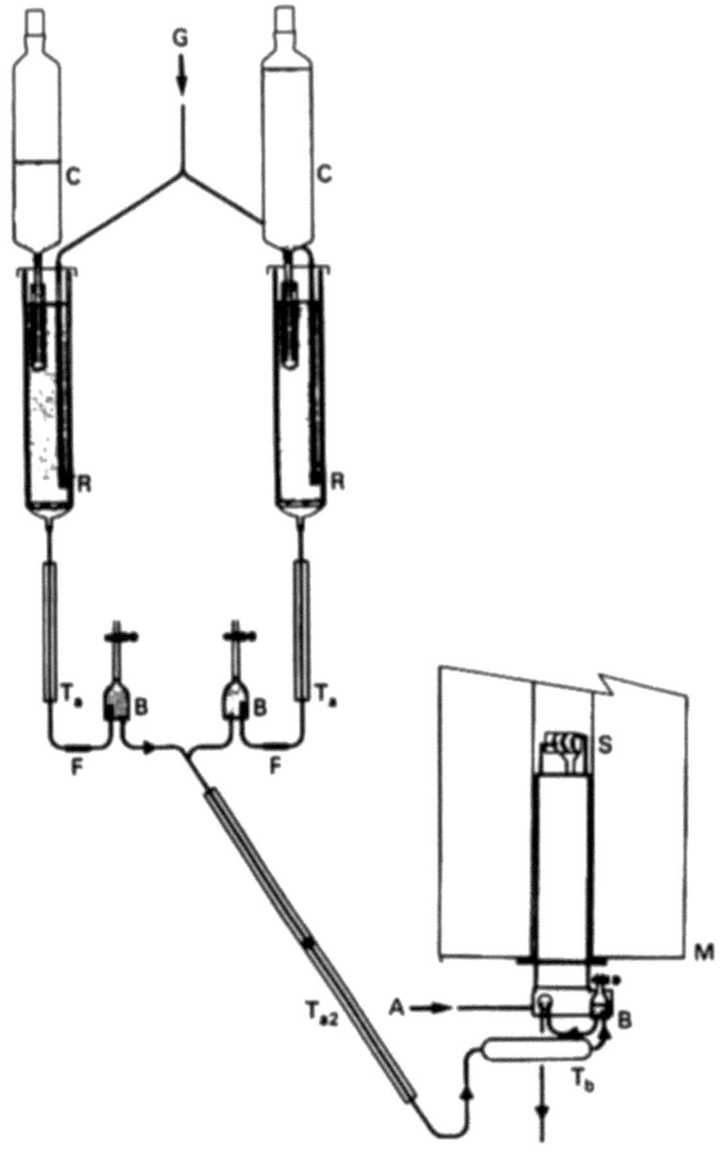

Figure 14. Apparatus used for Langendorff perfusion of rat hearts in the NMR spectrometer. Abbreviations: G, gas supply; C, constant-head device; R, thermostatically controlled glass reservoir with sintered glass in base; T_a and T_{a2}, thermostatically controlled glass tubes; B, thermostatically controlled bubble trap; F, flow control device; S, sample tube containing heart; M, wide-bore superconducting magnet (4.3 T); A, supply of thermostatically controlled air; T_b, thermostatically controlled helical glass tube.

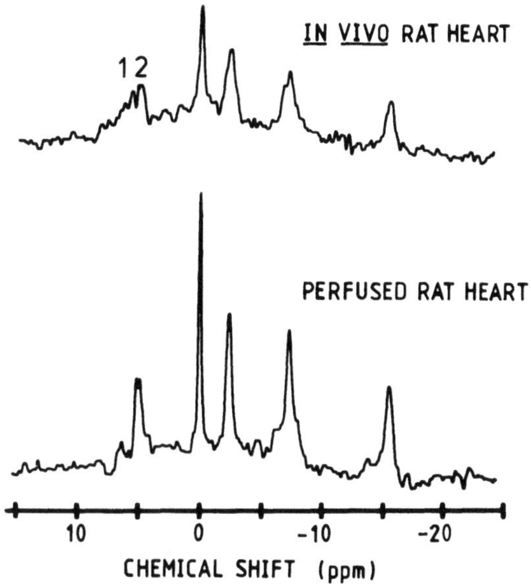

Figure 15. ^{31}P NMR spectra of *in vivo* (a) and perfused (b) rat hearts. Both spectra are of hearts from 300-g animals. Resonances are identified as in Figure 2 except for 1 and 2, which are assigned to the 2- and 3-phosphates of 2,3,-diphosphoglycerate in the blood.

system can be obtained with an RF coil placed around the exposed heart in an open-chested rat (Grove *et al.*, 1980). The animal, ventilated by a tube inserted into the trachea, can remain in a physiologically stable state in excess of 6 hr. The ^{31}P NMR spectrum (Figure 15) differs from that of the Langendorff perfused heart with glucose as a substrate in that the ATP/PCr ratio is about 30% lower. Presumably this is a consequence of the preferential utilization of fatty acids as the primary substrate in the whole animal (Matthews *et al.*, 1982b). The heart *in vivo* is, of course, perfused with blood, which has ATP, P_i, and, particularly, 2,3-DPG resonances in significant concentrations. The magnitude of the 2,3-DPG resonances in the spectrum of the *in vivo* rat heart may be diminished as a consequence of the blood flow, which rapidly moves the nuclear spins through regions of different field strengths in a way that may be expected to reduce significantly the size of the observed resonances (Singer, 1978; Jones and Child, 1976). Study of the *in vivo* preparation is of particular interest because the chemical work done by the heart even in the anesthetized animal is much greater than that in the Langendorff preparation. An important extension of these experiments has been the development of the techniques for chronically implanting a radiofrequency coil to allow monitoring ^{31}P NMR spectra around the *in vivo* rat heart over periods extending from days to weeks (Koretsky *et al.*, 1983). This approach is well suited to study of the pathogenesis of bioenergetic changes in cardiomyopathic models or long-term sequelae of myocardial infarction, to suggest only two problem areas. Although obviously a highly invasive method, it offers much higher inherent receiver sensitivity than the field-focusing or zeugmatographic methods noted in Section V.D.

C. Surface Coils

Both of the techniques described above receive signals from all areas of the heart. In many applications it would be desirable to receive signals from specifically defined regions of the heart. Surface coils can be used to determine bioenergetic parameters in roughly disk-shaped volumes as small as a few millimeters in diameter (Thulborn *et al.,* 1981). This allows, for example, a comparison to be made between cellular energetics within and outside of a localized ischemic region (Nunnally and Bottomly, 1981). With the advent of very-large-bore magnets, it has become possible to perform this type of experiment on the hearts of relatively large animals (P. Matthews and L. Chan, unpublished observations) *in vivo.*

D. Monitoring the Physiological State

In all of these preparations, it is important to be able to further characterize the metabolism and to assess the mechanical function of the heart. The primary goal should always be a correlation between the biochemical and functional states. A whole variety of measurements are obviously possible, including:

1. Coronary flow.
2. Aortic pressure.
3. Left ventricular pressure.
4. The rate of left ventricular pressure changes (dP/dt).
5. Spontaneous electrical activity (ECG).
6. Oxygen consumption.
7. Blood pressure in the whole animal.

The important message is that the experimenter should never feel as though the requirements of the NMR experiment preclude collection of desirable ancillary data.

V. WHAT CAN NMR TELL US?

The most important question that this chapter should begin to answer for the newcomer to NMR is "What types of information are potentially available from NMR studies of cardiac metabolism?" Nuclear magnetic resonance studies of hearts have been conducted for just a few years, so only a few of even those NMR techniques currently available have been applied. More techniques are being added to the repertoire of the spectroscopist with each issue of the specialist journals (see, for example, the *Journal of Magnetic Resonance*). The emphasis in this section is on possibilities rather than accomplishments in the hope that experimenters will be encouraged to extend the range of techniques that have been applied to whole-organ studies and the range of problems that can be addressed.

A. Identification and Quantitation of Metabolites

An important application of NMR is to the identification of metabolites present in a tissue sample. Nuclear magnetic resonance has a major advantage over most conventional analytical techniques in which the analyses must be directed towards the detection of specific compounds: NMR is a general probe for the presence of a particular nucleus in the sample, whatever compound it might be present in, provided only that the compound is relatively mobile. This advantage was demonstrated in early ^{31}P NMR observations of muscle, when high concentrations of unexpected metabolites were detected from rabbit muscle (Burt *et al.*, 1976), frog gastrocnemius (Dawson *et al.*, 1977), and dystrophic chicken muscle (Chalovich and Bárány, 1980) in the region where phosphodiester resonances are found. A similar compound has been observed in human forearm muscle ^{31}P NMR spectra from Duchenne dystrophy patients (Newman *et al.*, 1982). The compounds in the dystrophic chicken muscle were identified as glycerolphosphorylcholine and as L-serine ethanolamine phosphodiester. A reexamination of the literature provoked by these observations disclosed that the presence of high concentrations of phosphodiesters had been noted over 25 years ago in turtle tissue but, because of a lack of parallel studies in other tissue, "forgotten."

Identification of metabolites by NMR depends on a number of factors:

1. Presence of the particular isotope being observed.
2. Appropriate sensitivity of the nucleus (see Table I).
3. Sufficient molecular mobility to give rise to narrow resonance lines.
4. A large enough difference in chemical shifts to resolve multiple resonances.

The third point, that high-resolution NMR is limited to observation of freely mobile compounds, deserves emphasis. As a nucleus tumbles more slowly in solution, the spin–spin relaxation (characterized by the spin–spin relaxation time, T_2) becomes more efficient, and resonance lines broaden. Resonances from phosphodiesters in membrane phospholipids or DNA, for example, are not observed in the conventional ^{31}P experiment despite high concentrations in tissue because their line widths are tens of times broader than those of small molecules such as ATP. Special procedures are necessary to observe these broad resonances (Berden *et al.*, 1974). Binding of low-molecular-weight compounds to macromolecules may broaden their resonances to the point that they may no longer be observed under high-resolution data collection conditions. As Fisher (1971) discussed in an earlier volume of this series, this behavior is often exploited in NMR studies of ligand-binding to enzymes (Battersby and Radda, 1976).

Phosphorus has been easier to observe in living tissue than other nuclei because relatively few mobile metabolites are present in concentrations sufficient to give an identifiable resonance (~0.5 μmole/g wet wt. rat heart on the 73-MHz spectrometer in this laboratory) and because the chemical shift range for phosphate compounds generally encountered is large enough (~30 ppm) to resolve the major resonances well.

The NMR experiment is considerably more sensitive to protons, and, in principle, metabolites present in concentrations an order of magnitude lower should be observable. Although no ^{1}H NMR spectra of cardiac tissue have yet been reported, studies of the red blood cell (Brindle *et al.*, 1979), muscle (Pitkethly,

1979), and other tissues (Daniels *et al.*, 1976; Agris and Campbell, 1982) suggest that useful observations could be made.

One difficulty is resolution: the ubiquity of protons and the relatively small chemical shift range (14 ppm) can give rise to a difficult-to-interpret broad band of poorly resolved resonances. Metabolites in high concentrations may still be expected to be resolved by virtue of their relative intensities, however. Also, there is hope that the multipulse spin-echo technique (or some variant on the same theme; see Rabenstein and Nakashima, 1979), which has been used to simplify ^{1}H NMR spectra of red blood cells (Brindle *et al.*, 1979) and Friend leukemia cells (Agris and Campbell, 1982) by showing resonances from only the small, highly mobile metabolites, might be usefully applied to whole tissue.

A second problem lies in observing metabolites present in millimolar concentrations in the presence of water at 55 *M* because of limitations on the range of resonance intensities that the spectrometer computer can simultaneously represent in digital form (the "dynamic range" problem). A variety of methods have been proposed to overcome this difficulty. A traditional approach has been to apply a long, selective B_1 pulse at the water resonance frequency to completely saturate the water nuclei in order to eliminate the signal (Campbell and Dobson, 1979). At high fields, spin-echo pulse sequences may also reduce the water signal appreciably (Agris and Campbell, 1982). A different, very promising method is to use proton correlation spectroscopy, a technique that can be crudely described as rapid-sweep continuous-wave NMR (Ogino *et al.*, 1978).

General observation of carbon compounds using ^{13}C NMR is limited by the low natural abundance of ^{13}C (1.1%) as well as the relatively low sensitivity of the isotope (Wehrli and Wirthli, 1976; Table I). The situation can be improved by continuously irradiating the sample over the entire range of proton resonance frequencies ("broad-band decoupling"). Decoupling removes any spin–spin coupling between ^{13}C and nearby protons, simplifying the spectrum. It also enhances the signal intensity by a factor of about three (in favorable cases) because of the nuclear Overhauser effect, which arises from a change in the steady-state magnetization of the carbon nuclei following energy transfer to irradiated, spin-coupled protons. In consequence, broad-band proton-decoupled ^{13}C NMR is almost as sensitive as ^{31}P NMR on an atom-for-atom basis. Nontheless, the method is still limited to observation of natural abundance ^{13}C from compounds present in concentrations greater than about 0.2 *M*. An interesting application has been to the identification of the lipid composition of atherosclerotic lesions in isolated aortic strips (Hamilton *et al.*, 1979). The natural abundance ^{13}C NMR spectrum of isolated skeletal muscle has recently been described in some detail (Doyle *et al.*, 1981).

Recent studies of the perfused rat heart (Bailey *et al.*, 1981a) and the perfused mouse liver (Cohen *et al.*, 1979b) have demonstrated great potential for noninvasive metabolic studies of metabolites enriched by means of isotope-labeled substrates. Although the spectra may be more complex than those observed with ^{31}P NMR, spectral resolution is intrinsically higher: ^{13}C has a chemical shift range of 200 ppm, and inhomogeneity broadening will only be about one-half as severe as for phosphorus. Additional problems may be expected to arise in quantifying concentrations from the size of resonance signals because of uncertainties about the nuclear Overhauser enhancement observed for different carbons and variations in the degree of isotope enrichment at different sites within metabolites.

Because the area under an NMR peak is directly proportional to the number of nuclei in the particular chemical environment, NMR may be used to quantify metabolite levels in whole tissue (see, for example, Matthews *et al.*, 1982a). The constant of proportionality is determined by the conditions of pulsing and the relaxation properties of the nuclei. If experimental conditions are chosen so that the RF pulses are applied no more frequently than about five times the spin–lattice relaxation time, T_1, of the most slowly relaxing nucleus, the constant is equal to 1. Relative concentrations of metabolites are then easily determined for resonances having high signal-to-noise ratios either by mathematical integration or by the more "classical" method of cutting out the individual peaks and weighing them. The absolute concentrations of metabolites may be determined from the ratios of their resonance intensities to that of a standard compound of known concentration.

In addition to the considerations mentioned in earlier sections, the obvious point that the standard compound must be chemically stable should be noted. It is best to use a standard having the highest concentration compatible with the dynamic range of the spectrometer and the concentration of metabolites in the sample. This will minimize the random error introduced by spectral noise in determination of its area. If the standard compound is contained in a chamber that extends beyond the physical limits of the coil, it is necessary to determine the proportion of the standard that is actually detected in the NMR experiment. It is important to realize that the magnetic field generated by a current passing through a coil extends well outside of it and is attenuated with increasing distance from the coil in a complex manner. In this laboratory, we calibrate the "effective concentration" of methylene diphosphonate in the annulus of a sample chamber that extends beyond the limits of the coil by comparing its resonance intensity (under nonsaturating conditions) with that from a known concentration of a second standard compound (phosphoric acid) confined to a volume in the center of the coil.

The results of NMR determination of concentrations are possibly complicated by the inability to observe resonances having very broad lines in the high-resolution NMR experiment. It must be emphasized that the total extractable amount of even relatively small molecules may not be observed in whole-tissue spectra if the metabolites are immobilized by binding to macromolecules or membranes, experience large local field gradients (Brindle *et al.*, 1979), or are near paramagnetic sites. Consider, for example, that despite freeze-clamp data showing ATP/ADP ratios in the heart to be on the order of 5, no ADP can be observed in the ^{31}P NMR spectra of normoxic perfused hearts.

Bárány has proposed that the small proportion of the total ADP extractable from skeletal muscle that may be observed by ^{31}P NMR is a consequence of tight binding to the myosin ATPase (Bárány *et al.*, 1975). The high concentration of mitochondria in the heart (perhaps 35% of the intracellular volume; see Ottoway and Mowbray, 1977) may offer other mechanisms for broadening resonances beyond the detectable range:

1. Paramagnetic sites are abundant among the enzymes of oxidative phosphorylation.
2. The high protein content of the matrix (50–60%) may make it extremely "viscous" even for small molecules (Srere, 1981).
3. Rapid exchange between the mitochondrial matrix and the cytosol may broaden resonances if there is a significant difference in chemical shift between the two compartments.

Wong (1981) has reported significant differences between the adenine nucleotide concentrations of suspensions of liver mitochondria measured by ^{31}P NMR and those determined enzymatically on perchlorate extracts of the same suspension. However, suspensions of mitochondria pretreated with atractyloside before addition of adenine nucleotides show no discrepancy between concentrations measured by the two methods. Thus, it is possible that a proportion of the intracellular adenine nucleotides are "invisible" to NMR. However, this should not be expected to affect estimates of ATP concentration in the heart significantly, as less than 23% of total ATP is associated with the mitochondria (Kauppinen *et al.*, 1980).

Garlick (1979) has approached the problem of determining the proportion of the total ATP and phosphocreatine observable by ^{31}P NMR in the perfused rat heart by quantifying the high-energy phosphates in a given heart by NMR and then "freeze-clamping" the same heart to measure the total extractable concentrations. Preliminary results suggest that, within an error limit of about 20%, the NMR method observes the total extractable concentrations of ATP and phosphocreatine. Clearly, the amount is not very great for rat hearts; concentrations determined by NMR (Matthews *et al.*, 1982a) are in broad agreement with those measured by classical methods (see, for example, Randle and Tubbs, 1979). The proportion of ADP that is observed from heart tissue is less clear because the concentrations are too low in normoxic, perfused rat hearts for direct correlations to be attempted. Calculations based on the creatine kinase equilibrium (Veech *et al.*, 1979; Matthews *et al.*, 1981) suggest that only about 10% of the total ADP is free in the cytosol. The proportion of the total extractable orthophosphate that is observed by ^{31}P NMR has not been directly examined yet. The values obtained from ^{31}P NMR (Matthews *et al.*, 1982a) are generally lower than those reported from perchlorate extracts.

B. The Intracellular Environment

Among the unique contributions of whole-organ NMR has been the beginning of a description of the molecular environment within the cell. Phosphorus NMR allows the rapid determination of intracellular pH and assessment of the free divalent cation concentrations. In the near future, ^{13}C and ^{1}H NMR observations may be expected to offer means for corroborating and expanding the information already available.

Although microelectrodes have proven very effective with quiescent preparations, conventional methods for the measurement of intracellular pH in the beating heart are subject to disturbing experimental and theoretical complications (Gillies and Deamer, 1979; Poole-Wilson, 1978). Moon and Richards (1973) demonstrated that ^{31}P NMR may be used to measure intracellular pH noninvasively from the frequency of the intracellular inorganic phosphate resonance.

Inorganic phosphate exists mainly as HPO_4^{2-} and $H_2PO_4^-$ near neutral pH. Although the different electronic environments of the phosphorus nucleus in the two species would be expected to give rise to separate resonances, fast exchange ($\sim10^9$–10^{11} sec^{-1}) to the ionizable proton effectively averages their chemical shifts to give a signal with a chemical shift that is the weighted average of the chemical shifts of the protonated and unprotonated species. Figure 7 illustrates the chemical shift of orthophosphate as a function of pH. If it is determined with *in vitro* conditions similar to those *in vivo*, it may be directly used to determine intracellular pH.

To use such a titration as a "standard" curve for determination of intracellular pH, it is important to verify that it accurately describes the behavior of orthophosphate in the intracellular environment. In theory, chelation of metal ions, variation of ionic strength, and binding to macromolecules may all affect the pK_a (Gadian *et al.*, 1980). This point has been well illustrated in recent studies of the internal pH of chromaffin granules, catecholamine storage vesicles that contain high concentrations of catecholamines, ATP, and soluble proteins (Njus *et al.*, 1978). Another source of error is in determination of the chemical shift. An approach to estimation of the errors involved in determination of pH from chemical shifts has been proposed by Momsen *et al.*, (1979).

Determination of the pH from the orthophosphate chemical shift has been criticized in application to heart studies on the basis of these points and because of uncertainties about the intracellular distribution of orthophosphate (Poole-Wilson, 1978). Titrations in media having a range of ionic strengths (I = 0.12–2 M in NaCl or KCl) (far broader than might be encountered intracellularly) put the maximum error possible from a poor estimation of intracellular ionicity at only about 0.1 pH units (Gadian *et al.*, 1980; Roberts *et al.*, 1981).

Macromolecular interactions that might perturb the pK_a are unlikely because of the relatively narrow line width (on the order of 15 Hz) of the intracellular orthophosphate (Garlick *et al.*, 1979). Recently, intracellular 2-deoxyglucose-6-phosphate has been used as a pH marker in normoxic perfused rat hearts and during total global ischemia. The pH values determined from the intracellular 2-deoxyglucose-6-phosphate resonance are in excellent agreement with those simultaneously measured from the orthophosphate peak (Bailey *et al.*, 1981b). The intracellular distribution and interactions of the two molecules are unlikely to be identical, so it would appear as though there are no unanticipated interactions effecting pH measurements using orthophosphate. As measurements of the orthophosphate chemical shift may be made in less than a minute on current instruments, ^{31}P NMR may, in fact, be claimed to be the method of choice for intracellular pH determination in whole-heart studies. A special advantage of measuring intracellular pH by NMR is that it is possible to measure not only the main pH but also a distribution of pH values from nonexchanging (or slowly exchanging) compartments in the sample (Njus *et al.*, 1979; Ugurbil *et al.*, 1978b; Ogawa *et al.*, 1978).

In theory, the intracellular pH can be determined from the resonances of any compound that has a pK_a within about ± 0.4 units of the pH to be determined and a chemical shift that varies over a reasonable range with its state of ionization. For example, the intracellular pH of erythrocytes was measured from the ^1H NMR signals of hemoglobin histidine (F. Brown *et al.*, 1977).

Indirect observations of intracellular free Mg^{2+} concentrations have been made in skeletal muscle and in erythrocytes using ^{31}P NMR. Cohen and Burt (1977) found that Mg^{2+} binding to phosphocreatine increases the spin–spin relaxation rate although the spin–lattice relaxation rate is unaffected. By determining the dependance of the ^{31}P relaxation rate on the fraction of phosphocreatine bound by the Mg^{2+} *in vitro,* they were able to determine the free Mg^{2+} to be 3 m*M* from the T_2 measured for phosphocreatine in muscle. Gupta *et al.* (1979) used a different technique to measure free Mg^{2+} concentrations in glycolyzing eythrocytes: they correlated the amount bound to ATP, determined from the separation between the chemical shifts of intracellular ATP α and β phosphate resonances and the α–β and β–γ ^{31}P spin–spin coupling constants, with the total concentration of ATP and calculated the free $[Mg^{2+}]$ from the known affinity of ATP for Mg^{2+} *in vitro*. Significant differences in the free Mg^{2+} concentration were found between anaerobic and aerobic cells. Using a similar method, they estimated the free Mg^{2+} in skeletal muscle, concluding that the value is lower than that determined by Cohen and Burt (Gupta and Moore, 1980). A recent estimate made using ion-invasive microelectrodes supports the higher values, however (Hess and Weingart, 1982).

C. Intracellular Fluxes

Slow concentration changes that occur over a period of many minutes or a few hours are easily studied simply by taking a sequential series of spectra. The minimum interval between spectra is determined by the amount of time necessary to build up a signal-to-noise ratio sufficient for an accurate determination of peak areas or heights, whichever is being measured. Measurement of peak heights should be adequate for following concentration changes of a single metabolite provided there are no variations in line width. It takes longer to accumulate spectra having signal-to-noise ratio sufficient for following concentration changes than for following shifts in resonance frequency. Thus, for example, although pH can be determined from the inorganic phosphate signal frequency in well under a minute for an adult rat heart on our ^{31}P spectrometer, at least 1 min of collection is necessary to determine the phosphocreatine resonance intensity with reasonable precision. It is advisable to use an external concentration standard when observing time-dependent concentration changes to allow corrections for any time-dependent variations in spectrometer performance.

Extensive signal averaging to get a relatively high signal-to-noise ratio is the best data collection procedure only if the sample resonances are in a steady state or changing very slowly; signal-to-noise ratio is improved only at the cost of resolution in the real-time domain. An important type of experiment involves the observation of the time course of relatively rapid (i.e., $t_{1/2}$ of only a few minutes) concentration changes following some intervention, such as cessation of flow to induce total global ischemia. In such situations, it is desirable to collect many spectra with relatively few scans rather than fewer spectra with a greater number of scans for each one. The concentrations determined from any single spectrum will be subject to a greater random variation because of the relatively lower signal-to-noise ratio, but the time definition will be greater. The concentration information may be interpreted by determining the magnitude of the random scatter expected from data collected in a similar way when the sample is in a steady state.

The time resolution may be significantly improved if data collection is synchronised with a repetitive event. For example, if an event is repeated n times, an RF pulse may be applied at a time t after each of the n events, and the n FIDs summed to represent the response at time t with an acceptable ratio of signal to noise. An example of such "gated" NMR is synchronization of pulsing with electrical stimulation (pacing) of a heart so that an FID is collected only at the peak of systole for n heartbeats (Fossel *et al.*, 1980). The sum of the n FIDs will allow determination of metabolite concentrations during a short, precisely defined period of the excitation–contraction cycle. By accumulating a number of sets of FIDs at different times after an event, the time course of changes may be constructed with a time resolution eventually limited only by the time to collect a single FID (which may be conservatively estimated as about 100 msec).

Carbon-13 NMR may be used to study the kinetics of reactions by following the rate of isotope incorporation into metabolite pools or, subsequent to enrichment of a pool, by observing the rate at which the isotope is "washed out" during perfusion with unenriched substrates. The method, first applied in a study of soybean ovules (Schaeffer *et al.*, 1975), may be applied to reactions at equilibrium as well as those showing a net flux. Following work with *E. coli* suspensions (Ugurbil *et al.*, 1978a) and perfused livers (Cohen *et al.*, 1979b), the usefulness of this technique for elucidating fluxes and changes in the steady-state enrichment of metabolites in perfused hearts (Bailey *et al.*, 1981a) was also demonstrated. A significant advantage of ^{13}C NMR over classical ^{14}C isotope techniques is that information on the relative extents and rates of enrichment of different sites within a molecule is readily obtained.

A kinetic method unique to NMR is "saturation transfer," which allows the unidirectional rates of a reaction at equilibrium to be measured (Hoffman and Forsén, 1966; Forsén and Hoffman, 1963, 1964). The basis of saturation transfer is that an individual spin will "remember" any perturbation away from its equilibrium state for a time of the order of its T_1.

Consider a simple reaction in "slow exchange"

$$A \underset{k_{-1}}{\overset{k_1}{\rightleftharpoons}} B$$

in which nuclei in molecule A resonate at a different frequency than do those in B. If radiation is selectively and continuously applied so that the population differences between the upper and lower nuclear energy states in B disappears, the resonance intensity (because it depends on a net absorption of energy) falls to zero, and the magnetization is said to be saturated. Because of chemical exchange, however, nuclei at site B will move to site A at the exchange rate, and nuclei at A will move to B. Nuclei moving from B to A will "remember" the saturation and, if the rate of exchange is at least of the order of the spin–lattice relaxation rate, either show a reduced contribution to the magnetization at A or not contribute at all. Of course, because the system is at equilibrium, for every nucleus that moves from B to A, one will move from A to B and become saturated. The net effect is to reduce the equilibrium intensity of resonance A. The extent of the reduction in intensity for a given T_1 increases with the chemical exchange rate constant:

$$M_A^+/M_A^0 = 1/(1 + k_1 T_{1A}) \qquad (4)$$

(where M_A^+ is the equilibrium magnetization of A when B is saturated, k_1 is the unidirectional rate constant for chemical exchange from A to B, T_{1A} is the intrinsic spin–lattice relaxation time of nucleus A, and M_A^0 is the equilibrium magnetization of A in the absence of irradiation of B). Note that T_{1A} is not the relaxation time that would be measured in the usual way while chemical exchange is occurring; in the presence of exchange, the usual T_1 experiment will measure an apparent relaxation time that is a function of T_{1A} and the exchange rate.

Once a value is obtained for M_A^+/M_A^0, a further experiment must be performed to determine a unique value for k_1. The apparent spin–lattice relaxation time of resonance A (τ_A) measured at the same time the resonance B is fully saturated is related to the intrinsic T_{1A} and the rate constant k_1:

$$1/\tau_A = 1/T_{1A} + k_1 \qquad (5)$$

It follows from eqs. 4 and 5 that

$$k_1 = (1 - M_A^+/M_A^0)/\tau_A \qquad (6)$$

To illustrate the method, let us consider results from an experiment to determine creatine kinase fluxes in the isolated, Langendorff-perfused rate heart (11 m*M* glucose substrate, 37°C). For the purpose of analysis, the creatine kinase reaction,

$$\mathrm{PCr + ADP + H^+ \underset{k_{-1}}{\overset{k_1}{\rightleftharpoons}} ATP + Cr}$$

is considered as a simple unimolecular transformation:

$$\text{PCr} \underset{k_{\text{rev}}}{\overset{k_{\text{for}}}{\rightleftharpoons}} \text{ADP}$$

The pseudounimolecular rate constants (kf_{or}, k_{rev}) that will be calculated therefore cannot be interpreted to reflect properties of the true reaction rate constants k_1 and k_{-1}.

In order to determine the forward flux (which must be equal to the reverse flux if steady-state concentrations of ATP and phosphocreatine are maintained during the measurement), two spectra are initially accumulated, one with the ATP γ-phosphate resonance selectively irradiated and the other with irradiation of identical power and bandwidth applied downfield of phosphocreatine by an amount equal to the frequency separation between the phosphocreatine and the ATP γ-phosphate resonances. Enough time must be allowed between pulses to allow complete nuclear relaxation. The most efficient strategy is to use 90° radio frequency pulses and a delay period that is at least 3–5 times τ(PCr). The phosphocreatine magnetization in the first spectrum is M^+(PCr), and in the second it is M^0(PCr). A typical result gives the ratio $M^+/M^0(\text{PCr}) = 0.31 \pm 0.03$ ($n = 7$, ±S.E.M.; Matthews *et al.*, 1982b).

There are a great variety of FT NMR methods for determining the spin–lattice relaxation time (see, for example, Freeman and Hill, 1971; Levy and Peat, 1975; Canet *et al.*, 1975; Gupta, 1977). Particularly useful is the saturation recovery method (McDonald and Leigh, 1973). This apparent spin–lattice relaxation time of phosphocreatine with selective saturation of the ATP γ-phosphate resonance is 1.6 ± 0.2 sec ($n = 7$, ±S.E.M.). Thus, the pseudounimolecular rate constant,

$$k_{\text{for}} = (1 - 0.31)/1.6 \text{ sec} = 0.42 \text{ sec}$$

The flux may be calculated after quantitation of the phosphocreatine concentration:

$$\begin{aligned} \text{flux}_{\text{for}} &= k_{\text{for}} \text{ [phosphocreatine]} \\ &= 0.42 \text{ sec} \times 10.1 \text{ m}M \\ &= 4.6 \text{ m}M/\text{sec} \end{aligned}$$

The reverse flux may be determined by an analogous protocol with irradiation of the phosphocreatine resonance.

There are a number of potential sources of error in the saturation transfer experiment. An immediate concern is the stability of the preparation. As described, determination of the forward flux may take as much as a few hours, depending on the size of the sample, spectrometer sensitivity, and the signal-to-noise ratio necessary to measure values to the desired precision. Stability problems may be minimized by accumulating the M^+ and M^0 spectra (and, separately, different delay values for measurement of the relaxation time) as alternate small blocks of scans summed over the same time period.

It is important that irradiation of the exchange site be selective. Stray irradiation at the resonance being measured can introduce significant errors by altering the effective spin–lattice relaxation time. It may be advisable to estimate the amount of unwanted saturation of the resonance of interest by comparing the M^0 to the magnetization when the selective irradiation is applied a very long way off resonance (e.g., 10 MHz). Errors can also be introduced into the spin–lattice relaxation time measurement by increasing the offset of the resonance from the carrier frequency by B_1 field inhomogeneities (Sass and Ziessow, 1977; Levy and Peat, 1975). These effects can be minimized using the multipulse sequences proposed by Levitt and Freeman (1979).

As eq. 4 shows, with a given ratio of signal to noise (which determines the range of M^+/M^0 that can be measured), the magnitude of the pseudounimolecular rate constants that can be determined depends on the intrinsic relaxation time of the nucleus examined. In the rat heart, intrinsic relaxation times (at 73.836 MHz) are about 2 sec for orthophosphate (Matthews *et al.*, 1981), 1 sec for the ATP γ-phosphate, and 2.5–5.5 sec (depending on the contractile state of the heart) for phosphocreatine (Matthews *et al.*, 1982b). Thus, if M^+/M^0 values between 0.1 and 0.9 can be discerned, and $T_1(\mathrm{PCr}) = 4$ sec, one may crudely estimate that forward pseudounimolecular rate constants of between 0.2 and 2 sec^{-1} can be measured for the creatine kinase reaction.

Saturation transfer was first applied to rate analysis *in vivo* by T. Brown *et al.* (1977), who studied unimolecular exchange rates between orthophosphate and ATP catalyzed by the dicycloheximide-sensitive ATPase. It was later applied to measurement of creatine kinase reaction rates in skeletal muscle (T. Brown *et al.*, 1978; Gadian *et al.*, 1981a; Meyer *et al.*, 1982) and isolated, perfused hearts (T. Brown *et al.*, 1978; Nunnally and Hollis, 1979; Matthews *et al.*, 1982b). The steady-state ATP synthetase activity in the perfused rat heart has also been directly determined in this way (Matthews *et al.*, 1981).

Nunnally and Hollis (1979) made the interesting observation that the ratio of measured forward and reverse creatine kinase fluxes is greater than unity under certain conditions in the perfused heart. This has since been confirmed in our laboratory (Matthews *et al.*, 1982b) and was also noted in a study with isolated frog skeletal muscle (Gadian *et al.*, 1981a). In all cases, the time-averaged forward and reverse creatine kinase chemical fluxes must have been equal because phosphocreatine and ATP concentrations were maintained constant. An apparent flux ratio greater than unity is not inherent in the method, for the measured forward and reverse fluxes are equal when the reaction catalyzed by creatine kinase is examined *in vitro* (Meyer *et al.*, 1982). Nunnally and Hollis (1979) interpreted the flux discrepancy as evidence for intracellular compartmentation of ATP. However, consideration of the derivation of Eq. 4 (Matthews *et al.*, 1982b) shows that a low apparent reverse flux would also be measured if the ATP γ-phosphate were exchanging with sites other than phosphocreatine at rates comparable to that measured for the creatine kinase reaction.

D. Metabolite Compartmentation

One of the most exciting prospects afforded by whole-organ NMR is that the environmental sensitivity and noninvasive nature of the method might allow study of the compartmentation of metabolites, both within cells and from cell to cell across a tissue. In one of the first reports of the ^{31}P NMR observation of perfused rat heart, it was suggested that the increased acidity of ischemic areas should distinguish normal from damaged tissue and possibly allow measurement of infarct volumes from the relative magnitudes of signals arising from normal and acidotic regions (Garlick *et al.*, 1977). This hypothesis was later tested using rabbit hearts made regionally ischemic by ligation of the left anterior descending artery (Garlick, 1979; Hollis *et al.*, 1978). Although two orthophosphate signals from environments of different pH were observed, interpretation was complicated because of presumed phosphate washout by coronary arterial collateral flow. As noted earlier, Nunnally and Bottomley (1981) have described experiments in which they used a surface coil to study localized metabolism in small volumes of perfused rabbit hearts. They were therefore able to study time courses of metabolic changes in both infarcted and normally functioning regions of the same heart. The consequences of pharmacological interventions were easily observed.

Similar experiments with surface coils can also be performed *in vivo* using an open-chest preparation similar to that described by Grove and his colleagues (1980). The combination of B_0 field-focusing methods (Gorden *et al.*, 1980) and surface coils may allow study of metabolites in selected regions of hearts of larger animals (and, perhaps, eventually man) without the need for surgical placement of the coil. It has already proved possible to study the kidney in this fashion (Balaban *et al.*, 1981).

Zeugmatographic techniques (Lauterbur, 1973) that use precisely defined, nonuniform B_0 or B_1 fields to impart a spatial dimension to the resonance signals may eventually be applied to cardiac imaging. Lauterbur and co-workers (1978) first demonstrated the feasibility of this by mapping a regionally ischemic area in a dog heart on the basis of differences in water proton relaxation times after injection of Mn^{2+}: the ischemic regions did not absorb any of the injected Mn^{2+} and therefore had much longer relaxation times. Recent work has improved on this method (see progress reports in Witcofski *et al.*, 1982) and made ^{1}H zeugmatographic imaging of human hearts *in vivo* practical (Pykett, 1982). Although the metabolic information provided by this method is only indirect, the ability to monitor infarct size fairly precisely with a safe, noninvasive method could undoubtedly become important in cardiovascular pharmacology. In addition to allowing infarct sizing, "gated" images could provide important physiological information such as the ejection fraction.

Equally promising have been two types of experiments using ^{23}Na NMR. The first is simply a variation on ^{1}H zeugmatography that forms an image based on ^{23}Na distribution (Delayre *et al.*, 1981). The second method potentially provides a rapid method for quantitatively monitoring the redistribution of ^{23}Na between the intra- and extracellular spaces. Normally, resonances from intra- and extracellular ^{23}Na ions in a tissue sample occur at the same frequencies. However, through the use of a nonpermeant anionic complex of Dy^{3+}, the resonance signals from ^{23}Na in the extracellular space can be chemically shifted from those of ^{23}Na inside the cell (Gupta and Gupta, 1982).

Preliminary experiments have demonstrated that spatial imaging of the ^{31}P nucleus is possible but have also suggested that intracellular phosphate metabolite concentrations are too low for imaging on living tissue to be practical unless significant gains in sensitivity are made (Bendel *et al.,* 1980).

Intracellular compartmentation was first examined with NMR in isolated skeletal muscle. The observation was made that the line widths observed for orthophosphate and glucose-6-phosphate but not for phosphocreatine were appreciably broader than would be expected on the basis of their T_2s and the amount of inhomogeneity broadening. This was tentatively interpreted as evidence that orthophosphate was present in multiple intracellular environments, e.g., the sarcoplasm and the sarcoplasmic reticulum. On depression of the external pH with acetate, two inorganic phosphate and, in situations in which their concentrations were enhanced so as to be easily observed, two sugar phosphate peaks were detected (Busby *et al.,* 1978).

However, interpretation of such a study is not easy because it is difficult to eliminate the possibility that inhomogeneities among different cells in the tissue are giving rise to the effects observed. However, with a similar philosophy, Nunnally and Hollis (1979) cite an unpublished experiment in which they claim to have observed biphasic kinetics in the paramagnetic broadening of the ATP resonances in isolated rabbit hearts with uptake of Mn^{2+} from the perfusate. The main thrust of their report is to present saturation transfer measurements of the creatine kinase rates that show the apparent forward and reverse rates to be unequal in the Langendorff perfused heart but equal in the KCl-arrested heart or following an extended ischemic period (Nunnally and Hollis, 1979), consistent with compartmentation of ATP and redistribution of ATP between compartments under different conditions. As discussed in the previous section, however, other interpretations of the discrepancy between forward and reverse rates may be proposed. Finally, it should be considered that the more classical methods of isotope flux studies of compartmentation may soon be tried in a new way as ^{13}C NMR begins to be applied more generally to problems of heart metabolism.

The spin–spin and spin–lattice times are influenced by the environment of the molecule, particularly the local viscosity, pH, concentrations of counterions, and the nature of any specific intermolecular interactions such as binding to macromolecules. Thus, in principle, the T_1 and T_2 values for metabolites might be expected to be different for the same metabolites in different intracellular environments. Usually these relaxation processes are well described by a single exponential decay; compartmentation might be expected to give rise to more complex behavior. To date, however, no experimental evidence has been presented to support this proposal except spin-echo studies that can distinguish intra- and extracellular metabolites in erythrocyte suspensions (Brindle *et al.,* 1979).

E. The Unique Potential of NMR

The unique potential of NMR may be summarized in five points:

1. The method is dynamic and noninvasive, so all measurements may be related to those made at other times on the same tissue sample, e.g., before and after an intervention.
2. It offers a precise, general method for observing intracellular pH that can simultaneously discern multiple compartments of differing pH.
3. With saturation transfer, it allows the direct measurement of *in vivo* rates.
4. "Gated" NMR offers the possibility of concentration and perhaps even reaction rate measurements during very short, well-defined periods.
5. Stable-isotope-enriched studies with ^{13}C NMR provide the potential for dynamic observation and quantitation of specific site enrichments of metabolites.

VI. A VISION OF THINGS TO COME

Future developments will certainly see increases in spectrometer sensitivity for all nuclei, allowing further extensions of the approaches already discussed. The feasibility of whole-tissue ^{1}H and ^{13}C NMR demonstrated on other systems suggests that application to cardiac studies will soon follow. Spectrometer improvements are even opening up possibilities for observation of ^{15}N in isotope-enriched biological samples (Levy and Lichter, 1979; Lapidot and Irving, 1979). The low sensitivity of the ^{15}N nucleus no longer seems an insurmountable problem; protein synthesis has been followed in plant seeds (Schaeffer *et al.*, 1979) and leaves (Schaeffer *et al.*, 1981) using the technique of "nuclear cross polarization," which considerably enhances the sensitivity of the experiment for the low-sensitivity ^{15}N isotope.

Fluorine-19 is only slightly less sensitive in the NMR experiment than are protons. On the basis of results from an early application of ^{19}F NMR to a living system (Costa *et al.*, 1979), the possibility of using ^{19}F-labeled compounds in heart studies should be considered.

The recent dramatic growth in the literature of metal ion NMR suggests that the intracellular interactions and movements of biologically important ions such as Na^{+} and K^{+} might be amenable to further direct study in whole tissue by NMR (Shporer and Civan, 1977). A great incentive to development of metal ion NMR has been that the huge chemical shifts exhibited (up to several thousand ppm) promise high degrees of sensitivity to properties of the local environment. Recent developments in ^{23}Na NMR have already been described (see Section V.D). A number of ^{39}K NMR studies have been conducted in muscle and whole tissue, but potential for applications using the nucleus in cardiac studies is somewhat limited, as it is about 2000 times less sensitive than protons (Magnusson and Magnusson, 1973; Cope and Damadian, 1970; Bryant, 1970). Thallium NMR offers an intriguing alternative, as Tl^{+} substitutes for K^{+} in a number of systems, including the isolated frog heart (Hille, 1973; Rusznyak *et al.*, 1968; Mullins and Moore, 1960). Along with ^{1}H, ^{3}H, and ^{19}F, Tl is among the most sensitive nuclei in the periodic table. Because of this, it is perhaps more promising for heart studies than the other metal nuclei.

Two relatively new and sophisticated NMR techniques may eventually find applications relevant to whole-organ studies. The first is the powerful method of two-dimensional NMR, which can provide information concerning molecular structure and reaction kinetics and may be used to simplify the representation of complex spectra without sacrificing information (Freeman and Morris, 1979). The recent explosion of interest in solid–state NMR could also bring techniques relevant to cardiological studies. It has already been applied to studies of biological membranes and proteins (Mehring, 1974; Schaeffer *et al.*, 1981). The necessity for rapid spinning (perhaps at 2500–5000 revolutions per second) suggests, however, that such work will probably be confined to preparations maintained under rather unphysiological conditions.

The future for ^{1}H NMR zeugmatographic imaging in clinical medicine and pharmacology is certainly bright (see, for example, papers in Witcofski *et al.*, 1982). In stationary samples, cross-sectional spatial resolution approaching 0.4 mm was achieved some years ago (Hinshaw *et al.*, 1977). Because the image is determined by both ^{1}H concentrations and relaxation times T_1 and T_2, it can be made sensitive to a wide range of tissue changes. Use of selectively absorbed "contrast reagents" can enhance the discriminatory potential of the method. Proton imaging may soon be able to clearly characterize the distribution of necrotic, "blighted," and "jeopardized" tissue about an infarct *in vivo*.

With the recent advent of high-field magnets large enough to accomodate humans, high-resolution ^{31}P NMR may be expected to contribute to clinical cardiovascular pharmacology. Recent studies of skeletal muscle disease have demonstrated the potential for noninvasive study of metabolic lesions (Ross *et al.*, 1981; Gadian *et al.*, 1981b) and for characterization of generalized degenerative changes (Newman *et al.*, 1982). The greatest potential of this approach does not necessarily lie in improving clinical diagnosis so much as in defining new parameters for use in evaluation of long-term therapies. In principle, all of the information that can now be obtained with isolated organ or small animal preparations using ^{31}P NMR should eventually be available on the human heart *in vivo*. It will be exciting to watch how the promise that this affords will be realized over the next decade.

APPENDIX: SIGNAL-TO-NOISE RATIO AND COIL DESIGN

The basic ideas of a theory developed by Hoult (1978) to describe signal-to-noise detection in NMR are outlined in this Appendix. They may be used to guide the design and construction of receiver coils for specific physiological applications.

Recall Figure 8 diagramming the tuned circuit used in NMR probes. Note that there are two capacitors, one in parallel and one in series with the coil. The frequency at which the circuit resonates is determined by the inductance (L) of the coil and the parallel capacitance (C):

$$\omega_0 = 1/(LC)^{1/2}$$

A tuned circuit is selective in its frequency response, responding most strongly at the resonant frequency. Its selectivity to a particular frequency is expressed by the quality factor,

$$Q = \omega_0 L/R$$

(where ω_0 is the resonance frequency, L the inductance of the coil, and R the resistance of the circuit). The inductance is a measure of the energy stored in a coil, and, for a solenoid, it can also be used as a measure of the B_1 field within the sample volume. Thus, the Q can be used to describe the magnetic coupling between a solenoidal coil and a sample in its volume. This means that the Q of a solenoidal coil is a measure of the signal-to-noise ratio available. Hoult (1978) describes how the Q may be easily determined and used to assess the signal-to-noise ratio that may be achieved with a given solenoidal coil. Unfortunately, no such simple test is possible with Helmholtz coils.

It is the ratio of EMFs generated by the signal and the noise in a tuned circuit that determines the final signal-to-noise ratio. It may be shown that, for a fixed frequency, (1) EMF induced by nuclear spins $\propto B_1 V_s$, and (2) noise EMF $\propto (4kT_cR)^{1/2}$, where B_1 is the magnetic field generated in the coil by passage of unit current, V_s is the volume of sample within the coil, k is the Boltzmann constant, and T_c is the temperature. From these equations it follows that the ratio

$$\text{signal/noise} \propto CB_1V_s/R^{1/2}$$

(Gadian and Robinson, 1979), where C is the concentration of resonant nuclei in the sample. The resistance R includes contributions from the circuit components and the sample itself when a conducting sample is studied. In whole-tissue work, resistance from the sample may be the dominant term. If the sample resistance effectively determines the total resistance, $R \propto V_s^2$, and the signal-to-noise ratio should no longer be improved by using larger sample volumes. It also follows that $R \propto \omega_0^2$, so improvements in signal-to-noise ratio at higher B_0 field strengths should not be expected. When such conditions are reached, optimal coil design has been achieved.

ACKNOWLEDGMENTS

The authors would like to thank Drs. R. S. Balaban, D. G. Gadian, S. R. Williams, and Mr. R. Portous for their helpful comments on this manuscript and Drs. J. M. Salhany and R. G. Schulman for providing preprints of their work. Work in the Oxford laboratory has been generously supported by grants from the British Heart Foundation, Science Research Council, and Medical Research Council. P.M.M. acknowledges support from the National Science Foundation (U.S.A.) and receipt of a British Heart Foundation Junior Research Fellowship.

REFERENCES

Ackerman, J. J. H., Grove, T. H., Wong, G. G. Gadian, D. G., and Radda, G. K. 1980. Mapping of metabolites in whole animals by ^{31}P NMR using surface coils. *Nature, 283:*167–170.

Ackerman, J. J. H., Gadian, D. G., Radda, G. K., and Wong, G. G. 1981. Observation of ^{1}H NMR signals with receiver coils tuned for other nuclides. The optimization of B_0 homogeneity and a multi-nuclear chemical shift reference. *J. Mag. Reson., 42:*493–500.

Agris, P., and Campbell, I. D. 1982. Proton NMR studies of intact friend leukemia cells. *Science, 216:*1325–1327.

Bailey, I., Gadian, D. G., Matthews, P. M., Radda, G. K., and Seeley, P. J. 1981a. Studies of metabolism in the isolated, perfused heart using ^{13} C NMR. *FEBS LETT., 123:*103–109.

Bailey, I., Radda, G. K., Williams, S. R., and Gadian, D. G. 1981b. The activity of phosphorylase in total global ischemia in the rat heart: A ^{31}P NMR study. *Biochem. J., 196:*171–178.

Balaban, R. S., Gadian, D. G., and Radda, G. K. 1981. A ^{31}P n.m.r. study of the rat kidney *in vivo. Kidney Int., 20:*575–579.

Barany, M., Barany, K., Burt, C. T., Glonek, T., and Myers, T. C. 1975. Structural changes in myosin during contraction and the state of ADP in the intact frog muscle. *J. Supramol. Struct., 3:*125–140.

Bartholdi, T., and Ernst, R. R. 1973. Fourier spectroscopy and the causality principle. *J. Mag. Reson., 11:*9–19.

Battersby, M. K., and Radda, G. K. 1976. The stereospecificity of the glucose 6-phosphate binding site of glycogen phosphorylase *b. FEBS Lett., 72:*319–321.

Battersby, M. K., Garlick, P. B., Seeley, P. J., Sehr, P. A., and Radda, G. K. 1978. Phosphorus nuclear magnetic resonance studies in living tissue. In: *Biomolecular Structure and Function,* pp. 175–193. Ed. by Agris, P. F., Loeppky, R., and Sykes, B. Academic Press, New York.

Becker, E. D., Ferretti, J. A., and Gambhir, P. M. 1979. Selection of optimum parameters for pulse fourier transform nuclear magnetic resonance. *Anal. Chem., 51:*1413–1420.

Bendel, P., Lai, C. M., and Lauterbur, P. C. 1980. ^{31}P spectroscopic zeugmatography of phosphorus metabolites. *J. Mag. Reson., 38:*343–356.

Berden, J. S., Cullis, P. R., Hoult, D. I., McLaughlin, A. C., Radda, G. K., and Richards, R. E. 1974. Frequency dependence of ^{31}P NMR linewidths in sonicated, phospholipid vesicles: Effects of chemical shift anisotropy. *FEBS Lett., 46:*55–58.

Bracewell, R. 1965. *The Fourier Transform and Its Applications.* McGraw-Hill, New York.

Brindle, K. M., Brown, F. F., Campbell, I. D., Grathwohl, C. A., and Kuchel, P. W. 1979. Application of spin-echo nuclear magnetic resonance to whole cell systems. Membrane transport. *Biochem. J., 180:*37–44.

Brown, F. F., Campbell, I. D., Kuchel, P. W., and Rabenstein, D. C. 1977. Human erythrocyte metabolism studies by ^{1}H spin echo NMR. *FEBS Lett., 82:*12–16.

Brown, T. R., Ugurbil, K., and Schulman, R. G. 1977. ^{31}P nuclear magnetic resonance measurements of ATPase kinetics in aerobic *Escherichia coli* cells. *Proc. Natl. Acad. Sci. U.S.A., 74:*5551–5553.

Brown, T. R., Gadian, D. G., Garlick, P. B., Radda, G. K., Seeley, P. J., and Styles, P. 1978. Creatine kinase activities in skeletal and cardiac muscle measured by saturation transfer NMR. In: *Frontiers of Biological Energetics: Electrons to Tissues,* Volume 2, pp. 1341–1349. Ed. by Dutton, L., Leigh, J., and Scarpa, A. Academic Press, New York.

Bryant, R. G. 1970. Potassium-39 nuclear magnetic resonance. *Biochem. Biophys. Res. Commun., 40:*1162–1166.

Burt, C. T., Glonek, T., and Barany, M. 1976. Phosphorus-31 nuclear magnetic resonance detection of unexpected phosphodiesters in muscle. *Biochemistry, 15:*4850–4853.

Burt, C. T., Cohen, S. M., and Barany, M. 1979. Analysis of intact tissue with ^{31}P NMR. *Annu. Rev. Biophys. Bioeng., 8:*1–25.

Busby, S. J. W., Gadian, D. G., Richards, R. E., and Seeley, P. J. 1978. Phosphorus nuclear magnetic studies of compartmentation in muscle. *Biochem. J., 170:*103–114.

Campbell, I. D., and Dobson, C. M. 1979. The application of high resolution NMR to biological systems. In: *Methods of Biochemical Analysis,* Volume 25, pp. 1–134. Ed. by Glick, D. John Wiley & Sons, New York.

Campbell, I. D., Dobson, C. M., Williams, R. J. P., and Xavier, A. V. 1973. Resolution enhancement of protein PMR spectra using the difference between a broadened and a normal spectrum. *J. Mag. Reson.*, *11*:172–181.

Canet, D., Levy, G. C., and Peat, I. R. 1975. Time saving in ^{13}C spin–lattice relaxation measurements by inversion-recovery. *J. Mag. Reson.*, *18*:199–204.

Carr, H. Y., and Purcell, E. M. 1954. Effects of diffusion on free precession in nuclear magnetic resonance experiments. *Phys. Rev.*, *94*:630–638.

Chalovich, J. M., and Bárány, M. 1980. Serine ethanolamine phosphate in avian muscular dystrophy: Mechanism of accumulation in dystrophic muscle and relationship to phospholipid synthesis. *Arch. Biochem. Biophys.*, *199*:615–625.

Cohen, S. M., and Burt, C. T. 1977. ^{31}P nuclear magnetic relaxation studies of phosphocreatine in intact muscle: Determination of intracellular free magnesium. *Proc. Natl. Acad. Sci. U.S.A.*, *74*:4271–4275.

Cohen, S. M., Ogawa, S., and Shulman, R. G. 1979a. ^{13}C NMR studies of gluconeogenesis in rat liver cells: Utilization of labelled glycerol by cells from euthyroid and hyperthyroid rats. *Proc. Natl. Acad. Sci. U.S.A.*, *76*:1603–1607.

Cohen, S. M., Shulman, R. G., and McLaughlin, A. C. 1979b. Effects of ethanol on alanine metabolism in perfused mouse liver studied by ^{13}C NMR. *Proc. Natl. Acad. Sci. U.S.A.*, *76*:4808–4812.

Cooper, J. W. 1976. The computer in Fourier transform NMR. In: *Topics in Carbon-13 NMR Spectroscopy*, Volume 2, pp. 392–433. Ed. by Levy, G. C. John Wiley & Sons, New York.

Cope, F. W., and Damadian, R. 1970. Cell potassium by ^{39}K spin-echo nuclear magnetic resonance. *Nature*, *228*:76–77.

Costa, J. L., Dobson, C. M., Kirk, K., Poulson, F. M., Valeri, C. R., and Vecchione, J. 1979. Studies of human platelets by 19-F and 31-P NMR. *FEBS Lett.*, *99*:141–146.

Daniels, A. J., Williams, R. J. P., and Wright, P. E. 1976. Nuclear magnetic resonance studies of the adrenal gland and some other organs. *Nature*, *261*:321–322.

Dawson, M. J., Gadian, D. G., and Wilkie, D. R. 1977. Contraction and recovery of living muscle studied by ^{31}P nuclear magnetic resonance. *J. Physiol.* (*Lond.*), *267*:703–735.

Dawson, M. J., Gadian, D. G., and Wilkie, D. R. 1978. Muscular fatigue investigated by phosphorus nuclear magnetic resonance. *Nature*, *274*:861–866.

Dawson, M. J., Gadian, D. G., and Wilkie, D. R. 1979. Mechanical relaxation rate and metabolism studied in fatiguing muscle by phosphorous nuclear magnetic resonance. *J. Physiol.* (*Lond.*) *299*:465–484.

Delayre, J. L., Ingwall, J. S., Malloy, C., and Fossel, E. T. 1981. Gated ^{23}Na NMR images of an isolated perfused working rat heart. *Science*, *212*:935–936.

Doyle, D. D., Chalovich, J. M., and Bárány, M. 1981. Natural abundance ^{13}C NMR spectra of intact muscle. *FEBS Lett.*, *131*:147–150.

Ernst, R. R., and Anderson, W. A. 1966. Application of Fourier transform spectroscopy to magnetic resonance. *Rev. Sci. Instrum.*, *37*:93–102.

Ernst, R. R., and Morgan, R. E. 1973. Saturation effects in Fourier spectroscopy. *Mol. Phys.*, *26*:49–74.

Evans, F. E. 1979. Phosphorus-31 nuclear magnetic resonance studies on relaxation parameters and line broadening of intracellular metabolites of HeLa cells. *Arch. Biochem. Biophys.*, *193*:63–75.

Farrer, T. C., and Becker, E. D. 1971. *Pulse and Fourier Transform NMR*, Academic Press, New York.

Fisher, J. J. 1971. Nuclear magnetic resonance as applied to pharmacology. In: *Methods in Pharmacology*, Volume 1, pp. 431–453. Ed. by Schwartz, A. Meredith, New York.

Forsén, S., and Hoffman, R. A. 1963. Study of moderately rapid chemical exchange reactions by means of nuclear magnetic double resonance. *J. Chem. Phys.*, *39*: 2892–2901.

Forsén, S., and Hoffman, R. A. 1964. Exchange rates by nuclear magnetic multiple resonance. III. Exchange reactions in systems with several non-equivalent sites. *J. Chem. Phys.*, *40*:1189–1196.

Fossel, E. T., Morgan, H. E., and Ingwall, J. S. 1980. Measurements of changes in high-energy phosphates in the cardiac cycle by using ^{31}P nuclear magnetic resonance. *Proc. Natl. Acad. Sci. U.S.A.*, *77*:3654–3658.

Freeman, R., and Hill, H. D. W. 1971. Fourier transform study of NMR spin–lattice relaxation by progressive saturation. *J. Chem. Phys.*, *54*:3367–3377.

Freeman, R., and Morris, G. 1979. Two-dimensional Fourier transform NMR. *Bull. Mag. Reson.*, *1*:1–26.

Gadian, D. G. 1982. *Nuclear Magnetic Resonance and Its Applications to Living Systems*. Oxford University Press, Oxford.

Gadian, D. G., and Radda, G. K. 1981. N.m.r. studies of tissue metabolism. *Annu. Rev. Biochem.*, *50*:69–84.

Gadian, D. G., and Robinson, F. N. H. 1979. Radiofrequency losses in N.M.R. experiments on electrically conducting samples. *J. Mag. Reson.*, *34*:449–455.

Gadian, D. G., Radda, G. K., Richards, R. E., and Seeley, P. J. 1980. ^{31}P NMR in living tissue: The road from a promising to an important tool in biology. In: *Biological Applications of Magnetic Resonance*. Ed. by Schulman, R. G. Academic Press, New York.

Gadian, D. G., Radda, G. K., Brown, T. R., Chance, E. M., Dawson, M. J., and Wilkie, D. R. 1981a. The activity of creatine kinase in frog skeletal muscle studied by saturation-transfer nuclear magnetic resonance. *Biochem. J.*, *194*:215–228.

Gadian, D., Radda, G. K., Ross, B., Hockaday, J., Bore, P., Taylor, D., and Styles, P. 1981b. Examination of a myopathy by phosphorus NMR. *Lancet, 2*:774–775.

Garlick, P. B. 1979. *Molecular Studies of Cardiac Metabolism*. D. Phil. Thesis, University of Oxford, Oxford.

Garlick, P. B., and Radda, G. K. 1979. NMR and its applications to metabolic studies. In: *Techniques in Metabolic Research,* pp. 1–24. Ed. by Pogson, C. Elsevier, Amsterdam.

Garlick, P. B., Radda, G. K., Seeley, P. J., and Chance, B. 1977. Phosphorus NMR studies on perfused heart. *Biochem. Biophys. Res. Commun.*, *74:* 1256–1262.

Garlick, P. B., Radda, G. K., and Seeley, P. J. 1979. Studies of acidosis in the ischaemic heart by phosphorus nuclear magnetic resonance. *Biochem. J.*, *184*:547–554.

Gergely, J., and Maruyama, K. 1960. The binding of inorganic phosphate to myosin in the presence of adenosine triphosphate. *J. Biol. Chem.*, *235*:3174–3176.

Gillies, R. J., and Deamer, D. W. 1979. Intracellular pH: Methods and applications. *Curr. Top. Bioeng.*, *9*:63–87.

Gorden, R. E., Hanley, P., Shaw, D., Gadian, D. G., Radda, G. K., Styles, P., and Chan, L. 1980. Localisation of metabolites in animals using ^{31}P "Topical Magnetic Resonance." *Nature, 287*:367–368.

Grove, T. H., Ackerman, J. J. H., Radda, G. K., and Bore, P. J. 1980. Analysis of rat heart *in vivo* by phosphorus nuclear magnetic resonance. *Proc. Natl. Acad. Sci. U.S.A.*, *77*:299–302.

Gupta, R. K. 1977. A new look at the method of variable nutation angle for the measurement of spin–lattice relaxation times using Fourier transform NMR. *J. Mag. Reson.*, *25*:231–235.

Gupta, R. K., and Gupta, P. 1982. Direct observation of resolved resonances from intra- and extracellular sodium-23 in NMR studies of intact cells and tissues using dysprosium (III) tripolyphosphate as paramagnetic shift reagent. *J. Mag. Reson.*, *47*:344–350.

Gupta, R. K., and Moore, R. D. 1980. ^{31}P NMR studies of intracellular free Mg^{2+} in intact frog skeletal muscle. *J. Biol. Chem.*, *255*:3987–3993.

Gupta, R. K., Benovic, J. L., and Rose, B. 1978. The determination of the free magnesium level in the human red blood cell by ^{31}P NMR. *J. Biol. Chem.*, *253*:6172–6176.

Hahn, E. L. 1950. Spin echoes. *Phys. Rev.*, *80*:580–594.

Hamilton, J. A., Cordes, E. H., and Glueck, C. J. 1979. Lipid dynamics in human low density lipoproteins and human aortic tissue with fibrous plaques: A study by high field ^{13}C NMR spectroscopy. *J. Biol. Chem.*, *254*:5435–5441.

Hess, P., and Weingart, R. 1982. Free magnesium in cardiac and skeletal muscle measured with ion-selective micro-electrodes. *J. Physiol.* (*Lond.*), *318*:14P–15P.

Hille, B. 1973. Potassium channels in myelinated nerve. Selective permeability to small cations. *J. Gen. Physiol.*, *61*:669–686.

Hinshaw, W. W., Bottomley, P. A., and Holland, G. N. 1977. Radiographic thin-section image of the human wrist by nuclear magnetic resonance. *Nature, 270*:722–723.

Hoffman, R. A., and Forsén, S. 1966. Transient and steady state overhauser experiments in the investigation of relaxation processes. Analysis between chemical exchange and relaxation. *J. Chem. Phys., 45*:2049–2060.

Hollis, D. P., 1979. Nuclear magnetic resonance studies of cancer and heart disease. *Bull. Mag. Reson., 1*:27–37.

Hollis, D. P., Nunnally, R. L., Taylor, G. J., Weisfeldt, M. L., and Jacobus, W. E. 1978. Phosphorus NMR studies of heart physiology. *J. Mag. Reson., 29*:319–330.

Hoult, D. I. 1978. The NMR receiver: A description and analysis of design. *Prog. NMR Spect., 12*:41–77.

Hoult, D. I., and Richards, R. E. 1975. Critical factors in the design of sensitive high resolution nuclear magnetic resonance spectrometers. *Proc. R. Soc. Lond.* [*Phys.*] *344*:311–340.

Hoult, D. I., and Richards, R. E. 1976. The signal-to-noise ratio of the nuclear magnetic resonance experiment. *J. Mag. Reson., 24*:71–85.

Hoult, D. I., Busby, S. J. W., Gadian, D. G., Radda, G. K., Richards, R. E., and Seeley, P. J. 1979. Observation of tissue metabolites using ^{31}P nuclear magnetic resonance. *Nature, 252*:285–287.

Jacobus, W. E., Taylor, G. J., Hollis, D. P., and Nunnally, R. L. 1977. Phosphorus nuclear magnetic resonance of perfused working rat hearts. *Nature, 265*:756–758.

Jacobus, W. E., Pores, H., Lucas, S. K., Kallman, C. H., Weisfeldt, M. L., and Flaherty, J. T. 1982. The role of intracellular pH in the control of normal and ischaemic myocardial contractility: A ^{31}P n.m.r. and mass spectrometry study. In: *Intracellular pH: Its Measurement, Regulation, and Utilization in Cellular Functions*, pp. 537–565. Ed. by Nuccitelli, R., and Deamer, D. W. Alan R. Liss, New York.

Jones, D. W., and Child, T. F. 1976. NMR in flowing systems. *Adv. Mag. Reson., 8*:123–148.

Karplus, M. 1959. Contact electron-spin coupling of nuclear magnetic moments. *J. Chem. Phys., 30*:11–15.

Kauppinen, R. A., Hiltunen, J. K., and Hassinen, I. E. 1980. Subcellular distribution of phosphagens in the rat heart. *FEBS. Lett., 112*:273–276.

Koretsky, A. P., Wang, S., Murphy-Boesch, J., Klein, M. P., James, T. L., and Weiner, M. W., 1983. ^{31}P NMR spectroscopy of rat organs *in situ* using chronically implanted radiofrequency coils. *Proc. Nat. Acad. Sci.* (*U.S.A.*), *80*:7491–7495.

Lapidot, A., and Irving, C. S. 1979. Comparative *in vivo* ^{15}N NMR study of cell wall components of five gram-positive bacteria. *Biochemistry, 18*:704–714.

Lauterbur, P. C. 1973. Image formation by induced local interactions: Examples employing nuclear magnetic resonance. *Nature, 242*:190–191.

Lauterbur, R. C., Dias, M. H. M., and Rudin, A. 1978. Augmentation of tissue water proton T_1 rates by *in vivo* addition of paramagnetic ions. In: *Frontiers of Biological Energetics: Electrons to Tissues*, Volume 2, pp. 1341–1349. Ed. by Dutton, L., Leigh, J., and Scarpa, A. Academic Press, New York.

Lettvin, J., and Sherry, A. D. 1977. Gd (TTHA): An aqueous carbon-13 relaxation reagent. *J. Mag. Reson., 28*:459–461.

Levitt, M. H., and Freeman, R. 1979. NMR population inversion using a composite pulse. *J. Mag. Reson., 33*:473–476.

Levy, G. C., and Lichter, R. L. 1979. Nitrogen-15 Nuclear Magnetic Resonance Spectroscopy. John Wiley & Sons, New York.

Levy, G. C., and Peat, I. R. 1975. The experimental approach to accurate carbon-13 spin-lattice relaxation measurements. *J. Mag. Reson., 18*:500–521.

Magnusson, J. R., and Magnusson, N. S. 1973. NMR studies of sodium and potassium in various biological tissues. *Ann. N. Y. Acad. Sci., 204*: 297–309.

Matthews, P. M., Bland, J. L., Gadian, D. G., and Radda, G. K. 1981. The steady-state rate of ATP synthesis in the isolated perfused rat heart measured by ^{31}P n.m.r. saturation transfer. *Biochem. Biophys. Res. Commun., 103*:1052–1058.

Matthews, P. M. Williams, S. R., Seymour, A.-M., Schwartz, A., Dube, G., Gadian, D. G., and Radda, G. K. 1982a. A ^{31}P n.m.r. study of some metabolic and functional effects of the inotropic agents epinephrine and ouabain and the ionophore R02-2985 (X537A) in the isolated, perfused rat heart. *Biochim. Biophys. Acta, 720*:163–171.

Matthews, P. M., Bland, J. L., Gadian, D. G., and Radda, G. K. 1982b. A ^{31}P- NMR saturation transfer study of the regulation of creatine kinase in rat heart. *Biochim. Biophys. Acta, 721*:312–320.

McDonald, G. G., and Leigh, J. L. 1973. A new method for measuring longitudinal relaxation times. *J. Magn. Reson., 9*:358–362.

Mehring, M. 1974. *High Resolution and NMR Spectroscopy in Solids. NMR—Basic Principles and Progress,* Volume 11. Springer-Verlag, Berlin.

Meiboom, S., and Gill, D. 1958. Modified spin-echo method for measuring nuclear relaxation times. *Rev. Sci. Instrum., 29*:688–691.

Meyer, R. A., Kushmerick, M. J., and Brown, T. R. 1982. Application of ^{31}P NMR spectroscopy to the study of striated muscle metabolism. *Am. J. Physiol., 11*:C1–C11.

Momsen, G., Rose, Z. B., and Gupta, R. K. 1979. A reappraisal of ^{31}P NMR studies indicating enzyme complexation in red blood cells. *Biochem. Biophys. Res. Commun., 91*:651–657.

Moon, R. B., and Richards, J. H. 1973. Determination of intracellular pH by phosphorus nuclear magnetic resonance. *J. Biol. Chem., 248*:7276–7278.

Mullins, L. G., and Moore, R. D. 1960. The movement of thallium ions in muscle. *J. Gen. Physiol., 43*:759–773.

Navon, G., Ogawa, S., Schulman, R. G., and Yamane, T. 1977. ^{31}P Nuclear magnetic resonance studies of Ehrlich ascites tumor cells. *Proc. Natl. Acad. Sci. U.S.A., 74*:87–91.

Navon, G., Navon, R., Schulman, R. G., and Yamane, T. 1978. Phosphate metabolites in lymphoid, Friend erythroleukemia, and HeLa cells observed by high resolution ^{31}P nuclear magnetic resonance. *Proc. Natl. Acad. Sci. U.S.A., 75*:891–895.

Neely, J. R., Liebermeister, H., Battersby, E. J., and Morgan, H. E. 1967. Effect of pressure development on oxygen consumption by the isolated rat heart. *Am. J. Physiol., 212*:804–814.

Newman, R. J., Bore, P. J., Chan, L., Gadian, D. G., Styles, P., Taylor, D., and Radda, G. K. 1982. Nuclear magnetic resonance studies of forearm muscle in Duchenne dystrophy. *Br. Med. J., 234*:1072–1074.

Njus, D., Sehr, P. A., Radda, G. K., Ritchie, G. A., and Seeley, P. J. 1978. Phosphorus-31 nuclear magnetic resonance studies of active proton translocation in chromaffin granules. *Biochemistry, 17*:4337–4343.

Nunnally, R. L., and Bottomly, P. A. 1981. Assessment of pharmacological treatment of myocardial infarction by phosphorus-31 n.m.r. with surface coils. *Science, 211*:177–180.

Nunnally, R. L., and Hollis, D. P. 1979. ATP compartmentation in living hearts: A ^{31}P NMR saturation transfer study. *Biochemistry, 18*:3642–3646.

Ogawa, S., Rottenberg, H., Brown, T. R., Shulman, R. G., Castillo, C. L., and Glynn, P. 1978. High resolution ^{31}P nuclear magnetic resonance study of rat liver mitochondria. *Proc. Natl. Acad. Sci. U.S.A., 75*:1796–1800.

Ogino, T., Arata, Y., Fujiwara, S., Shoun, H., and Beppu, T. 1978. Use of proton correlation spectroscopy in the study of living cells. Anaerobic metabolism of *Escherichia coli. J. Mag. Reson., 31*:523–526.

Ottoway, J. H., and Mowbray, J. 1977. The role of compartmentation in the control of glycolysis. *Curr. Top. Cell. Reg., 12*:107–208.

Pieper, G. M., Todd, G. L., Wu, S. T., Salhany, J. M., Clayton, F. C., and Eliot, R. S. 1980. Attenuation of myocardial acidosis by propranolol during ischemic arrest and reperfusion of isolated, perfused hearts as determined by ^{31}P nuclear magnetic resonance spectroscopy. *Cardiovasc. Res., 14*:646–653.

Pitkethly, R. H. 1979. Part II Thesis, University of Oxford, Oxford.

Poole-Wilson, P. A. 1978. Measurement of myocardial intracellular pH in pathological states. *J. Mol. Cell. Cardiol., 10*:511–526.

Pykett, I. L. 1982. NMR imaging in medicine. *Sci. Am., 246*(5):54–71.

Rabenstein, D. L., and Nakashima, T. T. 1979. Spin-echo Fourier transform nuclear magnetic resonance spectroscopy. *Anal. Chem., 51*:1465A–1474A.

Radda, G. K., and Seeley, P. J. 1979. Recent studies on cellular metabolism by nuclear magnetic resonance. *Annu. Rev. Physiol., 41*:749–769.

Randle, P. J., and Tubbs, P. K. 1979. Carbohydrate metabolism of the heart. In: *Handbook of Physiology*, Section II, Volume 1, pp. 805–844. Ed. by Berne, R. M. American Physiological Society, Bethesda.

Roberts, J. K. M., Wade-Jardetsky, N., and Jardetsky, O. 1981. Intracellular pH measurements by ^{31}P n.m.r. Influence of factors other than pH on chemical shifts. *Biochemistry, 20:*5389–5394.

Ross, B. D., Radda, G. K., Gadian, D. G., Rocker, G., Esiri, M., and Falconer, J. 1981. Examination of a case of suspected McCardle's syndrome by ^{31}P n.m.r. *N. Engl. J. Med., 304:*1338–1342.

Rusznyak, I., Gyorgy, L., Omal, S., and Millner, T. 1968. On some potassium-like qualities of the thallium ion. *Experientia, 24:*809–810.

Salhany, J. M., Yamane, T., Shulman, R. G., and Ogawa, S. 1975. High resolution ^{31}P nuclear magnetic resonance studies of intact yeast cells. *Proc. Natl. Acad. Sci. U.S.A., 72:*4966–4970.

Salhany, J. M., Pieper, G. M., Wu, S., Todd, G. L., Clayton, F. C., and Eliot, R. S. 1979. ^{31}P nuclear magnetic resonance measurements of cardiac pH in perfused guinea-pig hearts. *J. Mol. Cell Cardiol., 11:*601–610.

Sass, M., and Ziessow, D. 1977. Error analysis for optimised inversion recovery spin–lattice relaxation measurements. *J. Mag. Reson., 25:*263–276.

Schaeffer, J., Stejskal, E. O., and Beard, C. F. 1975. Carbon-13 nuclear magnetic resonance analysis of metabolism in soybeans labelled by $^{13}CO_2$. *Plant Physiol., 55:*1048–1053.

Schaeffer, J., Stejskal, E. O., and McKay, R. A. 1979. Cross-polarisation NMR of ^{15}N labelled soybeans. *Biochem. Biophys. Res. Commun., 88:*274–280.

Schaeffer, J., Skokut, T. A., Stejskal, E. O., McKay, R. A., and Varner, J. E. 1981. Estimation of protein turnover in soybean leaves using magic angle double cross-polarization nitrogen-15 NMR. *J. Biol. Chem., 256:*11574–11579.

Shaw, D. 1976. *Fourier Transform NMR Spectroscopy,* Elsevier, Amsterdam.

Shporer, M., and Civan, M. M. 1977, State of water and alkali cations within the intracellular fluids: The contribution of NMR spectroscopy. *Curr. Top. Membr. Transport, 9:*1–69.

Shulman, R. G., Brown, T. R., Ugurbil, K., Ogawa, S., Cohen, S. M., and den Hollander, J. A. 1979. Cellular applications of ^{31}P and ^{13}C nuclear magnetic resonance. *Science, 205:*160–166.

Singer, S. T. 1978. NMR diffusion and flow measurements and an introduction to spin phase graphing. *J. Phys. E. Sciolnstrum., 11:*281–291.

Srere, P. A. 1981. Protein crystals as a model for mitochondrial matrix proteins. *Trends Biochem. Sci., 6:*4–7.

Sternlicht, H., Kenyon, G. L., Packer, E. L., and Sinclair, J. 1971. Carbon-13 nuclear magnetic resonance studies of heterogeneous systems. Amino acids bound to cationic exchange resins. *J. Am. Chem. Soc., 93:*199–208.

Styles, P., Grahtwohl, C., and Brown, F. F. 1979. Simultaneous multinuclear NMR by alternate scan recording of ^{31}P and ^{13}C spectra. *J. Mag. Reson., 35:*329–36.

Thulborn, K. R., du Boulay, G., and Radda, G. K. 1981. *In vivo* non-invasive measurements of energy metabolism and pH by ^{31}P n.m.r. in experimental stroke correlated with cerebral oedema. *J. Cereb. Blood Flow Metab., 1:*580–581.

Ugurbil, K., Brown, T. R., den Hollander, J. A., Glynn, P., and Shulman, R. G. 1978a. High resolution ^{13}C nuclear magnetic resonance studies of glucose metabolism in *E. Coli. Proc. Natl. Acad. Sci. U.S.A., 75:*3742–3746.

Ugurbil, K., Rottenberg, H., Glynn, P., and Shulman, R. G. 1978b. ^{31}P nuclear magnetic resonance studies of bioenergetics and glycolysis in anaerobic *Escherichia coli* cells. *Proc. Natl. Acad. Sci. U.S.A., 75:*2244–2248.

Ugurbil, K., Shulman, R. G., and Brown, T. R. 1979. High resolution ^{31}P and ^{13}C nuclear magnetic resonance studies of *Escherichia coli* cells *in vivo.* In: *Biological Application of Magnetic Resonance,* pp. 537–589. Ed. by Shulman, R. G. Academic Press, New York, London.

Van Putte, K. 1970. Elimination of H_1 inhomogeneity and spin-spin relaxation in the determination of spin-lattice relaxation times. *J. Mag. Res., 2:*174–180.

Veech, R. L., Lawson, J. W. R., Cornell, N. W., and Krebs, H. A. 1979. Cytosolic phosphorylation potential. *J. Biol. Chem., 254:*6538–6547.

Waugh, J. S., and Wang, C. H. 1967. Multiple spin echoes in dipolar solids. *Phys. Rev., 162:*208–216.

Wehrli, F. W., and Wirthli, T. 1976. *Interpretation of* ^{13}C *NMR spectra.* Hayden & Son, London, New York.
Witcofski, R. L., Karstaedt, N., and Partain, C. L. (Eds.). 1982. *NMR Imaging*. Bowman Gray School of Medicine, Winston-Salem, NC.
Wong, G. G. 1981. D. Phil. Thesis, University of Oxford, Oxford.
Wu, S. T., Pieper, G. M., Salhany, J. M., and Eliot, R. S. 1981. Measurement of free magnesium in perfused and ischaemic arrested heart muscle. A quantitative ^{31}P n.m.r. and multiequilibria analysis. *Biochemistry, 20:*7399–7403.

Index

MIX
Papier aus verantwortungsvollen Quellen
Paper from responsible sources
FSC® C105338

If you have any concerns about our products,
you can contact us on
ProductSafety@springernature.com

In case Publisher is established outside the EU,
the EU authorized representative is:
Springer Nature Customer Service Center GmbH
Europaplatz 3, 69115 Heidelberg, Germany

Printed by Libri Plureos GmbH
in Hamburg, Germany